Innovative Program Design for Individuals with Dual Sensory Impairments

Innovative Program Design for Individuals with Dual Sensory Impairments

edited by

Lori Goetz, Ph.D.
Department of Special Education
San Francisco State University
San Francisco

Doug Guess, Ed.D.
Department of Special Education
University of Kansas
Lawrence

and

Kathleen Stremel-Campbell, M.A.
Department of Special Education
University of Southern Mississippi
Hattiesburg

· P A U L · H ·
BROOKES
PUBLISHING CO.

Baltimore • London

Paul H. Brookes Publishing Co.
Post Office Box 10624
Baltimore, Maryland 21285-0624

Typeset by Brushwood Graphics Inc., Baltimore, Maryland.
Manufactured in the United States of America by
The Maple Press Company, York, Pennsylvania.

Library of Congress Cataloging-in-Publication Data

Innovative program design for individuals with dual sensory impairments.
Bibliography: p.
Includes index.
1. Hearing impaired children—Education. 2. Visually handicapped children—Education. I. Goetz, Lori. II. Guess, Doug. III. Stremel-Campbell, Kathleen.
HV2440.I56 1987 371.91′1 87-15132
ISBN 0-933716-84-2 (pbk.)

CONTENTS

Contributors ... vii
Foreword *Martha E. Snell* ... ix
Preface ... xiii

SECTION I INTRODUCTION

Chapter 1 Individuals with Sensory Impairments: Who Are They? How Are They Educated?
H.D. Bud Fredericks and Victor L. Baldwin ... 3

SECTION II CURRICULUM DEVELOPMENT

Chapter 2 Nonsymbolic Communication Development: Theoretical Concepts and Educational Strategies
Ellin Siegel-Causey and June Downing ... 15

Chapter 3 Share and Share Alike: Conventional Gestures to Emergent Language for Learners with Sensory Impairments
Charity Rowland and Kathleen Stremel-Campbell ... 49

Chapter 4 Functional Vision Programming: A Model for Teaching Visual Behaviors in Natural Contexts
Lori Goetz and Kathleen Gee ... 77

Chapter 5 Audiometric Assessment and Management
Paul S. Niswander ... 99

Chapter 6 Teaching Orientation and Mobility Skills within and across Natural Opportunities for Travel: A Model Designed for Learners with Multiple Severe Disabilities
Kathleen Gee, Rona Harrell, and Richard Rosenberg ... 127

Chapter 7 Integrated Programming for Students with Multiple Handicaps
Philippa H. Campbell ... 159

SECTION III INSTRUCTIONAL METHODS

Chapter 8 A Movement-Based Approach to the Education of Students Who Are Sensory Impaired/Multihandicapped
Jan Writer ... 191

Chapter 9 An Ecological Approach to Curriculum Development
John A. Nietupski and Susan M. Hamre-Nietupski ... 225

Chapter 10 Application of the Individualized Curriculum Sequencing Model to Learners with Severe Sensory Impairments
Edwin Helmstetter and Doug Guess 255

Chapter 11 Some Innovative Educational Applications of Advanced Technologies
Steven F. Warren, Eva H. Horn, and Everett W. Hill 283

SECTION IV SUMMARY

Chapter 12 Program Evaluation in Support of Program Development: Needs, Strategies, and Future Directions
Luanna H. Meyer and Joanne Eichinger 313

Index 355

CONTRIBUTORS

Victor L. Baldwin, Ph.D.
Teaching Research Division
Oregon State System of Higher Education
345 North Monmouth Avenue
Monmouth, OR 97361

Philippa H. Campbell, Ph.D.
Family Child Learning Center
Children's Hospital of Akron
1909 Third Street
Cuyahoga Falls, OH 44221

June Downing, Ph.D.
University of Arizona
Department of Special Education and Rehabilitation
Tucson, AZ 85721

Joanne Eichinger, M.S.
Division of Special Education and Rehabilitation
Syracuse University
805 South Crouse Avenue
Syracuse, NY 13244-2280

H.D. Bud Fredericks, Ph.D.
Teaching Research Division
Oregon State System of Higher Education
345 North Monmouth Avenue
Monmouth, OR 97361

Kathleen Gee, M.A.
Department of Special Education
San Francisco State University
1600 Holloway Avenue
San Francisco, CA 94132

Lori Goetz, Ph.D.
Department of Special Education
San Francisco State University
1600 Holloway Avenue
San Francisco, CA 94132

Doug Guess, Ed.D.
Department of Special Education
University of Kansas
377 East Haworth Hall
Lawrence, KS 66045

Susan M. Hamre-Nietupski, Ph.D.
Department of Special Education
Education Center
University of Northern Iowa
Cedar Falls, IA 50614

Rona Harrell, Ph.D.
Division of Special Education
Mobility Training Program
California State University at Los Angeles
5151 State University Drive
Los Angeles, CA 90032

Edwin Helmstetter, Ph.D.
Counseling Psychology
Washington State University
Pullman, WA 99614-2131

Everett W. Hill, Ed.D.
Department of Special Education
George Peabody College
Vanderbilt University
Nashville, TN 37203

Eva H. Horn, M.A.
Department of Special Education
George Peabody College
Vanderbilt University
Nashville, TN 37203

Luanna H. Meyer, Ph.D.
Division of Special Education and Rehabilitation
Syracuse University
805 South Crouse Avenue
Syracuse, NY 13244-2280

John A. Nietupski, Ph.D.
Department of Special Education
Education Center
University of Northern Iowa
Cedar Falls, IA 50614

Paul S. Niswander, Ph.D.
The Nisonger Center
The Ohio State University
Columbus, OH 43210

Richard Rosenberg, Ph.D.
Career Assessment and Placement Center
Whittier Union High School District
9401 South Pointer Avenue
Whittier, CA 90605

Charity Rowland, Ph.D.
Teaching Research Division
Oregon State System of Higher Education
345 North Monmouth Avenue
Monmouth, OR 97361

Ellin Siegel-Causey, Ph.D.
University of Kansas
Department of Special Education
3150 Haworth Hall
Lawrence, KS 66045

Kathleen Stremel-Campbell, M.A.
Department of Special Education
University of Southern Mississippi
Southern Station 5115
Hattiesburg, MS 39406

Steven F. Warren, Ph.D.
Department of Special Education
George Peabody College
Vanderbilt University
Nashville, TN 37203

Jan Writer, Ph.D.
School of Education
University of San Diego
Alcalá Park
San Diego, CA 92110

FOREWORD

THE "SHOES TEST"—that old idea of putting yourself into another's place—has been recently revived by Ann Turnbull and her colleagues at the University of Kansas. They have used this method to help parents and professionals consider the feelings and preferences of persons with severe handicaps. Taking the shoes test is tricky because there is no right answer, especially when you are trying to take the position of a person with significant loss of sensation through hearing and vision.

What is it like to have significant hearing and vision loss, and to have always been this way? With great difficulty, you would sort through and try to make meaning of the stimuli that you experience from movement, smell, taste, tactile sensation, and, to a lesser extent, sound and light. While it is likely that you would have some vision or some hearing or some of both, you might also have problems with thinking and remembering, or mental retardation. Making sense of one's environment and learning to operate in it would be difficult, in part, because the rest of the world functions with vision and hearing intact, and thus with language systems and rule-based interactions that come early and easily. Also, because the rest of the world speaks, hears, and sees, the shoes test is much harder for them to take. Very often the rest of the world does not understand you.

> Susan is hitting her head again, and pretty soon she will put her finger on her eyelid and push. I don't know what to do; I've tried lots of things: reprimands, three kinds of overcorrection, restraints, but nothing seems to work. Her mom and dad are afraid she will be completely blind if we can't get her to stop eye poking. We are not sure how much she can see, but we know she has light and dark discrimination. Her hearing appears to be functional, but she doesn't have a way to communicate, she hasn't learned much and she doesn't even walk without full assistance. If she loses all her vision, I think life will be even tougher for her.

What should be done? The school hired a vision specialist to examine Susan in the school and home setting. They learned that she did have some residual vision, and that no damage appeared to have resulted from her eye poking. The examination also revealed a potential explanation for the behavior: poking seemed to help her hold a focus, to keep her pupil fixed in one place. Next, an ophthalmologist examined Susan to check both her vision and any eye damage occurring since the last exam several years ago. Later, a functional analysis was carried out to check other reasons for the head hitting and the eye poking behaviors that were both judged potentially dangerous to Susan and targeted for reduction. Furthermore, her IEP was examined along with her current repertoire of skills. The teacher's efforts to unravel reasons for these behaviors were rewarded with the following information:

There had been no damage to the eye, and Susan still had the little vision that she had 3 and 6 years earlier.

The eye poking did have potential for reducing her residual vision and it also was unpleasant to view.

The eye poking probably helped stop or slow the strabismus.

Fairly simple eye surgery could reduce the strabismus, thereby lessening the tendency for Susan's eyes to move without control.

Head hitting was more frequent than eye poking, but both were rarely performed with force and left no marks on the skin.

Susan poked her eyes more when there were things to look at (people, materials) in perhaps an effort to hold her focus; eye poking occurred less during down time, when she tended to hit her head.

Susan poked her eyes and banged her head less when she was engaged in activities that appeared to interest her (using the music stick, playing "roll the ball" with a teacher or peer).

Susan poked her eyes and hit her head more when teachers called attention to the behaviors through reprimands than when teachers ignored them and differentially reinforced their absence with the presentation of interesting activities.

Susan didn't do much for herself; instead she waited for others to help her walk, eat, toilet, wash, and even play. She was good at waiting for help and usually got it.

Susan had not mastered a reliable means for communicating even though she had received training in manual signing and tactile communication board use; she did not (or was not asked to) choose activities or foods she wanted or decide whether activities would be terminated or repeated.

Susan did not walk without full support, even though there was no medical reason for being nonambulatory.

"Getting into Susan's shoes" meant taking a number of steps: obtaining more accurate information about her vision and her lack of walking and traditional communication, studying the variables that seemed to be maintaining her maladaptive behaviors, and contrasting her day-to-day flow of activities and behavior with that of other 11-year-olds who did not have her handicaps.

Now, 2 years later, Susan is walking around the school, in the community, and at home, either unassisted or with some help on uneven surfaces. She is making reliable choices during schooltime and at home. She has learned a variety of leisure skills and carries out routine grooming and eating tasks independently or with the partial assistance of another. Her eye surgery helped stop the eye movement but did not noticeably reduce the eye poking, so the teacher implemented a multifaceted program and keeps concurrent observational data on the two maladaptive behaviors. The elements of the intervention program involved: 1) teaching her functional skills that involved the use of her hands (including walking, which required the hands to balance), 2) reducing her "down time" and giving her choices about her activities throughout the day, and 3) using differential reinforcement to treat head hitting and eye poking. Students at school, who have helped teach Susan to walk, now speak to her instead of staring at her. "Susan is easier to understand now, because she walks," one fifth grader said. "She's more like me."

There is no doubt that students' sensory handicaps complicate the task of teaching them, even more so when they already have been identified as having mental retardation. Yet much of what we know about "best current practices" with students who have severe handicaps applies as well to students whose severe handicaps also include sensory impairments. We do not need to look toward faddish methods, nor do we need to begin from scratch in our efforts to devise intervention programs that work. Even with their serious impairments in vision and hearing, the students who are the focus of this volume behave and learn a lot like other students. Because of this, the contents of this volume rest on this premise—use the *simplest but still effective* strategies to teach skills identified to be meaningful or functional to the individual; rely on data (student performance and social validation data) to evaluate learning.

Based upon the expertise of the authors, many other themes emerge as one reads this volume:

1. Rather than bombard students with random stimuli (smells, temperature samples, varying tactile surfaces, strobe lights), as some "sensory stimulation" approaches advise, it is more reasonable to begin with the same proven strategies that we have used with other students having severe handicaps but without multiple sensory impairments. Thus, we start by targeting functional skills for individual students using an ecological inventory approach and then we teach the skills in useful clusters, while magnifying, enhancing, or bypassing natural task stimuli in ways suited to the student's ability to perceive those stimuli.
2. Total deafness and blindness are rare; most students have some residual vision and hearing that can be made more functional with instruction and aids.
3. Electronic travel aids, sensorimicrocomputer applications, and auditory and visual prosthetic devices can help some students, but only if these devices are selected to suit a given student, are functioning properly, are coupled with instruction, and enhance the accomplishment of functional life skills.
4. Communication means that the person at either end of the circuit can express and can be understood. Communication does not require a formal language system, but can be entered into with more expectation of success if the easier forms are used first. "Easier" forms include contingency awareness training (as long as it's useful to the student and suited to his or her age) and learning to anticipate by understanding nonverbal receptive cues. Also important is the identification of students' existing behaviors, adaptive or maladaptive, that communicate messages like: "I'm ready," "I need help," "I'm bored," "I want more," or "I want to get out of here!" To the extent that these messages occur and are reinforced by us (even if unintentionally), we have evidence of communication that can be used and expanded upon. Oftentimes, we will need to shift the contingencies and teach new communicative responses so that students do not use their inappropriate behavior as the means to communicate legitimate messages such as escape or boredom.

Proven teaching strategies occupy much of this volume. However, the research proof often has been derived from groups more able than many students with multiple sensory disabilities. The authors also address new combinations of existing techniques, novel variations of successful practices, and methods having a history of application but little supportive backing in research. Familiarity with these strategies is important for the teacher of students with multiple sensory impairments because proven techniques do not always work and because there is still much to learn about successful intervention with these individuals.

Part of the responsibility of being a teacher is to discover and use the methods that yield learning in students. This "discovery" relies heavily upon the collection of evidence (usually student performance data collected through direct observation) that reveals that one teaching method does not work and another method does. Perhaps more often with learners having multiple sensory handicaps, teachers must demonstrate responsible speculation—different ways to analyze the behaviors of their students and to teach them when "proven" methods fail. Researchers, in tandem with teachers, are responsible for further validating the success of teachers' discoveries or for sharing research discoveries with teachers. This cycle of responsible speculation followed by program change and data-based evaluation holds particular promise when students with multiple sensory disabilities fail to learn efficiently with typical methods.

Martha E. Snell, Ph.D.
University of Virginia

PREFACE

THIS VOLUME IS intended to address a perceived gap in the growing literature concerning educational services for persons with disabilities: the provision of "most promising practices" in education for persons with severe dual sensory impairments. In the 1980's, principles of integration and normalization have led to school programs aimed at achieving maximum independence and participation in multiple natural environments for individuals with severe disabilities. While empirical validation of effective practices for achieving these outcomes has been forthcoming, the particular needs of persons with dual sensory impairments, often in conjunction with other severe disabilities, have rarely been addressed. This book represents an initial effort to bridge that gap, with an emphasis upon the elementary and middle school years.

In addition to addressing the needs of a unique and often overlooked population, this volume also brings together a variety of approaches to curriculum development, program planning, and instructional delivery. Many of these approaches include empirical documentation. All of them reflect shared values of individualization and normalization. Educators, parents, and service providers are thus presented with a range of options for achieving elementary and middle school programs that are age-appropriate, teach functional skills that enhance independence across curriculum domains, maximize social participation, and respect the individual learner's preferences.

Within the first section, Fredericks and Baldwin define who individuals with dual sensory impairments are. They provide a historical perspective of service delivery systems for the population, and address current educational services trends. In addition, continuing needs for more integrated educational options are emphasized.

The second section of the book addresses program planning. Siegel-Causey and Downing provide an overview of early cognitive and communication behaviors for individuals with dual sensory impairments. They define specific content and procedures, emphasizing the importance of nonsymbolic communication intervention. The chapter by Rowland and Stremel-Campbell expands upon the early communication intervention theme, introducing the concept of emerging or "transitional" language content and procedures.

In Chapter 4, Goetz and Gee present a model for teaching functional use of residual vision. Their model details how to incorporate functional and age-appropriate curricular content, as well as learner motivation, into instructional programming to teach a sensory skill. Chapter 5 by Niswander provides a comprehensive discussion of audiometric assessment and considerations for selecting auditory prosthetics for children with both vision and hearing impairments. Next, Gee, Harrell, and Rosenberg, in Chapter 6, discuss an approach to teaching orientation and mobility skills to persons with multiple severe handicaps that emphasizes natural cues and utilizes natural travel opportunities in training. Specific lesson plans and data sheets are provided as examples. Finally, in Chapter 7, Campbell focuses upon a model for teaching basic motor and movement skills to students with multiple physical as well as sensory impairments. Goetz and Gee, Gee et al., and Campbell all present some empirical data in support of their approaches.

The third section of this book offers innovative, yet distinctly different instructional approaches and methods that are appropriate to the education of students with dual sensory impairments. This divergency of approaches reflects both a growing maturity in the field and the acknowledgment that educational and intervention practices for this population are necessarily complex and multifaceted. Writer begins this section in Chapter 8 with a movement-based approach to education that is derived from the writings and theoretical orientation of Jan van Dijk. In an organized and systematic fashion she discusses the basic child-centered derivations of this increasingly popular approach, and provides for the reader a wealth of practical instructional procedures for its implementation. Nietupski and Hamre-Nietupski next present in Chapter 9 a very thorough description of the ecological approach to the education of students with dual sensory impairments. Consistent with this orientation is a comprehensive format for designing and using community-based instructional procedures based upon functional, age-appropriate skill training. In Chapter 10, Helmstetter and Guess present a skill-cluster curriculum approach that has been adapted for students with multiple sensory impairments. They include in their chapter innovative considerations and procedures for allowing students to make choices and demonstrate preferences in their daily lives. Warren, Horn, and Hill, Chapter 11, conclude this section with a discussion of current and promising technological advances that are especially appropriate to the education and training of students with sensory impairments. Included in their chapter are the application of microcomputer technologies to the classroom setting, and an especially useful review of electronic travel aids.

Meyer and Eichinger, Chapter 12, conclude the book with a discussion of the role of evaluation in making ongoing revisions in educational services in order to improve program quality. Included in their chapter are initial results of a comprehensive survey to identify and provide social validation for potential "promising practices" from the perspectives of parents, educational experts, researchers, and direct service providers. The Program Quality Indicators checklist is included as an appendix and provides an appropriate and thought-provoking conclusion to the volume.

The increasing inclusion of learners with dual sensory impairments in classrooms serving students with other kinds of disabilities represents a unique challenge for all educators. Much remains to be done in order to provide maximally effective education for these individuals, including provision of secondary and postsecondary programs, and a range of employment and community living options. The contents of this volume represent only a beginning, but we believe it is a promising one.

Innovative Program Design for Individuals with Dual Sensory Impairments

SECTION I

INTRODUCTION

CHAPTER 1

Individuals with Sensory Impairments

Who Are They? How Are They Educated?

H. D. Bud Fredericks and Victor L. Baldwin

THE TITLE OF this book exemplifies an innovation in the world of special education that has been introduced in the past 5 years. The title reflects a change in the manner in which we refer to individuals with handicaps. No longer is it considered acceptable to refer to the "retarded child" or the "deaf-blind person." Instead, the person is represented first and then the disability. "The child with retardation," "the child who is retarded," or "individuals with multiple sensory impairments" are examples of the more acceptable description. This nomenclature has been officially adopted by The Association for Persons with Severe Handicaps (TASH) and the National Down Syndrome Congress (NDSC). The title of this book, *Innovative Program Design for Individuals with Dual Sensory Impairments,* represents a major departure from the common professional term of "deaf-blind." Federal legislation and regulations still refer to deaf-blind individuals. However, we shall refer to these same people as individuals with multiple sensory impairments.

POPULATION

The "deaf-blind" label, besides being an unacceptable appellation for those who are so handicapped, is inherently a misnomer. The "deaf-blind" label refers not only to those who are deaf and blind, but includes also those who are visually and auditorially impaired. Within the population defined as deaf-blind, the estimated distribution of the population across different levels of sensory impairment is shown in Table 1. Table 1 shows that only 6.1% of the population with multiple sensory impairments is deaf and blind. More than 90% of this population are categorized as either blind/severely hearing impaired or severely hearing impaired/severely vision impaired. An important fact for instructional purposes is that in 93.8% of this population there is either residual hearing or residual sight that can facilitate the instructional process.

An additional factor that must be considered with this population is that many students are either mentally retarded or are functioning as though they were retarded. The exact measurement of the level of retardation may be unattainable, and any score must be considered suspect, given the nature of the sensory deficits.

Table 1. Distribution by type of those with multi-sensory impairments

Group or population	Percentage (%)
Deaf/blind	6.1
Deaf/severely vision impaired	3.4
Blind/severely hearing impaired	48.0
Severely hearing impaired/severely vision impaired	42.4

Data extracted from Outlette, S. (1984), p. 14.

HISTORY OF SERVICE DELIVERY

The first child with multiple sensory impairments was educated at Perkins School in 1837. For the next 95 years, there was little federal recognition of this problem. Most children were not being educated and were found in institutional settings. In 1932, a specialized department for children with deaf-blindness was established at Perkins. Seven other such departments were established in institutional settings between 1937 and 1957.

A rubella epidemic occurred throughout the United States during 1963–1965, causing approximately 2,500 children to be born with multiple sensory impairments. The directors of the eight deaf-blind departments and other advocates convinced the federal government of the severity of the educational problem that would affect schools in 1969.

On January 2, 1968, federal legislation established centers and services for children with deaf-blindness. That legislation, administered by the Bureau of Education for the Handicapped (BEH), resulted in the establishment of 16 deaf-blind centers. These centers, as stated in the legislation, were "to develop and bring to bear upon such children, beginning as early as feasible in life, those specialized, intensive professional and allied services, methods, and aids that are found to be most effective to enable them (sic) (the children) to achieve their full potential for communication with, and adjustment to, the world around them, for useful and meaningful participation in society, and for self-fulfillment."

The growth of services for these children was phenomenal. In January, 1968, the best estimates were that 250 children were served. In 1980, the 16 centers reported serving 5,998 children through 300 service centers. At that time, the reported 0–12 population numbered 2,893.

Determining the actual number of children with both vision and hearing impairments has always been difficult. Part of the controversy regarding actual numbers stems from the counting procedures that are used across the various states and subsequently reported to the federal government. There are basically two sources of information to which the federal government has access that yield an aggregate count of these children.

The first source of information comes from the state director of special education in each of the states and territories. Each year, the state director is responsible for reporting the number of school-age children served in either the Public Law 94-142 (Education for All Handicapped Children) or the 89-313 (Title I/Chapter I: Aid to State Schools) program. Thus, in those states where educational services are not mandated for persons below 3 years of age or over 18 years of age, there would be no reporting of students within this age range who are vision and hearing impaired. Therefore, it is not hard to see why these numbers in the past have been fairly small.

The federal reporting form also requires the identification of students by handicapping category. Because some states do not have a deaf-blind category, additional difficulties are created in determining the accuracy of the numbers. In most of those states, the eligible students are counted under some other general category, such as multi-handicapped.

The second source of information to determine numbers of persons who are both vision and hearing impaired comes from the state coordinator for deaf-blind services (from individual states) or from the regional coordinator of a center for deaf-blind services that serves several states. In either case, these coordinators have established a registry. This registry identifies by name every student who is multiply sensory impaired. In most cases, the coordinator's sole job is to be concerned about service delivery to persons who are deaf-blind. Therefore, coordinators have records of nearly everyone who is brought to their attention as being classified as multiply sensory impaired. When the report from these coordinators is compared with the state directors' counts, there is considerable discrepancy. For example, in the 1984–85 reporting period, state departments of education identified 1,992 deaf-blind students age birth to 21, whereas coordinators of "deaf-blind" programs reported 4,270 students. Since "deaf-blind" programs are categorically funded by the Congress of the United States, these discrepant reports cause Congressional concerns about the actual numbers of children with multisensory impairments. Such concerns can put the "deaf-blind" program in potential jeopardy.

Staff from the Teaching Research (TR) Division of the Oregon State System of Higher Education have recently undertaken a nationwide study to rectify the differences between these two counts and to design procedures for obtaining accurate information. Generally, it was thought that the coordinators of deaf-blind programs probably had the best information on the actual numbers of students from birth to 21 because serving these students is one of the main functions of such programs. When asking these coordinators for specific counts of the children on their registries, it was also necessary to ask them to take an additional step, namely, to compare their findings with the report of their state director of special education. This required the coordinators to determine whether the students counted on their registries had also been reported by the state directors, either under the 94-142 or under the 89-313 funding authority, and to determine under which category the students were counted. This comparison determined whether the additional students actually existed, or were being counted more than once in some way.

The data for 1985–86 have been recently collected and are represented in Table 2. These data show that the numbers of children being identified at the lower age ranges (birth to 2) are quite small. After working closely with the persons responsible

Table 2. Summary of children and youth identified as deaf/blind by source of funding and age range for each state/territory

State/territory	Funding source: 142	Funding source: 313	Funding source: Unknown	Age grouping: 0–2	Age grouping: 3–5	Age grouping: 6–11	Age grouping: 12–17	Age grouping: 18–21	Age grouping: Unknown	Total
Alabama	10	24	56	0	0	0	0	0	90	90
Alaska	13	1	2	0	2	6	6	2	0	16
American Samoa	0	3	0	0	0	2	1	0	0	3
Arizona	32	14	17	0	8	15	24	16	0	63
Arkansas	15	54	1	2	10	23	24	11	0	70
California	200	29	89	2	21	74	118	97	6	318
Colorado	1	80	4	2	7	23	37	16	0	85
Connecticut	0	41	0	0	2	6	18	15	0	41
Delaware	0	33	1	3	6	13	8	4	0	34
District of Columbia	0	21	1	0	1	4	5	12	0	22
Florida	63	31	8	0	4	15	41	41	1	102
Georgia	39	25	63	0	2	15	26	21	63	127
Guam	0	7	0	0	0	2	3	2	0	7
Hawaii	8	18	0	0	0	0	0	0	26	26
Idaho	4	12	0	0	1	9	3	3	0	16
Illinois	0	181	0	0	0	0	2	0	179	181
Indiana	9	10	1	0	4	7	4	4	1	20
Iowa	12	30	0	0	2	7	14	19	0	42
Kansas	20	40	11	7	16	15	23	10	0	71
Kentucky	36	42	15	1	14	26	38	14	0	93
Louisiana	38	107	19	1	14	32	61	50	6	164
Maine	2	7	0	0	1	1	1	6	0	9
Maryland	15	37	1	0	6	4	23	20	0	53
Massachusetts	15	51	2	1	5	13	26	23	0	68
Michigan	2	110	24	2	16	35	39	32	12	136
Minnesota	0	0	81	3	14	20	19	24	1	81
Mississippi	0	45	5	0	0	7	20	23	0	50

Missouri	144	8	2	2	13	65	52	15	7	154
Montana	13	9	9	0	6	7	9	9	0	31
Nebraska	78	6	0	0	3	29	40	12	0	84
Nevada	2	0	1	0	0	0	0	0	3	3
New Hampshire	6	15	31	9	21	11	5	5	0	51
New Jersey	26	134	2	12	20	37	62	30	1	162
New Mexico	35	29	1	2	8	16	25	14	0	65
New York	104	236	1	2	26	74	115	106	18	341
North Carolina	16	14	4	4	4	3	17	6	0	34
North Dakota	1	20	0	0	1	6	6	8	0	21
Northern Mariana Is.	0	3	0	0	0	0	0	0	3	3
Ohio	17	18	1	1	0	5	10	20	0	36
Oklahoma	272	45	9	35	91	126	56	18	0	326
Oregon	0	82	7	0	6	26	28	27	2	89
Pennsylvania	11	85	1	0	5	12	28	37	15	97
Puerto Rico	21	0	18	0	0	0	0	0	39	39
Rhode Island	22	6	7	1	6	11	8	9	0	35
South Carolina	16	63	0	1	5	16	34	23	0	79
South Dakota	7	49	0	0	11	23	12	10	0	56
Tennessee	16	26	0	0	5	6	3	2	26	42
Texas	116	121	3	2	25	65	85	62	1	240
Utah	39	36	16	4	22	25	27	13	0	91
Vermont	0	10	0	0	1	3	3	3	0	10
Virgin Islands	0	14	0	0	0	0	0	0	14	14
Virginia	15	24	2	0	5	5	20	11	0	41
Washington	49	42	7	1	6	18	22	36	15	98
West Virginia	0	8	15	0	2	4	9	8	0	23
Wisconsin	7	17	0	0	0	4	6	14	0	24
Wyoming	12	3	6	0	0	0	0	0	21	21
Totals	1,567	2,159	537	100	448	971	1,266	963	515	4,263

142 = PL 94-142, the Education for All Handicapped Children Act of 1975; 313 = PL 89-313, Title I/Chapter I: Aid to State Schools.

for data collection, the TR staff found that there was a great deal of variation in the definitional process. Suggestions about that process occur later in this chapter.

The number of children identified varies from state to state, even when the states' populations are nearly equal. This discrepancy can best be illustrated by comparing Maine and Oregon, states with roughly equal populations. Maine reports 9 children and Oregon reports 89. The concerns about accuracy become more apparent if one compares a relatively populous state such as Indiana, which reports 20 children, with rural South Dakota, which reports 56 children. Consider also the case of Oklahoma, which reports 326 children, while California reports 318. No valid explanations for these differences can be offered at this time. Investigation into the discrepancies continues.

CURRENT TRENDS

A number of current events and situations have an impact on the delivery of services to this population. The first is the changing nature of federal support for the "deaf-blind regions or centers." Until 1982, the federal government funded services to the students primarily through 16 deaf-blind centers. From that time on, funding has been given not only to the centers, but also to individual states who have desired to provide and manage their own services for those who are multiply sensory impaired. The states assuming this responsibility frequently tend then to coordinate services for students who are deaf and blind with other services for students with severe impairments. Thus, in those states, the dichotomy of services between those with multiple sensory impairments and those with other severe impairments is beginning to disappear. This merger of services is especially apparent at the preschool level, where students with multiple sensory impairments are being included in programs serving students with other severe impairments.

Coupled with this changing emphasis from a regional to a state delivery system was a re-emphasis of priorities by the federal government during 1985 and 1986 to target monies funded under the Deaf-Blind Authorization (Title VI-C) toward those populations not being served. In most states, non-served populations included the population age birth to 2 and those over 18. In those states where services were mandated for those populations, access to Title VI-C dollars was further restricted.

An additional priority under Title VI-C was the provision of technical assistance to improve the quality of services for persons with multiple sensory impairments. Currently, the federal government has funded two national technical assistance centers to provide such assistance. One of these, The Association for Persons with Severe Handicaps (TASH) has responsibility for providing technical assistance to states and regional centers and to service providers and parents for the birth to 21 population. The Helen Keller National Center (HKNC) has responsibility for providing technical assistance to states and regional centers for the population over age 22. The major focus of these technical assistance efforts is to assist the individual states and the multi-state centers to improve the quality of services for those with multiple sensory impairments. For instance, TASH has focused much of their technical assistance on improving opportunities for students to be better integrated into more "normalized" community environments.

These changes represent a dramatic shift in funding patterns and put a greater burden on the states to provide quality services for persons who are multiply sensory impaired. Thus, the program has shifted from one of almost total federal support to a combination of federal and local (state/school district) support with a greater emphasis upon the local funding. This funding shift implies a reduction of federal responsibility for quality of services and a concomitant increase in state responsibility.

The second major impact on services has been the proliferation of early intervention services since the inauguration of Public Law 94-142. Since the passage of that law, approximately 20 states have mandated early childhood intervention services, some beginning at birth. These mandates have naturally included early intervention services for those children who were sensory impaired. In combination with the mandate of PL 94-142, which requires school districts to serve those of school age, these state programs have significantly reduced the need for federal support of the population with multiple sensory impairments in those states.

An interesting phenomenon relates to those early intervention mandates. The number of states that have mandated early childhood intervention services has remained relatively constant over the period from 1983 to 1986, although some states have rescinded previously mandated legislation and others have added it. This fluctuation of early childhood intervention mandates does have an impact on the population we are discussing. Populations receiving services previously mandated by states and therefore covered by state funding might, with the repeal of the state mandate, then have to receive more federal funding.

The recent passage of PL 99-457 amends PL 94-142, and will undoubtedly result in an expansion of services for young children with special needs. Specifically, this law extends the provision of services to the birth to 5-year age range. Title I provides for a discretionary grant program to states to plan and implement services to children from birth to 3 years and their families. Title II mandates services available through PL 94-142 for the 3- to 5-year age group.

The third impact on services for those with dual sensory impairments has been the tremendous growth in services since 1975 for those with severe handicaps. Not only has the number of services increased, but there have been significant changes in the types of programs and teaching techniques. Perhaps the greatest change has been in the emphasis on the least restrictive environment. More and more students who are severely disabled are being educated in environments that are integrated into public school buildings. Among the students so integrated are those with multiple sensory impairments. Although integration has, from one point of view, posed new problems in educating these students, it has more than compensated for these problems by the opportunities afforded these students to associate with and model after those students who are not handicapped, and to learn to function in the world of nonhandicapped students.

Three major philosophical constructs have also had an impact on the education of this population since 1975. The first of these philosophical constructs is the emphasis on functional curriculum versus developmental curriculum. Prior to 1980, the major emphasis of published curricula was to follow the growth patterns of nonhandicapped children and to teach skills in the order in which nonhandicapped children would normally acquire those skills. Since 1980, there has been a major emphasis on the teaching of skills that are functionally relevant to students with severe handicaps. In brief, this construct emphasizes teaching skills that are necessary for the student to survive in a nonhandicapped environment, and skills that will make him or her more independent in that environment. Frequently, this may mean skipping certain developmental steps, and teaching some skills that occur later in the developmental process prior to the teaching of other "earlier" skills. It also implies omitting the teaching of many skills that may not be functionally related to the daily performance requirements of the student.

The second philosophical construct that has had a significant impact on the education of students with severe handicaps is the emphasis on age-appropriate education. Prior to 1980, a visit to a classroom of adolescents with severe handicaps would probably show adolescent students working on tasks that were more suitable for elementary age or preschool age children. By emphasizing age-appropriate tasks, curricula are focusing on functional skills that are appropriate for the age of the individual. For instance, there are programs that teach skills to adolescents that will allow them to function better in the community, while elementary and preschool age students learn functional skills that will allow them to interact more effectively with their nonhandicapped peers.

The third philosophical construct that has had an impact on students with severe handicaps is the emergence of a more understanding philosophy and attitude toward parents of children with severe handicaps. In the 1970s, most parent training programs were designed to teach parents how to teach children. Lately, the emphasis on parent programs has been primarily to provide parents whatever support is necessary to allow them to maintain the child in the home (Benson & Turnbull, 1986). That support does not preclude teaching the parents skills that they can teach their children, but it also includes providing respite care, psychological support, or even monetary support in some cases. Thus, the impact on the family of a child with severe retardation and multiple sensory impairments is being better recognized by professionals. Many professionals have acquired or are being taught a greater sensitivity to the problems that these parents face. In addition, one of the major movements that has surfaced in the last 5 years has been the recognition of the problems that siblings face when coping with their brothers and sisters who are severely impaired.

NEEDS

There are many needs that still exist as quality programs for those with multiple sensory impairments are being developed. First, many of these students are still found in large institutional settings. Efforts to deinstitutionalize them and to being them into community-based programs have been slow and difficult because of the problems presented by their sensory impairments. Technology has not yet had a significant impact on this population, although we see the potential for technology to provide some solutions to assist in communication programming/intervention.

As more of these students are integrated into programs with other students with severe handicaps, a significant need for personnel preparation and inservice training arises, to inform teachers about how to utilize the students' residual sight and hearing in programming, as well as how to recognize and compensate for their auditory and visual deficits. Thus, the staff of programs serving those with severe handicaps need further training in dealing with students with sensory impairments. Not only does this training need to occur at the preservice level, but it is desperately needed at the inservice level as well. Until that training is more widely available at the preservice level, the difficulties with merging these programs or incorporating students with sensory impairments into programs for those with other severe handicaps will continue.

It is universally recognized that quality programs for those who are profoundly retarded and who have multisensory impairments are not readily available in most communities. Even quality programs that are serving those with severe impairments frequently are unable to extend that quality to those with profound impairments, such as persons who are nonambulatory, are not self-feeding, do not have self-help skills, have no language, and need daily physical, occupational, and communication intervention. The problems of educating these students are legion. Curricula specifically designed to be appropriate for those with profound handicaps have not been widely developed. In fact, there is rampant confusion as to what the nature of such a curriculum should be. Many problems still exist in integrating the medically fragile segment of this population in public schools. Moreover, there is still widespread rejection by many public schools of any population that is profoundly impaired or medically fragile.

After carefully reviewing the numbers of children who are reported year after year as deaf-blind, a question regarding definition becomes quite apparent. In the most traditional sense, our federal, and sometimes state, guidelines are established on the basis of the amount of deficit that must be identifiable under formalized testing procedures before a classification of *deaf-blind* can be made. In most cases, these guidelines refer to a specific level of visual and auditory acuity. A growing concern by the authors is that there may be a very large number of persons who are so severely handicapped that they are not readily assessable by formalized testing procedures to measure visual and auditory acuity. This group of people, however, are *functioning* as if they were having considerable difficulty in seeing and hearing. Because they cannot be formally identified does not mean that they should not receive the educational intervention strategies that have been documented as effective with persons of known visual and hearing deficits.

It can be argued that the educational prescription should drive the definition rather than the reverse. In other words, if it is determined that a student can benefit from instruction that utilizes exaggerated visual information (large print, positioning, etc.), additional auditory information (amplification, signing, etc.), or additional tactile information, then that student should be eligible for a deaf-blind registry. While the return to an era of labels is *not* desirable, the identification of these additional students and their names being added to some record-keeping system, might increase the probability that they will not go unnoticed and will be provided an appropriate educational program. As techniques are identified that are effective for teaching the person who is fully documented as having vision and hearing losses, why should other students who are functionally vision and hearing impaired *not* be afforded the same educational programs?

SUMMARY

Services for persons with multiple sensory impairments have, since 1968, moved from the status of primarily federal to primarily state programs, with the recognition that the responsibility for services for this population rests with the states, with some federal support. The need for early childhood intervention services has been recognized, but states have been slow in mandating those services nationwide. There has been difficulty in providing families the support that is necessary. Only partial deinstitutionalization and integration into public schools of this population has been achieved. Yet over the past 10 years there have been major strides in philosophy and educational techniques for teaching both those students with severe handicaps and those with multisensory impairments. The merging of these disciplines has benefitted the children and youth being served.

There is still much to do. Throughout the United States there are still too few programs that demonstrate quality services for those with multiple sensory impairments. Few programs are being integrated into public schools, and fewer still serve students with profound handicaps. However, progress has been made and problem areas have been identified. With hope, determination, and a high degree of professionalism, the quality of services over the next few years can be substantially improved. Many of the following chapters demonstrate how that improvement can be achieved.

REFERENCES

Benson, H.A., & Turnbull, A.P. (1986). Approaching families from an individualized perspective. In R.H. Horner, L.H. Meyer, & H.D. Fredericks (Eds.), *Education of learners with severe handicaps* (pp. 127–157). Baltimore: Paul H. Brookes Publishing Co.

Outlette, S. (1984). Deaf blind population estimates. In D. Watson, S. Barrett, & R. Brown (Eds.), *A model service delivery system for deaf-blind persons.* Little Rock: University of Arkansas.

SECTION II

CURRICULUM DEVELOPMENT

CHAPTER 2

Nonsymbolic Communication Development

Theoretical Concepts and Educational Strategies

Ellin Siegel-Causey and June Downing

IN RECENT YEARS, instructional strategies have been developed to supply service providers with procedures for teaching numerous skills to individuals with severe handicaps, including persons with dual sensory impairments. Communication skills training with these persons, however, continues to be an area of great challenge for educators and researchers (Bullis, 1985, 1986, 1987; Donnellan, Mirenda, Mesaros, & Fassbender, 1984; Musslewhite & St. Louis, 1982; Peck et al., 1984; Reichle & Keogh, 1986; Stillman & Battle, 1985b; Warren & Rogers-Warren, 1985).

Communication, viewed as the successful transmission of a message from one person to another, is of critical importance for all individuals. It is a skill within the capability of every individual, no matter how limited one's behavioral repertoire due to physical, sensory, and/or mental impairments (Fieber, 1977; Thoman, 1981; van Dijk, 1965a, 1965b, 1966, 1967, 1969, 1986). Difficulties in communication may especially arise when the social interaction involves one partner who has a dual sensory impairment, particularly if there is a concomitant mental and/or physical disability. These concomitant impairments may significantly reduce the individual's social interactions and environmental explorations. Consequently, the limited opportunity for exploration and interaction may affect the individual's communication and language progression due to the apparent relationship of cognition and social interaction for the development of language (Bates, 1976; Bruner, 1977; Carlson & Bricker, 1982; Schaffer, 1977; Schlesinger, 1977; Snow, 1984; Vygotsky, 1962). Many persons with dual sensory impairments do not use speech or other conventional symbol systems to convey their messages. These individuals may learn to understand what people communicate to them and to respond appropriately, but may have extreme difficulty developing a symbolic expressive communication system (speech, sign language).

The preparation of this chapter was supported in part by the U.S. Department of Education Contract #300-83-0237 and based in part on review of literature conducted by the first author. The information and opinions expressed herein do not necessarily reflect the position or policy of the U.S. Department of Education, and no official endorsement should be inferred.

The authors wish to extend appreciation to Carol Sims and Barbara Ernst who assisted in preparation of part of this chapter.

These individuals may instead use alternative nonsymbolic modes to communicate, such as gestures, vocal sounds, eye contact, body movements, and facial expressions.

A nonsymbolic interaction requires the listener to interpret the message received and to respond in a communicative manner. Ineffective communication frequently occurs when a nondisabled person fails to recognize and respond to the communicative expressions(s) of a person with a dual sensory impairment. Since communication involves the efforts of at least two people, there is a need to concentrate intervention efforts on the *interactive process* rather than to focus strictly on remediation of the limited repertoire of an individual. In addition, direct service providers, family members, and friends of individuals with dual sensory impairments should be provided training that involves facilitation of communication at a nonsymbolic level. Peck and Schuler (1984) note the critical need for this training emphasis because in most classrooms, service providers do not respond to students' basic nonsymbolic attempts at communication.

RATIONALE AND TARGET POPULATION

Considerable research has been done in the area of early language development (Bee et al., 1982; Bloom, 1970, 1973; Brown, 1973; Halliday, 1975), language disorders (Bloom & Lahey, 1978; Bricker & Carlson, 1981; Curcio, 1978; Curtis, Prutting, & Lowell, 1979; Goetz, Schuler, & Sailor, 1979, 1983), and social interactions (Bates, 1976; Bates, Benigni, Bretherton, Camaioni, & Volterra, 1979; Brazelton, Koslowski, & Main, 1974; Bruner, 1977; Chapman, 1981; Newson, 1979; Odom, 1983; Schaffer, 1977; Uzgiris, 1979; Vygotsky, 1962). In this chapter, there is no attempt to synthesize all available information on early communicative behavior; rather, this chapter limits its scope to behaviors identified in the literature as constituting nonsymbolic communication. *Communication at a nonsymbolic level* refers to the transmission of a message without the use of symbols (words, signs, graphics). The individual may use body movement, facial expression, eye gaze, vocal sound, etc. to convey a nonsymbolic message.[1]

Although it is generally recognized that individuals with dual sensory impairments are more dissimilar than alike, for this discussion the focus is on those persons who are severely limited in their ability to respond to auditory and visual stimuli and who need additional information from alternative sensory modes (tactile, vestibular, gustatory, olfactory, and kinesthetic) to communicate effectively. In addition, they may have severe mental and/or physical limitations, making it difficult for others to perceive and interpret their communicative messages. These individuals do communicate, but may not use speech or other symbols. Two descriptions in vignette form are presented in Table 1 to aid the reader in focusing on the person with dual sensory impairments who uses a nonsymbolic communication mode.

[1]The authors have chosen to use the term *nonsymbolic* as opposed to *presymbolic* or *prelinguistic*, since these latter terms connote a transition or development to symbolic communication. The authors of this chapter recognize that some individuals with dual sensory impairments will not use symbols but will communicate in a nonsymbolic manner.

Table 1. Description of two individuals with dual sensory impairments and additional disabilities

John is a 20-year-old adult with light vision, but no functional hearing. He also has a severe mental handicap. Though he does not use speech or sign to express his needs, he uses vocalizations intentionally to gain someone's attention. He responds to social and physical interactions by manipulating objects and also uses olfactory and gustatory modes to examine objects. John waits until others interact with him, but he does respond to those interactions with a smile, and will reach for another's hands if he wants more of something. To indicate displeasure he turns his head away, grimaces, and may push the object or person from him. John is very sensitive to another's touch and prefers to receive tactile stimulation with a towel or cloth on his skin (indirect touch). John responds with pleasure to a vibrator, to warm and soft textures, and to play with water. If ignored, John will bang his head and scream until someone interacts with him. John ceases these behaviors once the interaction begins and this seems to be an intentional and very effective means of gaining another's attention.

Ashley is 5 years old. Her muscle tone is tight and she displays an asymmetrical tonic neck reflex (ATNR) toward her left side. She has a mild hearing loss (40 dB). Although there are no structural abnormalities, Ashley does not display a directed gaze or follow visual stimuli. She is generally quiet and displays a neutral (not frowning, not smiling) expression. She often cries, whines, or screams when left alone for more than 2–5 minutes, when handled by new people, and through most of each meal. It does not appear that Ashley understands that her whining, screaming, or crying behaviors communicate a negative message to the adults around her. The familiar adults consistently respond to these messages as indications of displeasure or negation and try to provide alternate activities or adults, or other changes, according to the situation. Ashley continues to scream, whine, or cry after such accommodations have been made. In addition, she does not use briefer duration or less volume in negative expressions that would display more intentional communication. Further, Ashley does not appear to understand that positive behaviors (smiling, vocalizing, body movements, etc.) can produce communicative effects. Generally, Ashley's communication appears nonintentional in nature because she does not connect her expressions as having an effect on her physical or social environment.

There are numerous language intervention programs available that are derived from varying philosophical approaches, including: *cognitive* (Bloom, 1970; Bricker & Carlson, 1981; Brown, 1973; Miller & Yoder, 1974), *behavioral* (Deich & Hodges, 1977; Schiefelbusch & Bricker, 1981), *pragmatic* (Bates, 1976; Bruner, 1975; Halliday, 1975), and *ecological* (Mahoney & Weller, 1980; Ramey, Sparling, & Wasik, 1981). The majority of these programs, however, focus on the symbolic nature of communication and do not concentrate on the nonsymbolic communicative behavior that is characteristic of many persons having severe disabilities and/or dual sensory impairments. This chapter presents an interactional model (Bloom & Lahey, 1978; McCormick & Schiefelbusch, 1984) with emphasis on the importance of quality interactions with both the social and physical world. This particular approach recognizes the critical importance of the individual's manipulation of the environment and the role that social interactions play in achieving communicative competence.

Young children learn to communicate nonsymbolically with their eyes, gestures, facial expressions, and body movements prior to acquiring a formal language system such as speech or sign language. Many individuals with severe disabilities or dual sensory impairments function at a nonsymbolic communicative level and may not have a conventional way of expressing their needs, preferences, or ideas. Investigators in early communication development for children with disabilities (Bricker & Carlson, 1980; Brinker & Lewis, 1982; Odom, 1983; Rogow, 1984; Stillman & Battle, 1985b) recognize that individuals who communicate in a nonsymbolic manner need ways to express their likes and dislikes, to make choices and requests, and to indicate protest. The usual manner in which such communication occurs is through the individual's existing movements and behaviors. Despite the importance of these behaviors to immediate communication needs and in future language development, research and intervention strategies in communication facilitation for persons with disabilities has, for the most part, neglected to take into account the importance of these nonsymbolic communication behaviors.

ASSESSING COMMUNICATIVE BEHAVIOR AT THE NONSYMBOLIC LEVEL

The success of an intervention program will be influenced by the assessment procedure utilized to evaluate the skills and limitations of the targeted individual. The process of communication is a complex and multifaceted developmental skill. There is variability in the acquisition of nonsymbolic communication strategies, in communication environments, and in patterns of delay in nonsymbolic communication behaviors. In addition, the responsibility for assessment may vary, depending on the type of service delivery approach utilized and the professional staff available. Generally, nonsymbolic communication assessment is a shared responsibility between a communication specialist (usually a speech-language pathologist) and the primary service provider(s) (usually educators and parents).

An adequate evaluation of nonsymbolic communication skills must occur in conjunction with other assessments in the areas of vision, hearing, neurological status, perceptual motor skills, and social competencies. Assessment of nonsymbolic communication abilities must be done on an individual basis with consideration of the overall functioning level of each person. It is assumed that the recommendations from other chapters in this volume and other specific sources relevant to communication assessment will be integrated into an evaluation of nonsymbolic communication (Bullis, 1985, 1986, 1987; Siegel-Causey, Schulte, & Guess, in press; Stillman & Battle, 1985b; Stremel-Campbell, 1982).

Nonsymbolic Communication Assessment: Initial Acquisition (Birth–9-Month Developmental Level)

It is important that initial assessment focus on the individual's displays of nonsymbolic expressions (without words) of pleasure, displeasure, hunger, thirst, protest, request, gaining attention, greeting, and preference. Individuals who display nonsymbolic communication use their body movements, eyes, facial expression, touch, laughter, gestures, and sounds. An extensive review of the multifaceted behaviors included in this initial symbolic level is not possible within the format of this chapter. Siegel-Causey et al. (in press) provide a description of such behaviors and some of the potentially important aspects to assess, including:

Sensory responses: visually fixates and tracks; uses auditory discrimination and localization; gains attention through eye contact, facial expression, or sounds.
Social interactions: displays positive facial expression to familiar voice or presence; displays positive behavior (smile, laugh, relaxation) within pleasurable activities; participates in familiar routines; indicates displeasure; continues familiar patterns of movements.
Object interventions: increases/decreases activity level on seeing/touching interesting object; uses variety of actions on objects.
Expressive development—nonvocal: anticipates familiar event from context or whole body cues; associates familiar objects with specific actions; places adult's hands on object of desire.
Vocal: uses differentiated cry; vocalizes to indicate state, such as contentment, fear, anger.

These nonsymbolic behaviors develop approximately from birth to 9 months and may aid the evaluator in focusing on the scope and ontogeny of early nonsymbolic development.

Nonsymbolic Communication Assessment: Early Acquisition (9–12-Month Developmental Level)

At approximately the 8–10 month level, children have acquired intentional behavior and the ability to utilize nonsymbolic behaviors to produce desired responses or interactions (e.g., getting attention of others, indicating displeasure). From 9 months to approximately 12–15 months, the child continues to acquire further nonsymbolic behaviors on a continuum prior to using the first words (e.g., gesturing for "no"). The nonsymbolic behaviors on this continuum include the refinement of nonverbal (without words) behaviors to express wants, needs, feelings, and preferences. The communication evaluation at this early level of nonsymbolic development includes assessment of: 1) *expressive abilities:* a) refinement of nonverbal behaviors and b) additional vocal (production of sounds) behaviors; and 2) *receptive development:* a) verbal aspects (response to words) and b) nonverbal aspects (response to gestures, facial expression, and tactile cues).

Early nonsymbolic expressive and receptive processes allow the child to refine communication skills that develop from birth through approximately 9 months. A brief description (Siegel-Causey et al., in press) of nonsymbolic behaviors acquired between approximately 9–12 months includes:

Social interactions: responds to "no"; repeats behavior laughed at; uses gestures to direct attention; shows objects to elicit attention or display intention.

Object interactions: gives object on request; obtains hidden objects or objects on a string.

Expressive development—nonvocal: demonstrates social use of objects; shakes head "no"; gestures in context for yes, help, etc.; gives object to adult when action stops.

Vocal: displays five different babbling combinations; imitates nonspeech sounds (cough, tongue click, etc.); imitates sounds of adult.

Receptive development—nonvocal: ceases activity at "no" or "stop"; follows pointing cue; anticipates familiar events from contextual cues; responds to own name.

The behaviors included in this section may aid the evaluation process in focusing on the scope and progression of nonsymbolic development.

General Communication Assessment Considerations

A lack of visual acuity may have a crucial impact on the development of early communication. Visual impairments may interfere with the individual's ability to provide eye contact, follow another's gaze, and give a caregiver some clue as to the focus of attention. Hearing impairments may make it difficult for the individual to relate verbal descriptions of the environment to the corresponding physical items. When visual and auditory impairments are both present, these disabilities produce a multiplicative effect that alters the way in which the individual: 1) receives and sends information, and 2) interacts with the social and physical environment.

The assessment of the communicative abilities of individuals with dual sensory impairments who do not utilize symbols must focus on the nonsymbolic transmission and reception of a message. The assessment of communication should provide information regarding the following areas: 1) the current communicative performance of the child during communicative interactions, 2) the nature, extent, and potential reasons for communicative difficulties, and 3) the environmental factors involved in the individual's need for and use of communication. Communication is a highly complex skill, involving psychological, physiological, and social factors and, therefore, no single tool can provide a complete assessment and prescriptive guidelines for successful intervention. A combination of appropriate standardized assessment tools, behavioral checklists, ecological inventories, and observational tools is required to evaluate all aspects of the communication skills of the individual.

A selection of some of the assessment tools recommended for use with individuals who use nonsymbolic communication is provided in Table 2. Careful use of these instruments in conjunction with ecological inventories and thorough observational data may greatly enhance the ability of the direct service provider to intervene effectively with these individuals.

THE INFLUENCE OF SOCIAL INTERACTION IN NONSYMBOLIC DEVELOPMENT

The importance of social interaction and social context for early communication is promoted by the fact that infants and children learn their behavior has communicative significance and effect through the responses of others (Bakeman & Adamson, 1984; Bricker & Carlson, 1981; Carlson & Bricker, 1982; Masur, 1981; Murphy & Messer, 1977; Odom, 1983), as well as through the contribution of the caregiver in influencing the development of the child's appreciation of symbols (words) and their corresponding meanings (Schlesinger, 1977; Vygotsky, 1962). The progression of early communication development is centered within the interactions and relationships between the infant and the primary caregiver. Caregivers play a prominent role in early communicative development by displaying sensitivity to the nonsymbolic behaviors of infants and young children.

Sensitivity to Early Nonsymbolic Behaviors

Several authors view the influence of the primary caregiver during the preverbal/nonsymbolic stage as vital for the infant's future communicative ability and progress (Bakeman & Adamson, 1984; McClowry & Guilford, 1981; Odom, 1983; Snow, 1984). The importance of caregiver-infant interactions for the infant's future communicative growth is aptly stated by Odom (1983), "From birth, survival depends on the ability to interact with other human beings in a reciprocal manner. During the early months of life, environmental effects are mediated through the social interactive relationship between the infant and its caregiver" (p. 215). Through this stable, nurturing relationship with the caregiver, infants develop a feeling of security in their new world. This contributes to the infant's confidence in exploring the environment, and out of this confidence a firm base is established for future attempts at communication and other social skills.

The caregiver's ability to predict and interpret the infant's signals provide the infant with the feeling that his or her signals *do* elicit a predictable social response from the caregiver. In turn, this success in responding appropriately to the infant's signals produces a feeling of competence in the caregiver. These two aspects combined (the child's effective signals and the caregiver's relevant responses) result in the development of frequent, mutually satisfying interactions (Clark & Seifer, 1983; Goldberg, 1977). Carlson and Bricker (1982) maintain that the responsiveness of the caregiver can be directly related to the infant's success and/or failure in learning to communicate.

The preponderance of literature on the development of language focuses on the acquisition of *verbal* skills (Bloom, 1970, 1973; Goetz et al., 1979; Miller, 1981; Nelson, 1973). Some authors, however, who have studied the processes of language development assert that the prelanguage/nonsymbolic stage is a critical time for acquisition of linguistic *and* nonlinguistic skills (Schiefelbusch & Pickar, 1984; Snow, 1984; Sugarman, 1984). The thrust of recent developmental research shows: 1) infants do communicate before they talk, and 2) this communicative ability evolves during the first year of life (Bates et al., 1979; Bruner, 1975; Bullowa, 1979; Halliday, 1975; Hubley & Trevarthen, 1979; Sugarman, 1984; Wilkes, 1981).

The information compiled from research on the nonsymbolic stage is particularly relevant to the study of individuals who have dual sensory impairments because many of these individuals function at a developmental stage very similar to the

Table 2. Nonsymbolic assessment tools and screening guides

	Callier-Azusa Scale (H) Scales for the Assessment of Communicative Abilities (1985a) Stillman, R., & Battle, C. University of Texas at Dallas Callier Center for Communication Disorders Dallas, Texas 75235	*Communication Placement Assessment Manual* (1984) Stremel-Campbell, K., & Clark-Guida, J. Teaching Research Monmouth, Oregon	*Comprehensive Communication Curriculum Guide* (1981) Klein, M.D., et al. Early Childhood Institute University of Kansas Lawrence, Kansas 66045	*Nonverbal Prelinguistic Communication* (1983) Otos, M. Oregon Department of Education 700 Pringle Parkway SE Salem, Oregon 97310
Population designed for	Persons who are deaf-blind and severely/profoundly disabled	Individuals who have severe and/or profound handicapping conditions	Students who are severely/profoundly retarded, physically handicapped with little or no communication	Persons who are deaf-blind, multihandicapped, sensory impaired
Age range	Not specified; developmental levels birth–24 months	Younger range birth–30 months; older range not specified (estimate 4–6 mental age)	Not stated (birth–adolescent)	Birth–24 months
Criterion; norm referenced; developmental scale; other	Developmental scale	Developmental scale	Other (interview, questionnaire)	Developmental guide

Interpretation	Profile with approximate age equivalencies	Communication Assessment Profile (Developmental level) and IEP Planning Worksheet (Objectives)	Outcome is organized information of student's current communicative performance	Profile
Tool objective	Provide comprehensive, developmentally based framework for viewing communicative abilities	Instructional planning, establishing baseline functioning	Diagnostic assessment and establishing baseline functioning	Guide to assess current functioning level and plan future programs
Type of response	Observations of behavior in familiar environments, especially classroom settings	Direct observation, arranging situations, reports by familiar person/nonvocal and vocal child responses	Observation of child in *all* natural environments	Nonverbal and verbal (signed) responses in natural and structured situations
Assessment areas related to early communication	Representational and symbolic abilities, receptive communication, intentional communication, reciprocity	Responses to sensory input, interactions with objects, receptive and expressive communication, prelanguage	Attending behaviors, vocal development, communicative function and responses, prelanguage	Reactions to physical and social environments, attending behaviors, anticipatory behaviors, interactions with objects and people, nonverbal skills, gestures

Adapted with permission from Siegel-Causey, E., Schulte, E., & Guess, D. (in press). Psychological evaluation of speech and language disorders. In V.B. Van Hasselt & M. Herson (Eds.), *Psychological evaluation of the developmentally and physically disabled*. New York: Plenum.

nonsymbolic level of normal infants. Individuals with dual sensory impairments and normal infants functioning at a nonsymbolic level both rely heavily on gestural, vocal, and tactile means to communicate. Thus, the study of nonsymbolic interactions between infant and caregiver may provide important information relevant to nonverbal communication facilitation, for both the individual with dual sensory impairments and the normally developing child.

EARLY INTERACTIONAL PROCESSES WITH NONDISABLED INFANTS AND CHILDREN WHO ARE NONSYMBOLIC AND HAVE DUAL SENSORY IMPAIRMENTS

A complex, regulatory feedback system between the caregiver and infant is ready at birth. The newborn displays behaviors that facilitate predictable responses from the caregiver, and that provide the opportunity to develop patterns of negotiation, expansion, and differentiation (Als, 1979). Early nonsymbolic development is influenced by the context of social interactions (Bricker & Carlson, 1981; Cole & St. Clair Stokes, 1984; McCollum, 1984), as they provide "the major setting in which the infant practices and learns social, cognitive and communication skills" (McCollum, 1984, p. 301).

Infants are equipped with a repertoire of behaviors that function as communicative signals to the caregiver. These signaling behaviors include smiles, cries, facial expressions, gestures, vocalizations, and eye contact. Caregivers also respond to a young infant's behaviors as if these were intentional attempts to communicate (Fafouti-Milenkovic & Uzgiris, 1979; Hayes, Goodnow, & Murray, 1984; Hopkins, 1983; McClowry & Guilford, 1981). At the same time, caregivers gain and focus the infant's attention through exaggerated rhythmic speech, ritualized play, animated facial expression, consistent eye contact, and gestures (including patting, touching, holding, pointing, and tapping). Patterns of reciprocation that develop between caregivers and infants occur repeatedly throughout the day within natural routines (Newson, 1977). The infant begins to actively initiate, maintain, or terminate communicative exchanges (Lamb, Bell, & Borts, 1982; Newson, 1977). Early exchanges between caregivers and infants are important in establishing a dialogue-like structure within which the infant acquires communicative competence. Thus, the caregiver's role is critical in offering many opportunities for social exchanges and in providing the structure for early communicative interactions.

Some individuals with severe physical and/or mental disabilities and accompanying sensory impairments may function at similar developmental levels as the young infant. Their behaviors include many of the same reflexes, motor patterns, and nonsymbolic communicative levels observed in infancy. There are, however, some differences between the development of the nondisabled infant and that of the individual with dual sensory impairments. Differences occur in the development and use of visual and facial behaviors, and in vocal and other related expressive behavior. Visual deficits may result in lack of gaze behaviors and normal eye contact; visual behavior may also be tied to reflexes, and therefore not voluntarily controlled (Clark & Seifer,

1983; Langley, 1980). Smiling behaviors may be delayed (Brooks-Gunn & Lewis, 1984; Odom, 1983), may require different responses (e.g., tactile-kinesthetic contact) from the caregiver to elicit them (Langley, 1980; Walker & Kershman, 1981), or may be lacking (Odom, 1983). These early gazing and smiling behaviors are important in early interactions; the consequence of their absence may be disruptions within the interactional process, thus having an impact upon the infant's development of communicative competence. Their importance is emphasized by Langley (1980): "The two most significant factors in the development of a meaningful communication system appear to be the establishment of reciprocal gaze patterns between infant and primary caregiver, and the infant's subsequent smiling behavior" (p. 33). Clearly, the interactional process is affected if these behaviors fail to appear within the repertoire of the individual with dual sensory impairments.

Individuals with dual sensory impairments may also differ in terms of developing a sense of causality, appearing to be unaware that their behaviors have an impact. This lack of a sense of causality results in fewer repetitions of vocalizations or other behaviors (Langley, 1980), and therefore fewer opportunities for caregiver responses. In their study of children with deaf-blindness, Walker and Kershman (1981) found that fewer vocalizations, less distress, more neutral affect, and less predictability were exhibited by these children as compared to nondisabled infants. They also found that the children with dual sensory impairments offered fewer opportunities for caregivers to engage in interactive sequences. As a result, caregivers experienced difficulty in initiating and maintaining communication with their children who have dual sensory impairments. Signals that the child with dual sensory impairments or other disabilities is ready to interact are often "mixed" or unclear (Odom, 1983); the caregiver is less able to read them (Clark & Seifer, 1983) and therefore less able to respond to them appropriately. Odom (1983) observes that children or infants with disabilities may be less responsive to the caregiver, which in turn influences how the caregiver behaves toward the infant or child. Thus, caregiver interactions with infants who are disabled reflect unique issues in terms of sensitivity, timing, and contingency.

When a child is physically and/or mentally disabled and also has accompanying sensory impairments, the development of the interactional process is influenced. Children who function at the same nonsymbolic communicative level as young infants need to experience the same synchronous and predictable relationships with their primary caregivers. These children, however, may not be giving their caregivers readable signals (Clark & Seifer, 1983; Odom, 1983) and are not as predictable in their responses as the nondisabled, nonsymbolic infant (Walker & Kershman, 1981; Walker, Levine, & Grasse, 1982). Thus, the interactional process does not reflect contingent responsiveness by each dyadic member. Rather, the caregiver assumes responsibility for initiating and controlling interchanges (Bakeman & Brown, 1977; Brinker & Lewis, 1982; Brooks-Gunn & Lewis, 1984; Lamb et al., 1982), without the typical infant signals and cues to guide his or her responses. Consequently, the potential exists for asynchronous interchanges to disrupt the interactional process.

Caregivers (parents, teachers, service providers) of nonsymbolic children with dual sensory impairments assume a crucial role in the development of the child's communicative abilities. Caregivers need to be sensitive to the child's atypical responses and attempt to time their own responses to the unfamiliar and unresponsive interactive patterns of the child. Contingent interactions may be difficult for the caregiver to establish as a result of the less predictable responses of their child, as well as the influence of the disabling conditions on the interactional process. It is apparent that interchanges between caregivers and the child with dual sensory impairments reflect the same issues of sensitivity, timing, and contingency as interchanges between caregivers and nondisabled infants. At the same time, however, caregivers of children with dual sensory impairments experience more disruptions and uncertainties within the interactional process.

Comprehensive reviews of the processes of nonsymbolic development and the interactional context between the infant-caregiver dyad are available (Siegel-Causey & Guess, 1985; Siegel-Causey, Ernst, & Guess, 1987; Siegel-Causey, Sims, Ernst, & Guess, 1986). These sources also provide analysis of the process of communication development with caregivers and infants with disabilities and suggest related intervention strategies and research needs.

COMPONENTS OF NONSYMBOLIC COMMUNICATION

The following sections reflect a compilation of information obtained from literature and research on early communication development (Brazelton et al., 1974; Bullowa, 1979; Carlson & Bricker, 1982; Halle, 1982; McCormick, 1984; Miller, 1981; Schaffer, 1977; Schiefelbusch & Bricker, 1981; Schiefelbusch & Pickar, 1984; Siegel-Causey & Guess, 1985; Snow, 1984; Sugarman, 1984; Uzgiris, 1979; Ziajka, 1981). Modifications and adjustments in skill acquisition are included to accommodate the needs of the individual who does not receive normal sensory input. An effort has been made to consider sensory losses and the concomitant lack of behavioral responses that might result. Emphasis has been placed on tactile and kinesthetic behaviors as important to early communication skills and/or potential communicative behavior.

Four general categories are delineated to represent the basic components of nonsymbolic communication. These interrelated components are specified as: a) awareness, b) social interactions, c) physical interactions, and d) combined interactions. The identified components may aid the reader in recognizing the interrelated behaviors that form the basis for both nonsymbolic and symbolic communication (Bakeman & Adamson, 1984; Coggins & Carpenter, 1981; McClowry & Guilford, 1981; McCormick, 1984; Rice, 1984; Sugarman, 1984).

Overview of Nonsymbolic Skills

Although there is no existing research to verify that the suggested skills are prerequisites to symbolic behavior, there are sufficient data to strongly support the concept that the social and physical behaviors included consistently precede more symbolic communication (Als, 1979; Bakeman & Brown, 1977; Bullowa, 1979; Hayes, 1984;

McCormick, 1984; Newson, 1977; Piaget, 1959; Sugarman, 1984). The acquisition of intentional physical and social control over the environment may lead to a similar control of that same environment with the use of symbols. Our suggestions for communication programming reflect the concurrent emergence of the selected behaviors. The following nonsymbolic communication components provide the format for this section:

A. Awareness
   Reacts to physiological needs
   Reacts to environmental changes
   Engages unintentionally in cause and effect changes
   Recognizes familiar people
   Anticipates familiar events
   Intentionally acts on objects but not to communicate
B. Social interactions
   Rejects presence or actions of people
   Attends to social partner(s)
   Requests continuation of social or physical activity
   Demonstrates turn-taking
   Directs behavior intentionally to obtain presence of others
   Displays affection
   Shares joint attention
C. Physical interactions
   Uses objects to request continuation of physical or social activity
   Uses objects to reject events
   Uses objects to offer or comment
   Demonstrates anticipation of events by using representational objects
D. Combined interactions
   Gains other's attention prior to using objects to intentionally communicate
   Gains other's attention prior to using gestures or vocalizations to intentionally communicate

Awareness This category largely comprises behaviors that reflect awareness of oneself (e.g., biological needs, movement in space, physiological reactions to external influences); recognition of familiar people; display of basic preferences; and unintentional means/ends exchanges (i.e., accidental activation of a call signal). These behaviors are typical examples of the demonstration of awareness, and are not meant to exclude other similar behaviors.

Awareness of oneself and of environmental factors is fundamental to cognitive development (Piaget, 1966). It is also essential to communication, since awareness of the social and physical environment provides the substance for the message and for the intended recipient for the exchange. Awareness that stems from initial interactions with objects and people may be accidental in nature; for example, such awareness may arise from rolling over on a squeaky toy, tasting mud on one's hands, dropping something off a table. When actions (unintentional and intentional) toward an object or person are consistently perceived and acted on by others as intentional, these accidental or exploratory behaviors may later be used effectively by the individual to satisfy needs and desires. This is particularly true of interactions with objects that precipitate the appearance of a concerned other who then interacts with the individual in an anticipated or desired manner. Thus, the awareness that social partners (the caregiver, parent, teacher) react as a result of the individual's self-generated behavior aids in the progression from unintentional to intentional communication.

Social Interactions Behaviors directed toward another person comprise the category of social interactions. These behaviors include: rejecting the presence or actions of others; attending to a social partner (eye contact, smile, relaxed muscle tone); requesting continuation of social activity (crying when a partner leaves, body movements that serve to continue the interaction); taking turns during an interaction (patting someone's hand and waiting to be patted in return); intentionally obtaining the attention of others (grabbing someone's hand); displaying affection (touching an arm or leg); and joint attention (attending to some object or event with another person). These social elements of interactions are basic to communication (Bruner, 1977; Bullowa, 1979; Rice, 1984; Rogers-Warren & Warren, 1984; Snow, 1984) and indicate increased awareness of others in the immediate environment. An increased desire or willingness to interact with others may develop as social interactions satisfy personal needs. Recognizing others as a means to satisfy basic needs may be extremely reinforcing to the individual, thus strengthening attempts at communication. Therefore, random or isolated behaviors that accidentally draw the attention of another may later be repeated to intentionally draw attention and produce desired results of social interaction (banging an empty cup on a table until someone fills it with juice).

Physical Interactions This category is comprised of those behaviors that focus on the individual's interactions with the physical world, including interactions with others as objects rather than as social partners. Such interactions have the potential to communicate various messages, including: requesting continuation of an action (handing a wind-up toy back to someone but not obtaining that person's attention first); rejecting an activity (averting head, spitting out green beans, throwing clothes down); using objects to offer or comment (extending a cup but not toward another person); and anticipation of forthcoming events (grasping an empty spoon and extending it at mealtimes). The use of common objects (manipulating, looking at, pointing toward) directs the attention of a potential communicative partner toward the substance of the message, thus clarifying the intent. Initial physical interactions may be somewhat haphazard and may not produce the desired result (e.g., a child holding an empty cup receives additional milk, when he or she wanted juice). Given repeated experiences and an increased awareness of means/end relationships, the individual's skill in using objects as part of intentional communication may be enhanced. These nonsymbolic physical interactions enable the individual to clarify the message by using objects (e.g., the individual rejects the milk that was poured into the cup by pushing it away, and then leans toward the juice can). The individual gains greater control over the immediate environment by clarifying the intent of the communicative interaction through the use of objects, but may not display effective communication if the interaction is not *directed* toward another person. The individual is generally dependent on the other person's attentiveness and ability to interpret the situation as communicative.

Combined Interactions This category incorporates the communicative behavior that combines social interaction aspects (someone to communicate to) with physical interactions (intentional object use). When both of these general behaviors are used to communicate, the message is more direct, explicit, and easily interpreted. These combined interactions display the necessity of gaining the attention of the social partner prior to communicating. Behaviors included in combined interactions are communicating needs intentionally with objects used for clarification, and using consistent vocal sounds or gestures to communicate intent. Individuals are frequently taught to manipulate objects or even engage in symbolic behavior (signing, pointing to pictures) without including a partner in the interaction. Even the most sophisticated form of symbolic expression fails to communicate if it is performed in isolation. It is critical for an individual who has dual sensory impairments to learn that others exist in the environment, and that the *inclusion* of people in communicative interactions is essential for the successful transmission and reception of a message.

Facilitation of Nonsymbolic Acquisition

The remaining sections of this chapter will focus on practical instructional techniques to facilitate the development of nonsymbolic behaviors for communicative purposes. Emphasis has been placed on the tactile and kinesthetic behaviors of the individual as examples of early communication skills or potential communicative behavior. This does not mean that visual and auditory behaviors should be ignored. The service provider should incorporate these behaviors and adapt activities according to individual needs.

The techniques suggested are aimed at helping the individual with a dual sensory loss to acquire intentional control over physical and social environments. This control is easily recognizable at a symbolic level ("Hey, Mom, bring me a brownie!"), but is also evident at a nonsymbolic level (an individual extends a coffee cup toward a person pouring coffee). Unfortunately, such nonsymbolic behaviors are often overlooked and devalued due to the common educational expectation for traditional symbolic modes (Hopkins, 1983; Sachs, 1984; Shevin, 1979). To avoid reliance on symbolic communication modes and to devise ways of promoting the further development of behaviors that lead from unintentional to intentional communication at a nonsymbolic level, the following basic considerations are suggested.

Basic Considerations The proposed suggestions for facilitation of nonsymbolic communication include promoting behaviors that lead from unintentional to intentional communication at a nonsymbolic level. Direct service providers should recognize that communication involves at least two people and reflects the need/desire of one person to interact with another. This basic premise should remain a major consideration when developing classroom strategies to promote communicative competence. The use of this information and implementation of suggested activities should incorporate the following guidelines. Nonsymbolic communication activities should:

1. Occur within a variety of natural routines that are part of a meaningful daily schedule for a specific individual
2. Utilize materials that are age-appropriate, functional, and motivating for that individual
3. Utilize functional settings with nondisabled peers
4. Compensate for auditory and visual loss through alternative sensory input (tactile, kinesthetic, olfactory, vibratory)
5. Provide activities that promote communicative interaction frequently throughout the day

INTERVENTION STRATEGIES FOR SERVICE PROVIDERS AND CAREGIVERS

A common focus in describing language and communication intervention is the remediation of deficits in the person with disabling conditions. Since a communication interaction is a dynamic exchange involving at least two people, it is important for instructors to recognize that multiple sensory disabilities profoundly affect how others interact with that person. The willingness of persons without disabilities to communicate may be influenced by the limited behavioral repertoire of the individual with a dual sensory impairment. The social partner may not be sufficiently reinforced during interchanges that have limited visual behaviors (eye gaze toward objects or persons relevant to the interchange, eye contact, visual tracking), facial expressions, body movements, or vocal sounds.

Social interactions play a significant role in communication development (Bates et al., 1979; Brazelton et al., 1974; Newson, 1977; Nietupski, Schuetz, & Oakwood, 1980; Odom, 1983; Rogers-Warren & Warren, 1984; Rogow, 1984) and for this reason, dynamic, meaningful exchanges should occur frequently and with considerable effort on the part of the person without disabilities. Direct service providers need personal skills that accommodate the nonconventional or limited auditory, visual, and vocal displays of the person with dual sensory impairments. Facilitative interactions must incorporate kinesthetic, tactile, gustatory, vibratory, and olfactory stimulation to take the place of the customary dependence on visual and auditory modalities.

Nine general intervention categories have been devised to provide strategies that focus on intervention for service providers interacting with persons who display nonsymbolic behavior. These strategies have been drawn from the infant literature previously discussed and from extensive informal observation of effective communication instruction. The intervention strategies are:

1. Sensitivity to individual preferences and dislikes
2. Compensation for lack of distance senses
3. Responsivity to the individual's attempts to communicate

4. Consistency in instructional structure and format
5. Providing contingencies
6. Creating a need to communicate
7. Incorporating time-delay into adult responses
8. Establishing a cooperative social environment
9. Increasing expectations for communicative behavior

These adult intervention strategies are explained in the following section. In addition, examples from descriptions of John and Ashley (refer to Table 1), two hypothetical children who are nonsymbolic, are incorporated into the strategies. The relevant components of nonsymbolic communication (refer to page 27) are included at the end of each strategy example.

Sensitivity to Individual Preferences and Dislikes

A child-centered approach may produce the best results when interacting with an individual who displays limited interest in his or her social and/or physical world (van Dijk, 1966, 1967, 1986). Too frequently the instructional activities planned for a day are forced on an individual who may have little desire to participate and no way of expressing that disinterest. To encourage this individual to be involved with people and activities, it may be advisable to identify whatever interests that person has and build on those unique features. The physical and social world must appear pleasurable for the individual or there will be no reason to initiate or respond to interactions.

STRATEGIES: SENSITIVITY TO PREFERENCES

Nonintentional Communication

Ashley

A staff member rocks Ashley in a rocking chair holding her so that they face each other. This adult hums, sings, or rocks to a familiar tune. The activity continues with emphasis on encouraging a positive response (smile, giggle, decreased ATNR, relaxed muscle tone). If Ashley cries or screams, the activity is stopped and a different environment (warm pool, warm bed) is provided.

[Reacts to physiological needs; reacts to environmental events]

Intentional Communication

John

John is playing with a vibrating massage tool. A less handicapped peer from another room has been taught to interact with John by requesting a massage tool and applying it to John's back. This student stops the activity occasionally and waits for a response from John that indicates a desire for continuation (smile, grabbing for the tool, touching the student). Following the response, the student acknowledges John's request with a pat on his back and continues the massage.

[Requests continuation of social activity; communicates needs using objects for clarification]

GENERAL STRATEGIES:

— Physically interact with the individual in a manner that is pleasurable to that individual (rocking, swinging, giving a massage, tickling, foot bath, water play, twirling, etc.) and be attuned to any behavioral change.

— Make use of appropriate opportunities to hug, kiss, stroke, rub, and display a variety of affectionate behaviors to the individual. ("Appropriate" refers to the individual's age, the setting, situation, etc.)
— Establish play activities in which you can imitate the individual's unintentional or intentional behavior (e.g., follow the individual's movements, copy object manipulations, repeat vocalizations).
— During interactions with things and people in the environment, note specific actions that the individual uses. Imitate the action observed in that context so that this behavior can be considered a gesture. Be consistent in using this gesture in similar contexts, provided it parallels the individual's behaviors.
— Allow the individual to make choices whenever possible (type of food, clothing, activity, object, person to be placed by). This demonstrates respect for the individual's preferences and helps to develop decision-making skills (Guess, Benson, & Siegel-Causey, 1985).

Compensation for the Lack of Distance Senses

When hearing and vision are diminished or lacking, the individual's exploration of the world may be severely restricted, and care must be taken to bring environmental stimuli (both physical and social) into nearer proximity so that interaction may occur. This is particularly true for the individual with dual sensory impairments and physical disabilities. In addition to decreasing the distance between the stimulus and the individual, the size, shape, color, and sound produced by an object (or person) should be considered. Many toys and other objects have been analyzed for their effectiveness with children who have dual sensory impairments (Langley, 1985). Activities and objects that can be enjoyed without vision or hearing are preferable. Choosing appropriate activities that do not require vision or hearing is a challenging exercise for the creative service provider. The assumption that the tactile mode will "take over" for the input from the sensory modes should be avoided. The assessment of the individual's tactile preferences and processing abilities must be discerned on an individual, ongoing basis.

STRATEGIES: COMPENSATION FOR DISTANCE SENSES

Nonintentional Communication

Ashley

Ashley is positioned in a variety of ways so that she can move her limbs or other body parts. A mobile of brightly colored and sparkling objects and bells or wind chimes is placed where she can see and touch it with an accidental or reflexive movement. Social interactions with Ashley occur as she activates the mobile.

[Engages unintentionally in cause and effect exchanges]

Intentional Communication

John

When working on a task, John sits close to someone so he can feel that person and have a recipient for any messages. John must touch that person prior to receiving help (additional materials, assistance in the bathroom, etc.). An adult or peer who will respond appropriately and consistently is placed next to John, to be a communication partner and provide reinforcement

[Attends to social partner]

GENERAL STRATEGIES:

- Find comfortable positions that involve body contact with adults and other individuals during a day's activities.
- Manipulate the environment so that small physical movements create unexpected results (tower of blocks to tumble down, limb movement causes a mobile to activate, loosening the knot of a balloon causes it to deflate).
- Assist the individual in recognizing familiar people by tactually and visually exploring commonly worn items (watch, jewelry, glasses) on that person.
- Adapt toys to include long, durable extensions that can be easily used by the individual. Items should be within access of the individual, but should require some manipulation of the extension.
- Have other students in close proximity participate in highly exciting, pleasurable, motivating situations. Make sure that the targeted individual is aware the activity is occurring. This targeted individual must obtain someone's attention in order to be included in the activity.
- Teach a natural gesture for "I want," and model the desired behavior when interacting with the individual by extending an open palm to the individual (use tactile input as appropriate) to indicate that something is desired from the individual.

Responsivity to the Individual's Attempts to Communicate

Being responsive to the behaviors of an individual, whether intentional or nonintentional, is critical if these potentially communicative behaviors are to increase and develop greater sophistication (Bates, Olson, Pettit, & Bayles, 1982; Clark & Seifer, 1983; Elliott, 1984). The service provider must be sensitive to small, basic behaviors elicited by the individual, and must respond to these behaviors as if they were communicative. For some individuals, such behaviors may be difficult to identify. These behaviors may include increased respiration, eye blink, change in body tone, or the movement of a limb that may be reflexive. Given attention to even these topographically minute behaviors, the individual with dual sensory impairments may develop a greater awareness that it is possible to influence his or her immediate social and physical environment. These early attempts at communication can then be shaped into more intentional forms as the individual develops an awareness of the contingencies in his or her environment.

STRATEGIES: RESPONSIVITY TO COMMUNICATION ATTEMPTS

Nonintentional Communication

Ashley

Occasionally, the staff engage Ashley in an activity they believe she does *not* like (for example: bouncing up and down). When she cries, they immediately stop, letting her know that they have stopped because she cried. She

Intentional Communication

John

When John wants to go to the bathroom, he grabs his belt buckle and shakes it. Upon seeing this behavior, an adult approaches John and asks him if he has to go to the bathroom while imitating John's gesture (shaking is then engaged in an activity she does like (listening to a tape of her mother). A staff member stays in close physical contact, watching for any sign of enjoyment. Occasionally, the staff member stops the tape and observes Ashley. If she looks at, moves toward the sound, decreases/increases movement, etc., these behaviors are acknowledged (verbally and tactilely) and the recorder is turned on again.

[Rejects actions of people; requests continuation of activity]

his belt buckle). John is then assisted to go to the bathroom. (All interactions with John incorporate touch, so that John feels the other person making use of his [John's] gestures).

[Communicates needs intentionally, using objects for clarification]

GENERAL STRATEGIES:

- Reinforce *any* effort (movement, pounding on the floor or object, grimace) on the individual's part to draw your attention. Make sure each individual has some external method of obtaining adult attention (interface child to a switch that activates a call signal, bell, or other noisemaker, or light).
- Respond to the individual's behavior (body movements, change in activity level, facial expressions, change in muscle tone, etc.) in a consistent manner. Assume intentionality for behaviors that occur frequently.
- Recognize the communicative value in stereotypical behavior (hand flapping, hair twirling, light gazing) and aggressive behaviors (hair pulling, tantrums, screaming, hitting). The individual may be trying to communicate boredom with a program or dislike of an activity. Before attempts are made to rid the individual of these behaviors, it may be advisable to examine the potential message within these behaviors (Donnellan et al., 1984).
- Provide an activity that is not particularly appealing to the individual to allow the individual an opportunity to control the adult by rejecting the activity. Then change to a different activity that the individual prefers.
- Provide a model or hand-over-hand instruction to assist the individual in seeking attention from an adult or peer (use of call signal, tapping on the shoulder, making a noise, waving a hand, etc.). Providing activities should be contingent on the individual using the attention-getting behavior.
- Engage the individual in a variety of pleasurable activities (swimming, swinging, rocking, wrestling, back rubs, etc.), and frequently stop the activity. A signal from the individual (splashing, body movement forward, kicking legs out, increasing muscle tone, etc.) determines the continuation of the same activity. When there is no response or negative response (cry, frown, push way, grimace, etc.) discontinue the activity.
- Make sure all care providers are consistent in using the individual's own gestures and/or vocalizations. All adults should respond to the individual's gestures.
- Avoid using abstract symbols (signs, print) with an individual who does not have a consistent use of gestures or vocalizations.

Consistency in Instructional Structure and Format

Consistent routines and structure in daily events may prepare the individual to anticipate forthcoming events and future activities. Consistent routines enhance the individual's interpretation of messages and may increase self-initiated expressions related to the upcoming event. Interactions with the individual need to be consistent both within routines and in the manner of communication.

Once routines have been established and the individual begins to anticipate the sequence of steps, a break in a routine can provide an opportunity for a communicative interaction. It may be the occasional unexpected and irregular occurrences that most effectively trigger an initiation from a student who normally does not initiate any interactions. The routine must be well established, however, before the individual can be expected to notice disruptions or peculiarities in a sequence of events.

STRATEGIES: CONSISTENCY IN STRUCTURE AND FORMAT

Nonintentional Communication

Ashley

Every time Ashley is repositioned, each service provider engages in following routine:

1. Greets Ashley
2. Touches her shoulder and waits 5–10 seconds for attention to social partner
3. Places one arm under Ashley's knees and the other around her shoulders and back; exerts slight pressure and release
4. Tells Ashley "up" (verbal)
5. Waits 5–10 seconds to allow her the opportunity to indicate readiness, anticipation, awareness, etc., by tensing her muscles or leaning forward slightly
6. Lets Ashley know verbally that the signal was "interpreted" as intentional
7. Picks Ashley up

[Engages unintentionally in cause and effect exchanges]

Intentional Communication

John

The adaptive physical education instructor greets John by saying "Hi!" and placing John's hands on the whistle that always hangs from his neck. The instructor waits until John gets tennis shoes (always kept in the same place) before going together to the gym.

[Attends to social partner; demonstrates anticipation of events]

GENERAL STRATEGIES:

— Develop the prosodic (rhythmic) elements of communication by engaging in simple pleasurable repetitive actions and watching for anticipation behavior from the individual ("Peek-a-Boo" game of putting a cloth on a young child's face, taking it off and saying, "Boo!" while kissing or blowing on the child's face; lifting the child's arm or leg up in the air, saying "Up!", setting back down, pausing, then repeating).

— Within daily events (diapering, feeding, repositioning, dressing, fine motor tasks, etc.), establish clearly differentiated steps that are consistent.

— Provide the individual with consistent tactile, auditory, and/or visual information prior to the actual start of the activity (e.g., stimulate oral musculation prior to mealtime; provide tactile and auditory cues prior to lifting; allow individual to sniff deodorant prior to using it).

— In preparation for forthcoming events, assist the individual in obtaining necessary objects and materials immediately preceding the activity (gather meal utensils, food, etc.; obtain swimsuit and towel; gather cassette recorder and tape, etc.). A sequence or calendar box with separate compartments that hold objects representing activities may be helpful for some individuals.

— Have all caregivers (OT, PT, adaptive physical education, speech therapist, paraprofessional, etc.) begin intervention sessions in a manner unique to themselves. Intermittently throughout the session, the adult should draw attention to any unique personal and/or activity-specific characteristics (e.g., paraprofessional draws individual's attention to necklace that she wears daily; adaptive PE person moves individual's arms forward and back to mimic a throwing motion).

— After a routine has been well established, interrupt that routine by occasionally introducing unfamiliar people, new or too few items, a slightly different sequence of events, etc.

Providing Contingencies

To help develop an individual's potential as an active learner and to develop contingency awareness, it is important to emphasize the relationship between behaviors and their effects. The individual is reinforced for behavior when a positive result occurs (leaning forward gets more pushes on a swing). At a nonsymbolic level, the individual must be provided contingent experiences to learn that his or her expressions have predictable outcomes. The individual's cry brings a staff member to find the reason for the distress. The individual's smile at lunch time is interpreted as wanting another bite of food. The service provider learns that his or her responses have certain effects on other individuals—positive and negative. Both the individual and the service provider need to participate in mutual contingency experiences. The individual may begin to understand that his or her actions have predictable effects on others, and this enables that person to anticipate subsequent responses. Being able to predict these effects may lead to more intentional communicative acts (Clark & Seifer, 1983; Rogow, 1984). In addition, contingent responding allows the individual to develop some control over the immediate environment, which may enhance the desire to communicate, and may also lead to increased self-esteem.

STRATEGIES: PROVIDING CONTINGENCIES

Nonintentional Communication

Ashley

Staff members position Ashley so that a random or reflexive action will depress a switch that activates a tape recorder. The tape recording is a repeating message for someone to

Intentional Communication

John

During free-time, John is offered a choice between investigating a variety of seashells or manipulating a brailler (both activities are ones he enjoys). Both objects are placed become to her. Each time the tape recording is activated, someone attends to Ashley by stopping the tape player and asking her what she wants. A pleasurable social event is also provided.

[Engages unintentionally in cause and effect exchanges]

fore him and he is encouraged to explore them for recognition. John is asked to choose which item he wants to use. The item he chooses represents the activity he will do.

[Demonstrates intentional behavior to obtain objects]

GENERAL STRATEGIES:

— Position the individual and/or the switch so that unintentional movements activate motivational objects (vibrator, fan, toy, music, heating pan, etc.).
— Engage the individual in a variety of pleasurable activities that can be easily interrupted (e.g., wind-up music or mechanical top, watching TV or movie that is controlled by a minute-relay switch; finishing a game at the video arcade; rolling a ball).
— During play activities, assist the individual in a variety of building and stacking activities. Place desired object(s) on top and demonstrate how to knock down the tower to obtain the object.
— During mealtimes, provide the individual with two choices. The choices can be between two preferred items (juice and yogurt; cookie and cracker) or one preferred and one nonpreferred food or drink. Occasionally offer something to eat or drink that is distasteful to that individual. Accept any "no" response and offer a more appealing food item.
— During regularly scheduled periods, provide the individual with two-choice activities. Provide two different types of switches that activate two different objects, noisemakers, etc. Occasionally provide the individual with a choice that involves something that he or she distinctly dislikes. Pair this activity/object with a specific switch to indicate rejection.
— Require the individual to obtain needed items before engaging in a familiar activity (no juice until the individual obtains his cup, no outing until the individual begins to put her shoes on, no trip in the van until the individual obtains the keys).

Creating a Need to Communicate

There is no need for individuals to attempt to communicate if: 1) they have no control over their environment, 2) nothing happens (in a positive way) as a result of their communicative efforts; and 3) if everything they need or want is provided without any effort or request. In addition, individuals who do not clearly see or hear others fulfilling their needs may require extra motivation to initiate interactions. Individuals not only need a reason to communicate and something to communicate about, but they also need a reason to communicate (Bloom, 1970; Bloom & Lahey, 1978). By anticipating and satisfying potential needs before they become apparent to the individual, the motivation or reason to interact with another person is greatly diminished. For individuals who do not initiate interactions for social reasons, taking advantage of basic human needs can provide the necessary impetus for communication interactions.

STRATEGIES: CREATING A NEED TO COMMUNICATE

Nonintentional Communication	Intentional Communication
Ashley	*John*
Ashley is normally changed at regular intervals so she does not often remain in soiled diapers. Her teacher begins to wait until Ashley indicates discomfort (usually a moan) before attending to her needs. When Ashley moans, her teacher makes her aware that she has come to help Ashley as a result of the moaning.	John enjoys snack time and waits quietly for his juice. One day at snack time the other students are given their cups, but John's is withheld. A staff member pours the other students a drink, while making sure that John is aware of what is happening and can smell the juice. If John screams or bangs his head, staff acknowledge this initiation, but pair it by displaying a more appropriate "I need help" behavior (tapping someone on the shoulder and then touching the juice container).
[Reacts to physiological needs]	[Gains another's attention prior to using objects to intentionally communicate]

GENERAL STRATEGIES:

— Provide only limited amounts of specific social interaction or of an item (1 minute lotion rub, pleasurable movement that is interrupted, tickling for a few seconds, half a cookie, two pushes on a swing, 5 minutes in the pool, timer turns off music after 1 minute, etc.).

— Retain an object that the student desires until that individual attends to the adult holding the object (moves closer to, puts hand on the adult, taps adult, provides eye gaze, etc.). Interfere with an individual's play with a favorite toy by placing it out of reach or with something slightly obstructing its use.

— Create minor obstacles/distractions in the individual's customary path to a desired outcome (place chairs in front of a refrigerator for an individual who often goes to obtain his or her own food; someone stands between the individual and a favorite person; etc.).

— Create situations in which individuals must initiate adult/peer attention in order to obtain/participate in a desired activity (a pitcher of juice is handed to an individual but a peer has his cup; it's time to go swimming but her suit is not available; lunch is set-up but the adult who feeds the individual is not attending to her; after going to the bathroom the individual needs help buckling his belt).

Incorporating Time Delay into Adult Responses

This intervention strategy complements the prior strategy of creating a need situation. Once a need to communicate has been established, the individual requires sufficient time to respond. Often individuals are placed on the instructor's hectic time schedule, overlooking the possibility that the individual may require a longer latency period in which to respond. The length of time provided to respond will depend on the activity and the individual student. Knowledge of the individual's abilities and the situation will help to determine the appropriate time to wait for a response before providing a prompt. Since many individuals with severe disabilities become dependent on cues or prompts before responding, using prompts after a specified delay period, and then fading specific prompts to more general ones, may help to create greater self-generated or independent behavior on the part of the individual.

STRATEGIES: INCORPORATING TIME DELAY

Nonintentional Communication

Ashley

While swinging with Ashley on the playground, the assistant stops and holds Ashley at the top of the arc and waits (20 seconds) for a response. This somewhat uncomfortable position along with the time delay tends to precipitate a response from Ashley (kicking a leg or vocalization). Ashley's responses are interpreted by the assistant as intentional and the swinging is resumed.

[Requests continuation of activity]

Intentional Communication

John

While taking a bath, John is prompted to wash various parts of his body by an adult touching each body part. John has learned to wait until he is touched before proceeding. Those touch prompts are now delayed and faded to a more general pat on the back ("You're doing fine, John") until John keeps washing without individual prompts prior to each step. When he finishes in a reasonable length of time, he is rewarded by a favorite snack or activity. If he does not finish in a reasonable length of time, the consequence is ending his bathing in rather chilly bath water.

[Attends to social partner; demonstrates anticipation of events]

GENERAL STRATEGIES:

— Refrain from immediately responding to the individual's needs before that need becomes critical (e.g., feeding the individual when he or she indicates hunger, rather than according to a specific time schedule).
— Refrain from engaging in the activity that the individual desires until the individual displays an attending response.
— Prior to prompting the initial steps of a routine activity, allow the individual a chance to demonstrate at least part of those steps.
— Act hesitantly or reluctantly, as if unsure what the individual wants. Try to require a more obvious and persistent response from the individual.

Establishing a Cooperative Social Environment

A competitive situation or one in which the individual has no opportunities to interact with peers diminishes the potential for communication. With individuals who have severe impairments, there is a tendency to establish a one-to-one, student/teacher ratio for most instructional activities. This technique may be particularly disadvantageous to those individuals who cannot see or hear their classmates, and hence may not be aware of their presence. To increase the opportunities for incidental social interactions, pair or group individuals for activities (both structured and unstructured) whenever possible. When individuals are grouped in close proximity to one another, and are encouraged to share materials and cooperate in one activity instead of several different activities, there are more opportunities for peer interactions and, therefore, more opportunities to practice basic communication skills.

STRATEGIES: COOPERATIVE SOCIAL ENVIRONMENTS

Nonintentional Communication

Ashley

At recess Ashley is paired with a nondisabled or less disabled peer who is instructed to help her with her coat and assist in maneuvering her travel chair to the playground. The teacher encourages other students to show Ashley their toys, hold her hand, bring her leaves and stones they collect, etc. These students have been trained to respond in a very positive manner to Ashley when she is not crying, and to leave her alone when she does cry. This intervention has provided enough structure that now Ashley is perceived as just "one of the gang," and students interact with her during recess without adult prompting.

[Recognizes familiar people]

Intentional Communication

John

Prior to leaving on an educational trip to a public laundromat, John is shown the car keys and assisted in gathering his dirty laundry. Before leaving, John chooses the student who will be his sighted guide by touching one of two students who are in close proximity to him. After making his choice of a guide, he is assisted in gripping that person's arm appropriately. The guide is periodically instructed about proper guidance techniques. This choice and pairing of students is repeated prior to many excursions. The guides enjoy their time with John and are disappointed when they are not chosen.

[Recognizes familiar people; communicates needs intentionally]

GENERAL STRATEGIES:

— Establish situations for peer interaction that incorporate turn taking *and* physical contact during the individual's play/recreational periods (mutual back rubs, scratching each others' backs, brushing each others' hair, etc.).

— As much as possible, encourage the individual to participate in reciprocal roles of an activity (pushing/pulling a wagon and riding in a wagon, hammock, etc.; washing and drying dishes; one individual stops and another starts electronic/mechanical objects).

— Develop a buddy system, pairing individuals with different abilities for a variety of activities. The nondisabled individual or person with milder disabilities is able to assume a leadership role, while prompting responses from an individual with severe disabilities more effectively and naturally than occurs in a teacher/student relationship.

— Create play or work situations that require two or more people to achieve a common goal (e.g., building a tower with several individuals/adults sequentially contributing individual blocks; planting a flower with each individual being responsible for one step in the process; cooking a meal with each individual having certain utensils and foods necessary to complete a recipe; going outside with one individual giving a coat to a peer to put on, and then having the peer reciprocate).

Increasing Expectations for Communicative Behavior

Raising expectations for communicative actions does not necessarily mean that the display of symbolic behavior (written words, speech, sign language) is the only intended goal. Parents and instructors can consistently encourage nonsymbolic communication by expecting occurrences in a variety of situations, with different people, and across many different activities and settings. It is also critical to expect communicative behavior to increase in frequency and complexity while utilizing a nonsymbolic mode. Therefore, if it is determined that an individual may potentially "never" acquire symbols for communication, progress in communication skill development can proceed horizontally. The individual can be taught to refine existing nonsymbolic techniques with a greater audience to ensure a growing control over the environment and a greater expression of needs, wants, and interests.

STRATEGIES: INCREASING EXPECTATIONS FOR COMMUNICATIVE BEHAVIOR

Nonintentional Communication

Ashley

Initially Ashley would receive some juice if she reduced the muscle tone of her facial muscles and did not cry. After achieving this goal successfully, she is now required to also move her head forward as an indication of wanting juice.

[Requests continuation of activity]

Intentional Communication

John

When John wants to eat, he usually grabs his spoon and taps on his plate. Staff members sit next to John but do not respond to him until he touches them first. In this way he is being required to include a communication partner in the interaction.

[Attends to social partner; gains other's attention prior to gesturing to intentionally communicate]

GENERAL STRATEGIES:

— Make use of frequent natural gestures in interactions with individuals who do not use symbols. Make them aware that gestures and not just signs or spoken words are acceptable and expected in all settings.
— Ignore primitive attempts by the individual to communicate (such as standing near a desired toy or a general vocalization used for all wants). Turn away from the individual and require a more persistent response from the individual before acting.
— Shape different gestures, movements, and vocalizations to resemble distinct intentional communicative actions.
— Communicate your expectation of communication and wait for an expression/response.

CONCLUSION

In summary, this chapter stresses the importance of nonsymbolic behaviors in the development of communication for persons who do not make use of symbols. An attempt has been made to focus on the basic communicative behavior of individuals with severe multiple sensory and/or mental impairments. Communicative behaviors that are nonsymbolic in nature (cries, body movements, grasping an object, smiles) provide the individual with a means of communicating basic needs and wants. These behaviors do not have the same precise connotations as symbolic behavior (speech, sign language, writing); thus, the burden of the communication interaction falls on the conversational partner. For effective communication to occur, the nondisabled partner must be attentive, responsive, and accepting of a wide variety of seemingly unconventional behaviors as communicative. The display of sensitivity, timing, and contingency are important facilitative aspects for nonsymbolic development.

The nonsymbolic behaviors described throughout this chapter are a valuable means (and for some, the sole means) of interacting with another person. For this reason, these behaviors should be viewed and accepted as a legitimate mode of communication, especially for the individual who may never use symbols. Use of the term *presymbolic* was avoided because it may imply an inevitable transition to a symbolic mode of communication. The authors recognize that some persons may not develop a symbolic system. Lack of symbolic behavior, however, does not mean that an individual cannot communicate (a common misconception), but merely that an individual has an alternative way of expressing needs and desires. Although this mode of nonsymbolic communication may require somewhat more effort and interpretation from a communicative partner, this effort is both necessary and well worth the time spent if the end result is improved communication for those who have so often been misunderstood and ignored.

REFERENCES

Als, H. (1979). Social interaction: Dynamic matrix for developing behavioral organization. In I.C. Uzgiris (Ed.), *Social interaction and communication during infancy* (pp. 21–38). San Francisco: Jossey-Bass.

Bakeman, R., & Adamson, L.B. (1984). Coordinating attention to people and objects in mother-infant and peer-infant interactions. *Child Development, 55*, 1278–1289.

Bakeman, R., & Brown, J.V. (1977). Behavioral dialogues: An approach to the assessment of mother-infant interaction. *Child Development, 48*(10), 195–203.

Bates, E. (1976). *Language and context: The acquisition and pragmatics.* New York: Academic Press.

Bates, E., Benigni, L., Bretherton, I., Camaioni, L., & Volterra, V. (Eds.). (1979). *The emergence of symbols: Cognition and communication in infancy.* New York: Academic Press.

Bates, J.E., Olson, S.L., Pettit, G.S., & Bayles, K. (1982). Dimension of individuality in mother-infant relationship at 6 months of age. *Child Development, 53*, 446–461.

Bee, H.L., Bernard, K., Eyres, S., Gray, C., Hammond, M., Spietz, A., Snyder, C., & Clark,

B. (1982). Prediction of IQ and language skill from perinatal status, child performance, family characteristics, and mother-infant interaction. *Child Development, 53*, 1134–1156.

Bloom, L. (1970). *Language development: Form and function in emerging grammars.* Cambridge, MA: MIT Press.

Bloom, L. (1973). *One word at a time: The use of single-word utterances before syntax.* The Hague: Mouton.

Bloom, L., & Lahey, M. (1978). *Language development and language disorders.* New York: John Wiley & Sons.

Brazelton, T.B., Koslowski, B., & Main, M. (1974). The origins of reciprocity: The early mother-infant interaction. In M.L. Lewis & L.A. Rosenblum (Eds.), *The effect of the infant on its caregiver* (pp. 49–77). New York: John Wiley & Sons.

Bricker, D., & Carlson, L. (1980). An intervention approach for communicatively handicapped infants and young children. *New Directions for Exceptional Children, 2*, 33–48.

Bricker, D., & Carlson, L. (1981). Issues in early language intervention. In R.L. Schiefelbusch & D.D. Bricker (Eds.), *Early language: Acquisition and intervention* (pp. 477–515). Baltimore: University Park Press.

Brinker, R.P., & Lewis, M. (1982). Discovering the competent handicapped infant: A process approach to assessment and intervention. *Topics in Early Childhood Special Education, 2*(2), 1–16.

Brooks-Gunn, J., & Lewis, M. (1984). Maternal responsitivity in interactions with handicapped infants. *Child Development, 55*, 782–993.

Brown, R. (1973). *A first language: The early stages.* Cambridge: Harvard University Press.

Bruner, J. (1975). The ontogenesis of speech acts. *Journal of Child Language, 2*, 1–19.

Bruner, J. (1977). Early social interaction and language acquisition. In H. Schaffer (Ed.), *Studies in mother-infant interaction* (pp. 271–289). London: Academic Press.

Bullis, M. (Ed.). (1985). *Communication development in young children with deaf-blindness: Literature review I.* Monmouth, OR: Communication Skills Center for Young Children with Deaf-Blindness, Teaching Research Division.

Bullis, M. (Ed.). (1986). *Communication development in young children with deaf-blindness: Literature review II.* Monmouth, OR: Communication Skills Center for Young Children with Deaf-Blindness, Teaching Research Division.

Bullis, M. (Ed.). (1987). *Communication skills development in young children with deaf-blindness: Literature review III.* Monmouth, OR: Communication Skills Center for Young Children with Deaf-Blindness.

Bullowa, M. (Ed). (1979). *Before speech: The beginning of interpersonal communication.* New York: Cambridge University Press.

Carlson, L., & Bricker, D.D. (1982). Dyadic and contingent aspects of early communicative intervention. In D. Bricker (Ed.), *Intervention with at risk and handicapped infants: From research to application* (pp. 291–308). Baltimore: University Park Press.

Chapman, R.S. (1981). Mother-child interaction in the second year of life, its role in language development. In R.L. Schiefelbusch & D.D. Bricker (Eds.), *Early language: Acquisition and intervention* (pp. 291–308). Baltimore: University Park Press.

Clark, G.N., & Seifer, R. (1983). Facilitating mother-infant communication: A treatment model for high-risk and developmentally-delayed infants. *Infant Mental Health Journal, 4*(2), 67–81.

Coggins, T., & Carpenter, R. (1981). The communicative intentions inventory: A system for observing and coding children's early intentional communication. *Applied Psycholinguistics, 2*, 235–251.

Cole, E.B., & St. Clair Stokes, J. (1984). Caregiver-child interactive behaviors: A clinical procedure for the development of spoken language in hearing-impaired children. *British Journal of Audiology, 18*, 7–16.

Curcio, F. (1978). Sensorimotor functioning and communication in mute autistic children. *Journal of Autism and Childhood Schizophrenia, 3*, 281–292.

Curtis, S., Prutting, C., & Lowell, G. (1979). Pragmatic and semantic development in young children with impaired hearing. *Journal of Speech and Hearing Research, 23*, 534–553.

Deich, R., & Hodges, P. (1977). *Language without speech*. New York: Brunner/Mazel.

Donnellan, A.M., Mirenda, P.L., Mesaros, R.A., & Fassbender, L.L. (1984). Analyzing the communicative functions of aberrant behavior. *Journal of the Association for Persons with Severe Handicaps, 9*(3), 201–212.

Elliott, N. (1984). Communicative development from birth. *Western Journal of Speech Communication, 48*(2), 184–196.

Fafouti-Milenkovic, M., & Uzgiris, I.C. (1979). The mother-infant communication system. In I.C. Uzgiris (Ed.), *Social interaction and communication during infancy* (pp. 41–56). San Francisco: Jossey-Bass.

Fieber, N. (1977). *Sensorimotor cognitive assessment and curriculum for the multihandicapped child*. Omaha, NE: Media Resource Center, Meyer Children's Rehabilitation Institute.

Goetz, L., Schuler, A., & Sailor, W. (1979). Teaching functional speech to the severely handicapped: Current issues. *Journal of Autism and Developmental Disorders, 9*(4), 325–343.

Goetz, L., Schuler, A., & Sailor, W. (1983). Motivational considerations in teaching language to severely handicapped students. In M. Hersen, V. Van Husselt, & J. Matson (Eds.), *Behavior therapy for the developmentally and physically disabled* (pp. 57–77). New York: Academic Press.

Goldberg, S. (1977). Social competence in infancy: A model of parent infant interaction. *Merrill-Palmer Quarterly, 23*(3), 163–177.

Guess, D., Benson, H.A., & Siegel-Causey, E. (1985). Concepts and issues related to choice-making and autonomy among persons with severe disabilities. *Journal of The Association for Persons with Severe Handicaps, 10*(2), 79–86.

Halle, J. (1982). Teaching functional language to the handicapped: An integrative model of natural environment teaching techniques. *Journal of The Association for the Severely Handicapped, 7*(4), 29–37.

Halliday, M.A.K. (1975). *Learning how to mean: Explorations in the development of language*. New York: Elsevier North-Holland.

Hayes, A. (1984). Interaction, engagement, and the origins and growth of communication: Some constructive concerns. In L. Feagans, C. Garvey, & R. Golinkoff (Eds.), *The origins and growth of communication* (pp. 136–161). Norwood, NJ: Ablex Publishing.

Hayes, A., Goodnow, J., & Murray, J. (1984). Analyzing states in the behavior of mother and infant. In R.A. Glow (Eds.), *Advances in the Behavioral Measurement of Children* (pp. 1–27). Greenwich, CT: JAI Press.

Hopkins, B. (1983). The development of early non-verbal communication: An evaluation of its meaning. *Journal of Child Psychology and Psychiatry, 24*(1), 131–144.

Hubley, P., & Trevarthen, C. (1979). Sharing a task in infancy. In I.C. Uzgiris (Ed.), *Social interaction and communication during infancy* (pp. 57–80). San Francisco: Jossey-Bass.

Klein, M.D., Wulz, S.V., Hall, M.K., Waldo, L.J., Carpenter, S.A., Lathan, D.A., Myers, S.P., Fox, T., & Marshall, A.M. (1981). *Comprehensive communication curriculum guide*. Lawrence: Early Childhood Institute, University of Kansas.

Lamb, D.L., Bell, D., & Borts, M.K. (1982). Infant-caregiver interactions: Assessment and intervention. *Monographs of Project Finis* (Whole #2), Marshalltown, IA.

Langley, M.B. (1980). *The teachable moment and the handicapped infant*. ERIC Clearinghouse on Handicapped and Gifted, Council for Exceptional Children, Reston, VA.

Langley, M.B. (1985). Using toys as learning tools with the deaf-blind child. In J. Goodrich & P. Kinney (Eds.), *Adaptips: Adapting curricula for students who are deaf-blind and who function in the sensorimotor developmental stage* (pp. 92–11). Lexington: University of Kentucky.

Mahoney, G., & Weller, E. (1980). Ecological approach to language intervention. In D. Bricker & L. Carlson (Eds.), *New directions for exceptional children* (pp. 17–32). San Francisco: Jossey-Bass.

Masur, E.F. (1981). Mothers' responses to infants' object-related gestures: Influences on lexical development. *Journal of Child Language, 9*, 23–30.

McClowry, D.P., & Guilford, A.M. (1981). Normal and assisted communication development. In D.P. McClowry, A.M. Guilford, & S.O. Richardson (Eds.), *Infant communication: Development, assessment, and intervention* (pp. 9–19). New York: Grune & Stratton.

McCollum, J.A. (1984). Social interaction between parents and babies: Validation of an intervention procedure. *Child Care, Health, and Development, 10*, 301–315.

McCormick, L. (1984). Review of normal language acquisition. In L. McCormick & R. Schiefelbusch (Eds.), *Early language intervention* (pp. 35–88). Columbus, OH: Charles E. Merrill.

McCormick, L., & Schiefelbusch, R.L. (1984). An introduction to language intervention. In L. McCormick & R. Schifelbusch (Eds.), *Early language intervention* (pp. 1–34). Columbus, OH: Charles E. Merrill.

Miller, J.F. (1981). Early psycholinguistic acquisition. In R.L. Schiefelbusch & D.D. Bricker (Eds.), *Early language: Acquisition and intervention* (pp. 329–338). Baltimore: University Park Press.

Miller, J.F., & Yoder, D. (1974). An ontogenetic language teaching strategy for retarded children. In R.L. Schiefelbusch & L.L. Lloyd (Eds.), *Language perspectives—acquisition, retardation and intervention* (pp. 505–528). Baltimore, MD: University Park Press.

Murphy, C.M., & Messer, D.J. (1977). Mothers, infants and pointing: A study of gesture. In H.R. Schaffer (Ed.), *Studies in mother-infant interaction* (pp. 325–354). London: Academic Press.

Musslewhite, C.R., & St. Louis, K.W. (1982). *Communication programming for the severely handicapped: Vocal and nonvocal strategies*. Houston: College–Hill Press.

Nelson, K. (1973). Structure and strategy in learning to talk. *Monographs of the Society for Research in Child Development, 38*(1-2), 1–135.

Newson, J. (1977). An intersubjective approach to the systematic description of mother-infant interaction. In H.R. Schaffer (Ed.), *Studies in mother–infant interaction* (pp. 47–61). New York: Academic Press.

Newson, J. (1979). The growth of shared understandings between infant and caregiver. In M. Bullowa (Ed.), *Before speech: The beginning of interpersonal communication* (pp. 207–222). London: Cambridge University Press.

Nietupski, J., Schuetz, G., & Oakwood, L. (1980). The delivery of communication therapy services to severely handicapped students: A plan for change. *Journal of The Association for Persons with Severe Handicaps, 5*, 13–23.

Odom, S.L. (1983). The development of social interchanges in infancy. In S.G. Garwood & R.R. Fewell (Eds.), *Educating handicapped infants. Issues in development and intervention* (pp. 215–254). Rockville, MD: Aspen Systems.

Otos, M. (1983). *Nonverbal prelinguistic communication: A guide to communication levels in prelinguistic handicapped children*. Salem: Oregon Department of Education.

Peck, C.A., & Schuler, A.L. (1984). Instructional techniques. In C.A. Peck, A. Schuler, C. Tomlinson, K. Theimer, T.G. Haring, & Semmel, M.I. (Eds.), *Social competence curriculum project: A guide to instructional programming for social and communicative interactions* (pp. 182–194). Santa Barbara: Special Education Research Institute, University of California.

Peck, C.A., & Schuler, A., Tomlinson, C., Theimer, K., Haring, T.G., & Semmel, M.I.

(1984). *Social competence curriculum project: A guide to institutional programming for social and communicative interactions.* Santa Barbara: Special Education Research Institute, University of California.

Piaget, J. (1959). *The language and thought of the child.* London: Routledge.

Piaget, J. (1966). *Origins of intelligence in children.* New York: International University Press.

Ramey, C., Sparling, J., & Wasik, B. (1981). Creating social environments to facilitate language development. In R.L. Schiefelbusch & D.D. Bricker (Eds.), *Early language: Acquisition and intervention* (pp. 447–476). Baltimore: University Park Press.

Reichle, J., & Keogh, W.J. (1986). Communication instruction for learners with severe handicaps: Some unresolved issues. In R.H. Horner, L.H. Meyer, & H.D. Fredericks (Eds.), *Education of learners with severe handicaps: Exemplary service strategies* (pp. 189–219). Baltimore: Paul H. Brookes Publishing Co.

Rice, M. (1984). Cognitive aspects of communicative development. In R.L. Schiefelbusch & J. Pikar (Eds.), *The acquisition of communicative competence* (pp. 143–184). Baltimore: University Park Press.

Rogers-Warren, A.K., & Warren, J.F. (1984). The social basis of language and communication in severely handicapped preschoolers. *Topics in Early Childhood Special Education, 4*(2), 57–72.

Rogow, S. (1984). The uses of social routines to facilitate communication in visually impaired and multihandicapped children. *Topics in Early Childhood Special Education, 3*(4), 64–70.

Sachs, J. (1984). Children's play and communicative development. In R.L. Schiefelbusch & J. Pikar (Eds.), *The acquisition of communicative competence* (pp. 109–135). Baltimore: University Park Press.

Schaffer, H.R. (1977). Early interactive development. In H.R. Schaffer (Ed.), *Studies in mother-infant interaction* (pp. 3–16). London: Academic Press.

Schiefelbusch, R.L. & Bricker, D.D. (Eds.). (1981). *Early language: Acquisition and intervention.* Baltimore: University Park Press.

Schiefelbusch, R.L., & Pickar, J. (Eds.). (1984). *The acquisition of communicative competence.* Baltimore: University Park Press.

Schlesinger, I.M. (1977). The role of cognitive development of linguistic input in language acquisition. *Journal of Child Language, 4*, 153–169.

Shevin, M. (1979, June). *Crying as effective verbal behavior: The descriptive analysis of crying in various settings.* Paper presented at the Association for Behavior Analysis convention, Dearborn, MI.

Siegel-Causey, E., Ernst, B., & Guess, D. (1987). Elements of nonsymbolic communication and early interactional processes. In M. Bullis (Ed.), *Communication development in young children with deaf-blindness: Literature review III* (pp. 57–102). Monmouth, OR: Communication Skills Center for Young Children with Deaf-Blindness, Teaching Research Division.

Siegel-Causey, E., & Guess, D. (1985). Early development of prelinguistic communication. In M. Bullis (Ed.), *Communication development in young children with deaf-blindness: Literature review I* (pp. 61–77). Monmouth, OR: Communication Skills Center for Young Children with Deaf-Blindness, Teaching Research Division.

Siegel-Causey, E., Schulte, E., & Guess, D. (in press). Psychological evaluation of speech and language disorders. In V.B. Van Hasselt & M. Herson (Eds.), *Psychological evaluation of the developmentally and physically disabled.* New York: Plenum.

Siegel-Causey, E., Sims, C., Ernst, B., & Guess, D. (1986). Elements of prelanguage communication and early interactional processes. In M. Bullis (Ed.), *Communication development in young children with deaf-blindness: Literature review II* (pp. 59–83). Monmouth, OR: Communication Skills Center for Young Children with Deaf-Blindness, Teaching Research Division.

Snow, C.E. (1984). Parent-child interaction and the development of communicative ability.

In R.L. Schiefelbusch & J. Pickar (Eds.), *The acquisition of communicative competence* (pp. 69–107). Baltimore: University Park Press.

Stillman, R., & Battle, C. (1985a). *The Callier-Azusa Scale (H) Scales for the Assessment of Communicative Abilities*. University of Texas at Dallas, Callier Center: South Central Regional Center for Services to Deaf-Blind Children.

Stillman, R.D., & Battle, C.W. (1985b). Developmental assessment of communicative abilities in the deaf-blind. In D. Ellis (Ed.), *Sensory handicaps in mentally handicapped people* (pp. 319–335). London: Croom Helm.

Stremel-Campbell, K. (1982). The development of language in the mentally retarded, hearing impaired child: Instructional methods. In D. Tweedie & E.H. Shoyer (Eds.), *The multiply handicapped hearing impaired: Identification and instruction* (pp. 211–248). Washington, DC: Gallaudet College Press.

Stremel-Campbell, K., & Clark-Guida, J. (1984). *Communication placement assessment manual* (Contract No. 300-81-0411). Monmouth, OR: Teaching Research Division.

Stremel-Campbell, K., Johnson-Dorn, N., Clark-Guida, J., & Udell, T. (1984). *Communication curriculum*. Monmouth, OR: Teaching Research Publications.

Sugarman, S. (1984). The development of preverbal communication: Its contribution and limits in promoting the development of language. In R.L. Schiefelbusch & J. Pickar (Eds.), *The acquisition of communicative competence* (pp. 24–67). Baltimore: University Park Press.

Thoman, E.G. (1981). Affective communication as the prelude and context for language learning. In R.L. Schiefelbusch & D.D. Bricker (Eds.), *Early language: Acquisition and intervention* (pp. 181–200). Baltimore: University Park Press.

Uzgiris, I. (Ed.). (1979). *Social interaction and communication during infancy*. San Francisco: Jossey-Bass.

van Dijk, J. (1965a). Motor development in the education of deaf-blind children. *Proceedings of the Conference on the Deaf-Blind, Refsnes, Denmark* (pp. 41–47). Boston: Perkins School for the Blind.

van Dijk, J. (1965b). The first steps of the deaf-blind children towards language. *Proceedings of the Conference on the Deaf-Blind, Refsnes, Denmark* (pp. 47–50). Boston: Perkins School for the Blind.

van Dijk, J. (1966). The first steps of the deaf-blind children towards language. *The International Journal for the Education of the Blind, 15*(4), 112–114.

van Dijk, J. (1967). The non-verbal deaf-blind child and his world: His outgrowth towards the world of symbols. *Proceedings of the Jaaverslag Institute voor Doven*, 1964–1967 (pp. 73–110). Sint-Michielsgestel, The Netherlands: Institute for the Deaf.

van Dijk, J. (1969). Educational approaches to abnormal development. *Proceedings from the Institute for the Deaf* (pp. 15–25), Sint-Michielsgestel, The Netherlands: Institute for the Deaf.

van Dijk, J. (1977). What we have learned in 12½ years: Principles of deaf-blind education. In M.R. Jurgens (Ed.), *Confrontation between the young deaf-blind child and the outer world* (pp. 1–10). Sint-Michielsgestel, The Netherlands: Swets & Zeitlinger, B.V.

van Dijk, J. (1986). An educational curriculum for deaf-blind multihandicapped persons. In D. Ellis (Ed.), *Sensory impairments in mentally handicapped people* (pp. 375–382). London: Croom-Helm.

Vygotsky, L.S. (1962). *Thought and language*. Cambridge, MA: MIT Press.

Walker, J.A., & Kershman, S.M. (1981, April). *Deaf-blind babies in social interaction: Questions of maternal adaptation*. Paper presented at the meeting of the Society for Research in Child Development, Boston, MA.

Walker, J.A., Levine, M.H., & Grasse, D.M. (1982). Maternal language in teaching and play interactions with handicapped babies. *Journal of the Division for Early Childhood, 5*, 86–96.

Warren, S.F., & Rogers-Warren, A.K. (Eds.). (1985). *Teaching functional language: Generalization and maintenance of language skills*. Baltimore: University Park Press.
Wilkes, E.M. (1981). A description of language development for parents. *Volta Review, 83*(6), 394–403.
Ziajka, A. (1981). *Prelinguistic communication in infancy*. New York: Praeger Publishers.

CHAPTER 3

Share and Share Alike

Conventional Gestures to Emergent Language for Learners with Sensory Impairments

Charity Rowland and Kathleen Stremel-Campbell

COMMUNICATION, SINCE IT requires at least two partners, is necessarily shared behavior. The communicating partners typically share several aspects of communication. First, the communication form or mode, whether it is speech, sign language, gesture or print is generally shared. Second, the communicator attempts to share a topic, and his or her own perspective on the topic, with a partner. Third, the communicator will attempt to share a specific intent with the partner. Finally, conversational roles will be shared, with one partner taking the speaker's role and then providing a bid to the listening partner to take a turn as speaker. It is easy to see how these aspects of communication are shared in the typical exchange between speaking partners. However, it is often difficult to see this sharing in an interaction involving a person with severe handicaps who does not communicate via conventional modes. No matter how sincerely functional and natural training strategies are espoused, the initial stages of communication training for a person with severe physical, sensory, or cognitive impairments are likely to take on a strained and artificial quality. Sharing fully in a communicative exchange is difficult under these circumstances, yet sharing is an essential goal if the learner[1] is to realize the full power of two-way communication.

The theme of sharing will be emphasized throughout this chapter as communication strategies for learners with sensory impairments are discussed. First, however, the research that has shaped communication intervention for learners with sensory impairments will be reviewed.

BACKGROUND

The great preponderance of research on language acquisition has involved observations and experimental investigations of nondisabled children.[1] Interventions have

The preparation of this chapter was supported in part by the U.S. Department of Education Contract #300-83-0237. The information and opinions expressed herein do not necessarily reflect position or policy of the U.S. Department of Education, and no official endorsement should be inferred.

[1]The term *learner* is used to refer to children and youth with dual sensory impairments and/or severe handicaps. The term *children* is used to refer to studies involving children without apparent handicaps.

been based, in part, on this research and have reflected what is known of the "normal" sequence of language development. In the future, it may be concluded that a model of communication based upon "normal" sequences is inappropriate for one population or another. However, at this point, the best guess is to assume that duplication or adaptation of the "normal" sequence facilitates communicative development.

This chapter reviews aspects of prelanguage development that may be necessary before communication via a symbolic language is developed. Additionally, adaptations to assist the learner in the "transition" from prelanguage to language will be discussed.

Over the past 20 years, the concept of communication has changed radically. Before the 1970s, communication was widely viewed as a behavior that could be realized only through formal language. The current, more liberal, perspective on communication dictates that language is the culmination of a communicative competence that begins early in a child's life. This perspective is the result of convergent trends in the literatures of language acquisition and developmental psychology. The first trend derives from an abundance of developmental research (Bateson, 1975; Condon & Sander, 1974; Lewis & Rosenblum, 1977; Schaffer, 1977) describing the sophisticated receptive and signaling abilities of the human infant that are demonstrated in vocal and visual exchanges between parents and neonates. The second trend derives from a revival of interest in the pragmatic aspects of language introduced by Austin some years ago (Austin, 1962). The pragmatic perspective emphasizes the uses or functions of language. Dore (1974) and Halliday (1975), for instance, have examined and categorized the functions or intents evident in the early speech acts of young children. Bates (1976), Bates, Benigni, Bretherton, Camaioni, and Volterra (1977) and Sugarman-Bell (1978) have extended pragmatic analyses to the preverbal behaviors of infants and found that many of the functional properties of language are realized in these behaviors. It appears from such research that the nondisabled infant successfully uses a variety of preverbal behaviors to affect the social environment even before any formal language appears. A request, for instance, may be realized very effectively through such strategies as fussing, reaching or pointing.

This preverbal gestural repertoire allows the child to reference objects, persons, and activities in the immediate environment by pointing, touching or looking at them. Symbols are necessary, however, to reference environmental entities that are not immediately present. The first symbols acquired bear a rather obvious perceptual relationship to their referents—perhaps a depictive gesture such as patting a chair to represent "sit down" or an "mmm" to represent food. Later, more abstract symbols—spoken words that bear an arbitrary relationship to the perceptual properties of the referent—appear. According to Werner and Kaplan (1963), the conventional symbols that eventually replace these early symbols retain a vestigial perceptual relationship to the actual referent, at least from the child's perspective. Eventually, the child begins to combine these conventional symbols in a rule bound fashion to produce formal language according to syntactic conventions.

Werner and Kaplan (1963) view symbol formation as a process founded in the relationship between infants, mothers and objects or events in the environment. The physical and conceptual distance between mother, infant, and object/event (or referent) becomes progressively greater as symbolic vehicles (gestures, speech) acquire referential properties. The distancing between these elements is described through the dual processes of "decontextualization" and "denaturalization." *Decontextualization* refers to both spatial and temporal distancing between the elements of communication. As the sophistication of communication increases, the child may communicate a message while spatially removed from the referent (for instance, the child may reference an object in another room by labeling it with a word, rather than actually touching or pointing to it). The child may also communicate about a referent that is temporally distant (for instance, an event that occurred yesterday or will occur tomorrow). *Denaturalization* refers to decreasing material similarity between the symbol and its referent. Whereas early symbols bear a strong perceptual similarity to their referents, later ones bear an arbitrary relationship. These concepts are critical as the learner with sensory impairments develops a communication system that can be shared with another person.

Communication has two distinct and powerful aspects to it: *reception* and *expression*. Receptive communication refers to the learner's comprehension or understanding of communicative *input*. Expressive communication refers to the learner's production or use of communicative *output*. In terms of spoken language, speech production is the expressive form that relies on the complex coordination of breath control and oral-motor movements; speech perception is the receptive form that relies upon fine discrimination and analysis of auditory input. Unlike the nondisabled child, many learners with sensory impairments will use different modes for receptive and expressive communication. In this chapter, receptive and expressive communication are discussed separately. Separate consideration of expressive and receptive communication helps one to analyze them as potentially separate systems for individual learners with sensory impairments. In order to share a communication system with a learner who has multiple impairments, it is necessary to carefully consider the *input* system as well as the *output* system.

THE DEVELOPMENT OF EXPRESSIVE COMMUNICATION

The current perspective on communication and language development is very optimistic in terms of its implications for the remediation of severe communication impairments. It is now possible to examine and potentially remediate the development of *generic* communication skills that may be demonstrated through *either* nonsymbolic or symbolic means. A sequence of expressive communication development appears in Table 1. This sequence covers seven levels of communication from nonintentional behavior through early language behavior.

This sequence is intended to serve as an organizational framework that will allow practitioners to analyze: a) the level at which the learner currently functions, b) the next logical level of development to target, and c) expectations beyond the

Table 1. Sequence of communicative competence

Level	Salient behavior
Level I: Pre-intentional behavior	Pre-intentional or reflexive behavior that expresses the *state* of the subject. State (e.g. hungry, wet) is *interpreted* by observer.
Level II: Intentional behavior	Behavior is intentional, but is not intentionally communicative. Behavior functions to affect observer's behavior, since observer *infers* intent.
Level III: Nonconventional presymbolic communication	Nonconventional gestures are used *with intent* of affecting observer's behavior.
Level IV: Conventional presymbolic communication	Conventional gestures are used with intent of affecting observer's behavior.
Level V: Concrete symbolic communication	Limited use of concrete (iconic) symbols to represent environmental entities; one-to-one correspondence between symbol and referent.
Level VI: Abstract symbolic communication	Limited use of abstract (arbitrary) symbols to represent environmental entities. Symbols are used singly.
Level VII: Formal symbolic communication (language)	Rule-bound use of arbitrary symbol system. Ordered combinations of two or more symbols according to syntactic rules.

immediate future. The assessment of a learner's current performance should be used only as a starting point from which to push the learner toward a higher level of communication. By attempting a rather fine-grained analysis of the early stages of expressive communication, practitioners are encouraged to *push ahead*, in a logical fashion, and to *look ahead* beyond current efforts, so that communication planning is a foresightful process.

In the typical nondisabled child, the seven levels of development presented in Table 1 would occur between birth and 24 months of age. This sequence is also applicable for learners with sensory impairments. Level I represents reflexive or reactive behaviors that are not under the learner's voluntary control. Those behaviors that are reliably associated with specific states of the learner's well-being (such as hunger, comfort, pain) come to be interpreted by the caregiver as communicative, although the behavior itself is not intentional, much less intentionally communicative. At Level II, the learner is capable of intentional behavior, but does not intentionally attempt to affect another person's behavior. The learner has voluntary control over many behaviors, but is not aware of the communicative impact of these behaviors. Certain behaviors function communicatively, however, because caregivers interpret them as communicative. At Level III, the learner becomes aware that his or her behavior may affect another person's behavior, and the learner begins to use primitive or nonconventional means to *intentionally* communicate a limited variety of messages. Such clues as eye contact, persistence, and substitution of means (Bates, Camaioni, & Volterra, 1975; Dore, 1974) provide clear evidence of the intentionality of the communicative behavior. The means that the learner uses to communicate at this stage (pushing away, tugging at people, shrieking, whining) are effective, but are not acceptable means of communication in older individuals. These first three levels of communication are the focus of the previous chapter (Siegel-Causey & Downing, Chapter 2, this volume).

The next four levels in the sequence involve intentional communication through conventional means and are distinguished by the degree of abstractness of the communicative behavior. At Level IV, the learner substitutes conventional gestures, such as pointing, giving, showing, waving, and nodding the head for the nonconventional gestures of Level III. These conventional gestures convey specific meanings according to conventions agreed upon by the learner's society and culture. They remain in the learner's repertoire throughout adulthood as an acceptable and informative augmentation to formal language (McNeill, 1985). Finally at Level V the learner begins to communicate via *symbols*. At this level, the learner begins to pair concrete symbolic representations with specific referents in the environment, acquiring the critical concept of a one-to-one correspondence between a symbol and referent. These representations are "concrete" in the sense that they share one or more perceptual features with their referents. For instance, a learner may pat the floor to indicate "sit down," or may make an "mmm" sound to indicate "eat." At Level VI, the learner acquires the use of a limited number of *abstract* symbols as communicative vehicles. These symbols are abstract in that they bear an arbitrary relationship to their referents; they are not tied to the perceptual features of the referent. At this stage, the learner is able to use single words (or signs) that approximate adult speech forms to refer to a limited number of entities that are highly salient to his or her experience. Finally, at Level VII, the learner begins to acquire the rules of a formal language system—rules that dictate the order in which the arbitrary symbols, or words, may be combined. At this stage, the child may produce two- or three-word utterances, varying the word order purposefully to produce different meanings.

The transitional stages between presymbolic communication and formal symbolic communication (true language) are critical and difficult ones for many learners with dual sensory impairments. The child without disabilities appears to move virtually overnight from preverbal communication to the use of a few words. Indeed, Level V, communication via concrete symbols, does not seem to emerge as a distinct stage of development for most children who are not disabled, but is intermixed with the use of conventional gestures and early language. The transition from communication via conventional gestures to the use of abstract symbols is frequently not made by learners with sensory impairments. Many learners with sensory impairments have been the premature subjects of literally years of training in a formal language system such as manual sign language (Level VI or VII) before they have acquired the ability to use a symbol with a one-to-one correspondence to a specific referent (Level V). Not surprisingly, the language training has been fruitless. Learners may have a vocabulary of 3–5 signs that they use indiscriminately; one day they will produce "candy" whenever a sign is required, and another day they will run through their entire repertoire—"candy," "eat," "bathroom," "more," under similar circumstances. Or they may appear to acquire the use of very nonspecific signs such as "more" and "eat," which are appropriate at any time of day, in any context, but they do not acquire specific signs that are appropriate in only very limited circumstances. These learners appear to lack the critical concept of a one-to-one correspondence between a symbol and a specific referent. The gestures that are used at Levels III and IV, after all, are nonspecific in their application and do not impart the concept of a one-to-one correspondence between symbol and referent.

Thus far, this chapter has presented a sequence of expressive communication development and pinpointed some of the more difficult stages for learners with sensory impairments. Now it further analyzes the process and looks at the components of expressive communication. Three critical components of expressive communication—form, function, and content—are discussed.

Forms of Expressive Communication

Communication and language may be achieved through a wide variety of forms (or modes) in addition to speech. Since many learners with dual sensory impairments may not use speech, the selection of an appropriate communication form is critical to communication intervention efforts. A number of nonspeech symbolic systems have been developed for use by nonspeaking clients. These are reviewed by Fristoe and Lloyd (1979), Musselwhite and St. Louis (1982), Schiefelbusch (1980), and Silverman (1980). Increasingly, these non-speech symbol systems have been used to stimulate communication by nonverbal persons with severe disabilities, with generally encouraging results (Kiernan, 1983; Lloyd & Karlan, 1984). Certain forms of communication correspond somewhat to different levels of communication development. Preverbal vocalizations and gestures allow the communication of basic needs, for instance, but do not permit symbolic referencing. Table 2 illustrates how five major forms or modes of communication are differentially appropriate at the seven levels of expressive communication discussed earlier. The shaded areas represent the communication forms (vocal and motor/gestural) typically observed in nondisabled infants. Vocal communication will not be discussed further, since it is the least likely form to emerge in learners with dual sensory impairments. The four alternative forms are discussed below, emphasizing conventional and symbolic forms of communication.

Motor/Gestural Systems Siegel-Causey and Downing (Chapter 2, this volume) discuss the importance of consequating early body movements as intentional behavior. As these intentional behaviors are responded to repeatedly "as having communication value," they have the potential to be used as intentional presymbolic communication behaviors or forms. Many learners will spontaneously use nonconventional (Level III) gestures, such as pushing away unwanted objects and manipulating people (tugging, hand guiding), to communicate basic needs. Some learners will easily make the transition from the use of primitive gestures to the use of conventional gestures, such as giving and waving (Level VI). However, many of these conventional gestures (e.g., pointing, showing, alternating gaze) require visual referencing and may not be appropriate for learners with severe vision impairments.

Gestures may also be used as early symbols. Depictive gestures (such as the gesture for "come"; the gesture/sign for "eat") may be used to reference specific objects or events. The learner with good manual dexterity, memory, and representational skills may be able to move on to more symbolic forms by acquiring the use of abstract manual signs.

Two-Dimensional Symbols (Pictures) Some learners may not use gestures or signs due to fine motor or memory limitations. For those learners who use limited concrete symbols and who have some functional vision, two-dimensional symbol systems may be the symbolic choice. Two-dimensional symbols include photographs, line drawings, abstract graphics, print, and some symbol systems that incorporate pictographs and can be used according to a formal syntactic system. Major advantages of two-dimensional systems are that they demand only a selecting or an indicating response and that they are permanent symbols, unlike speech or sign language. Because the learner has access to a permanent display of symbols, he or she need only recognize the correct one rather than recall the symbol from memory. Careful pretesting is necessary, however, to determine whether a learner can associate photos or line drawings with referents. Two-dimensional symbols may be presented in a variety of ways, depending upon the learner's ability to make an indicating response. Learners with good fine motor ability may flip the pages of a picture book, or may shuffle through a deck of picture cards. Learners with more limited fine motor abilities may point to or tap individual pictures included in a display on a wheelchair tray or in a book. Others may need to use microswitch technology to enable the scanning and selection of picture symbols.

Some concrete picture systems are commercially available (Johnson, 1981), and other concrete systems include Rebus (Woodcock, Clark, & Danes, 1969) and Pic-Syms (Carlson & James, 1980). Many parents and teachers choose to take photographs or draw their own simple pictures of the salient people/objects/locations/activities for each learner. At the concrete symbolic stage (Level V), vocabulary is limited to entities that can be meaningfully represented by a photo or line drawing. Abstract concepts (yes, no) are difficult to represent concretely. A number of symbol systems (Level VI) utilizing abstract pictures are also commercially available, among them Blissymbolics (McNaughton & Kates, 1980) and Rebus (Woodcock et al., 1969), which include both concrete and abstract symbols. Abstract graphics, printed letters, or words may also be used for learners with adequate cognitive and visual discrimination skills.

Table 2. Communication forms (mode) associated with each level of communication

Communication level	Vocal	Motor/ gestural	Electronic technology	Three-dimensional symbols	Two-dimensional symbols
Level I: Pre-intentional behavior	Cry Gurgle Coo	Head movements Postural change Limb movements Facial expression			
Level II: Intentional behavior	Fuss	Regard object Smile Avert head Approach Move away Reach toward Push away	Contingency awareness		
Level III: Nonconventional presymbolic communication	Laugh Non-speech sounds	Above behaviors + Eye contact Manipulate person	Calling device		

Level IV: Conventional presymbolic communication	Intonated sound patterns Vocalization accompanies gesture	Alternating gaze Extend object Touch object Touch person Open palm Shrug Hands up/out Point Wave Nod/shake head Kiss/hug/pat Raise hand	Two-choice option Yes/no option		
Level V: Concrete symbolic communication	Mimic sounds of objects	Depictive gestures (mine, come, sit) Pantomime	Selection of concrete 2-dimensional symbols	Concrete objects	Photos Line drawings
Level VI: Abstract symbolic communication	Single spoken words	Single manual signs	Selection of abstract 2-dimensional symbols	Abstract shapes Single brailled forms	Abstract graphics Single printed forms
Level VII: Formal symbolic communication (language)	Combination of 2+ spoken words	Combinations of 2+ manual signs	Selection of combinations of 2+ symbols	Combinations of 2+ 3-dimensional symbols (NonSLIP, braille)	Combinations of 2+ 2-dimensional symbols (BLISS, print)

Three-Dimensional Symbols Unfortunately, two-dimensional symbols are not appropriate for learners without functional vision or for learners who do not understand the association between pictures and referents. Such learners may use three-dimensional symbols, which have the same advantages as two-dimensional symbols, but which are also tactually discriminable. Three-dimensional symbols may vary from the use of: a) miniature objects to represent life-size objects; to b) the use of the Non-SLIP system (Carrier & Peak, 1975), which incorporates a limited set of abstract plastic shapes into an artificial grammar; to c) braille, which of course mirrors the semantic and grammatical potential of spoken or written languages.

Three-dimensional symbol systems, with the exception of braille, are new to the special education literature and not well-researched—yet the use of objects as symbols seems to have been an outgrowth of van Dijk's work (1964, 1966, 1967) with children who have dual sensory impairments. Van Dijk, in turn, bases his approach on the theories of Werner and Kaplan (1963). Stillman and Battle (1984) have described the use of concrete objects as symbols within the context of "concrete calendar systems" that utilize objects initially as receptive cues within a time-management system. Three-dimensional objects may also be used as an expressive communication system.

Designing an expressive communication system using three-dimensional symbols requires systematic planning and foresight. Critical parameters of the symbols and the symbol array must be considered, and, once in use, the system must be constantly monitored and modified to foster steady progress toward higher levels of communication. The major parameters to consider are: a) the frequency with which the symbols may be used in the natural environment, b) the number of symbols included in the array of symbols, and c) the perceptual or functional iconicity of the symbol (i.e., the degree to which it reflects the physical or functional properties of the referent). During the initial stages of concrete symbol use (Level V), symbols would be selected that can be used frequently throughout the day within a small array, and that are related functionally or perceptually to their referents. Figure 1 illustrates examples of symbols in a progression of decreasing perceptual iconicity (or increasing arbitrariness) for a person with functional vision. For the learner who must discriminate between symbols tactually, the iconicity progression may be quite different, however.

One system using abstract three-dimensional symbols is the Non-SLIP system (Carrier & Peak, 1975), a series of abstract shapes that may be combined according to the rules of the system's own miniature grammatical system. Teachers may create their own three-dimensional shapes to be used as symbols at Level VI, however. A block shaped like a "t" may represent "toilet," for instance. Braille letters and words constitute three-dimensional symbols suitable for use by persons with extremely good tactile discrimination skills and high cognitive skills.

Electronic Technology For the learner who suffers extreme orthopaedic handicaps, microswitch/electronic technology may be necessary to afford a means of expression. Various switching devices may be connected to reinforcing stimuli or to a symbol display that can be activated by a minimal physical response, such as a slight head

	Iconic Relationship	Symbol	Referent
Level V: Concrete Symbol	MINIATURE OBJECT	TOY PHONE	PHONE
	PARTIAL OBJECT	SEAT BELT BUCKLE	CAR/ OUT
	ASSOCIATED OBJECT	COAT HOOK	COAT
	ONE SHARED FEATURE	BASKETBALL FABRIC (Shared Texture) OR PING PONG BALL (Shared Shape)	BASKET-BALL
Level VI: Abstract Symbol	ARBITRARY	ABSTRACT 3-D SHAPE	FINISHED

Figure 1. Examples of three-dimensional symbols that show a decreasing degree of iconicity for the learner with functional vision.

turn, a kick, or a swipe of the hand. Learners with lower cognitive skills may initially use switches connected to simple sensory reinforcement objects to enable them to gain an awareness of environmental contingencies or a sense that they have some control over the animate and inanimate environment (Brinker & Lewis, 1982). Steps toward a communication system may then include the use of switches to activate a "calling device" (simply to gain the attention of another person), the use of a two-choice switch through which a learner may indicate a choice, and the use of switches to indicate "yes" versus "no." A learner in this category who has higher cognitive skills and social motivation may simply need to be provided with a means of making a selection of symbols in order to communicate through a device such as a Zygoboard, Dial Scan or Touch Talker. One of the most pressing research needs in the area of communication for persons with severe handicaps is an examination of the progression from contingency intervention to the establishment of expressive communication via microswitch technology. See Schweigert (1986) for a review of this issue.

Selecting the Appropriate Form for Expressive Communication The selection of an expressive communication form will depend largely on the learner's motor and sensory capacities. The learner's cognitive abilities, including memory and representational level, are also a significant factor in this decision. Romski, Sevcik and Joyner (1984) discuss many of the pros and cons of nonspeech symbol systems. It is not necessary, however, to reduce the options to one. It is quite appropriate to work with two, or even three, expressive systems simultaneously with a given learner, provided that the approach is designed to push the learner systematically to higher levels of communication. For instance, learners may use a wide repertoire of conventional gestures to express basic needs, and also use concrete objects as symbols to enable them to communicate more specifically than they can through gestures. In addition, the teacher might require that the same learners pair manual signs with several of the concrete objects, in an attempt to move them on to a more abstract symbol system. A learner will use different expressive modes as his or her communicative abilities develop. The learner must be taught and encouraged to use increasingly abstract and conventional communication systems based upon his or her social and cognitive development. If a learner must use a highly artificial communication system, it must be made accessible and understandable to peers and non-classroom personnel. Two- and three-dimensional symbols should be labeled so that family and friends understand what they represent. If a high-technology system is only available at school, a low-technology system must be available for use in non-school environments.

Sharing Forms of Communication Learners with severe handicaps may be observed to utilize a unique form of communication—such as a picture communication system, or an electronic device—that is not shared by any other learner or teacher in the classroom. The learner is required to use this form, but because no other learner does, it fails to function as a two-way communication system. To realize the full communication potential of an alternative system, the learner must understand that it can be used by another person, too. The onus then falls on the teacher or parent to *share* this unique communication system with the learner. Sharing this system will accomplish two ends. First, correct use of the system is modeled by the teacher. Second, the learner is taught that communication *is* a two-way affair.

The Function of Expressive Communication

The pragmatic perspective on communication development has focused on its social functions. The basic functions of language and communication are defined by their effects within social interchanges. The communication forms discussed in the previous section may express many different communication functions. Carpenter, Mastergeorge and Coggins (1983) followed the acquisition patterns of the nonverbal, intentionally communicative behaviors of six infants, ages 8 to 15 months. They found a significant trend for communication functions to emerge in the following sequence: a) protest, b) request for action, c) request for object, d) comment on action, e) comment on object, and f) answering.

The basic communicative functions (such as protesting, requesting, attracting attention) may be realized through presymbolic means such as touching, extending objects, and pointing; forms that are effective only in the presence of the object. The acquisition of concrete and abstract referencing abilities broadens the communicative functions available to the learner, adding two very powerful functions to the learner's repertoire. First, the learner is able to name or label objects, people, and activities.

Second, the ability to label enables the learner to communicate about entities that are temporally or spatially distant.

Intervention Techniques All too often, learners with sensory impairments use only communicative functions that attract attention, request more (generally food), and protest. Curcio (1978) found that children with autism display request, refusal, and greeting, but do not demonstrate pointing or showing to express comments or to direct another's attention to referents. Donnellan, Mirenda, Mesaros, and Fassbender (1984) have observed that many of the "inappropriate" behaviors displayed by persons with severe handicaps (e.g., tantrums, self-abusive behaviors, stereotypies) serve communicative functions. They have catalogued some of these behaviors and the range of functions that these behaviors may express. Donnellan et al. suggest that practitioners attend closely to the communicative intent of such behaviors and present strategies for eliminating them, including replacing the inappropriate behavior with more conventional communicative behavior.

The practitioner's job is to expand the learner's repertoire of communicative functions in addition to expanding specific communication forms or vocabulary items. The small amount of research that is available on the training of communicative functions (Reichle, Rogers, & Barrett, 1984) has used the technique of creating an environment that provides obligatory contexts for the production of specific functions, similar to the language assessment techniques indicated by Chapman (1981), Craighead (1984), and Snyder-McLean, Solomonson, McLean, and Sack (1984). To train a protest function, for instance, one might occasionally present the learner with an object that he or she is known to dislike. To train a learner to request more of an activity, one might engage in a highly preferred activity, stop and refuse to resume it until an appropriate signal is made. A number of learners with sensory impairments seem to request *continuation of an action* or to request *more* of an object prior to initiating a request for a new action or object. This "continuation of action" function may be a form of decontextualization (Werner & Kaplan, 1963) that a learner with more severe impairments needs to go through. That is, the learner may have to be engaged directly in an activity in order to know that an opportunity for requesting is available. After repeated opportunities for the "requesting more" function are provided and presymbolic forms are consequated, the learner must eventually learn to request without first being engaged in the activity. In many cases, the more primitive functions (protesting, requesting) may not require training beyond the provision of adequate opportunities to express the functions. It is the training of more sophisticated functions such as offering, commenting, questioning, and answering questions, that requires a significant effort beyond merely providing opportunities in the natural environment. This is an area of intervention requiring extensive research.

Sharing Communicative Intent or Function The restricted range of functions expressed by the learner seems to parallel the restricted range of functions on the part of caregivers. Often a typical interaction with a learner who has severe impairments involves a large number of commands and praise or feedback for motor behaviors from the teacher. Teachers and caregivers must learn two things: first, to utilize a wide range of communicative functions themselves; and second, to provide the learner with opportunities to use a similarly wide range of functions. An extremely useful exercise to set the groundwork for sharing a full range of functions is to collect a sample of the teacher's or parents' verbal behavior and the preverbal or verbal behaviors of the learner, and to categorize the different communicative functions exhibited by both partners. Most learners will not be capable of producing the full range of functions that the teacher can, but a more equal sharing of communication functions may be possible.

The Content of Expressive Communication

Content refers to the meaning of communication, or in more conventional terms, semantics. A number of authors have studied the initial meanings communicated by children without handicaps and have classified initial lexicons into different sets of categories (Bloom, 1973; Guillaume, 1978). Not surprisingly, the first topics of conversation, as expressed at the one-word stage, are topics of high interest to the child—topics such as people (Mom, Dad), objects and food (favorite toys, leisure items, toys), and words related to actions or wants (more, no, up, down). Furthermore, children seem to be very economical in their choice of words, saving words for contexts where nonverbal means are insufficient to communicate their message (Moerk, 1977). Foster (1985) has examined the development of topics in children's communication on a broader level than the lexical studies provide. In a longitudinal study of topic development in five children (ages 1–30 months), Foster found that the earliest topics of communication were "self topics" (focusing on the child), followed by "environmental topics" (directing attention away from the child), that in turn were followed by "abstract" or "displaced" topics that generally require linguistic behavior.

When practitioners find themselves in the position of dictating the vocabulary of a learner's communication system, they have two major spheres of influence. First, they must decide upon the initial lexicon, which dictates the range of meaning about which the learner may communicate. A number of authors have presented strategies and parameters for initial lexicon selection for manual signs (Griffith, Robinson & Panagos, 1983; Karlan & Lloyd, 1983; Luftig, 1984) and graphic symbols (Wilson, 1980). According to Luftig (1984), the parameters that must be considered in the choice of an initial sign lexicon are: a) production variables (those related to ease of production), b) psycholinguistic variables (such as abstractness, frequency), and c) socio-pragmatic variables (such as functionality, saliency to the individual). Ideally, the socio-pragmatic parameters would be considered first, resulting in the selection of a lexicon of high salience to the individual based upon an analysis of the individual's current functioning combined with data from initial vocabularies of children who are nonhandicapped. The chosen lexicon would then be further narrowed to exclude items that are rated difficult in terms of production variables or psycholinguistic variables.

The second way in which one may have an impact upon content is by giving learners interesting environments so that they will have something to communicate about. The learner who is confined to a sterile and monotonous environment is not likely to have much to communicate about. Though this is a difficult problem for a teacher or therapist to redress, it is a highly salient area of remediation. Halle (1984) and Snyder-McLean et al. (1984) provide general strategies for enhancing the communication content-value of a learner's environment.

Sharing Communicative Content By providing interesting environments that stimulate the learner to communicate, teachers also provide topics to be "discussed" with the learners. Sharing the learner's interests allows communication about shared content. The typical learner functioning at an early level of expressive communication is probably more interested in obtaining mobility in his or her environment (down, outside) than in naming animals. Eventually, of course, the young communicator must learn to communicate about content that is not entirely self–centered. With severely delayed communicators, however, one must make the prospect of communicating extremely motivating, and the caregiver may have to follow the learner's lead for much longer than one would with a child who is not disabled.

RECEPTIVE COMMUNICATION DEVELOPMENT

The emphasis on a shared system of communication must also be addressed as *the teacher* communicates with the learner. Criteria for the choice of receptive communication systems must include an assessment of whether exchanges are *successful*. Mahoney (1975) proposes that for language to develop effectively, learners must be able to detect meaning by some nonverbal means. The literature on child development contains numerous studies demonstrating that young children respond to intonational contours, suprasegmental features, facial expressions, and manual gestures prior to words (Chapman, 1981; Folger & Chapman, 1978; Moerk, 1975; Rondal, 1978). Parents must modify their communication input to the learner so that he or she will understand increasingly complex nonlinguistic and linguistic messages.

Studies of mothers' nonverbal communication indicate that mothers of young children (15 months) use literal cue markers, such as tapping the child, or tapping or manipulating the object, in addition to conventional gestures and verbal directives (Allen & Shatz, 1983; Murphy & Messer, 1977; Schaffer & Crook, 1979). Mothers pair these literal cues with their verbal utterances. The use of these literal markers paired with verbal directives seems to increase the child's compliance to attention-getting directives (Schaffer & Crook, 1980). Parents must also be able to determine from the learner's nonlinguistic cues that their attempts to communicate are not too complex for the learner. There is a lack of extensive research specific to the role of the mother's nonlinguistic behavior in receptive communication development (Schaffer, Hepburn, & Collis, 1983).

Learners who are sensory impaired will have difficulty understanding someone's message if they do not perceive facial and gestural cues, or hear the intonation patterns or pauses in the turn-taking routines. Thus, the variables of form, function, and content must also be considered in developing interventions for receptive communication, taking into account the learner's sensory, motor and cognitive limitations.

Forms of Receptive Communication

As with expressive communication, a wide variety of receptive communication forms exist that are appropriate to specific learners according to their sensory abilities. Many learners will not comprehend even the simplest speech or manual sign language, so that practitioners must consider alternate forms of receptive communication, such as the use of environmental and literal cues within ongoing routines. The use of literal markers and language input through the learner's tactile sense must be explored and developed through more systematic interventions. Special types of literal cues will need to be used as adaptations for the learner with sensory impairments if the learner is to understand the messages of others. These literal cues must be used routinely in ongoing interactions and must have specific meaning (content) as well as specific functions. Three types of nonverbal receptive cues will be discussed below: a) object cues, b) touch cues, and c) gesture cues.

Object Cues Object cues are everyday objects used consistently to provide specific information. Initially, object cues or class cues (McInnes and Treffrey, 1982) simply provide information about what is about to happen to the learner (i.e., "here's another bite"; "I'm taking you out of the wheelchair"). These early cues have the potential to reduce startle behavior and forms of inappropriate behavior, since they let the learner know what is to happen to him or her. Since many learners cannot utilize their vision or hearing to obtain cues within interactions, the object cues serve as adaptations for receptive input. Early object cues are those that are closely tied to personal need routines (bottle feeding, spoon feeding, diaper changing, moving positions, movement to new locations). Initially, added properties of smell, temperature, and texture may be emphasized to increase the amount of sensory input. Subsequently, the learner should be given an opportunity to make a specific and active response to the object cue, such as opening his or her mouth when the spoon is presented as a cue within the eating routine. Object cues may also provide information about gaining access to or moving to different locations. For example, car keys may be given to the learner to indicate that Mom and he or she are going for a ride in the car. The object cues that are selected should be dependent on the learner's age, preference, and specific environmental opportunities for activities and interactions. Many of the objects that are initially used as receptive or "input" cues can later be used by the child as expressive forms, thus allowing the learner to share the communication system. A list of suggested functional object cues is presented in Table 3.

Touch Cues Touch cues are signals executed on the learner's body to provide a specific message (such as tap on the shoulder to indicate "sit down"). Touch cues are often used in conjunction with object cues. Early touch cues would include touching the learner to let him or her know that someone is present for an interaction. Activities that do not involve objects are often signaled with a touch cue. For instance, a cue for "I'm going to pick you up/put you down" would be given prior to simply acting on the

Table 3. Functional object cues

Meaning	Object cue
Personal needs/locations	
Person identification	Specific to an individual (ring/hair/bracelet)
Eat	Spoon
Drink	Bottle
Change	Pants or diaper
Go	Walker
Finished	Tub to put objects in
Bed/sleep	Blanket, small pillow or bed toy
Down on mat	Piece of the mat/carpet
Going to play area	Specific toy
Going to the gym	Wrist band
Bath	Washcloth or sponge
Dress	Small shoe
Outside	Astroturf or small brick piece
Drive in car	Car keys
Swimming	Swim suit/cap
Work activity	Time card
Store/community	Wallet/I.D. card
Specific Materials	
Music	Audio tape
Bubbles	Bubble wand
Swing	Piece of chain or rubber
Drink	Cup
Vibration pad	Piece of plastic
Yogurt	Yogurt container
Cracker	Cracker wrapper
Snack	Small Tupperware container
Toy truck	Wheel
Exercise bike	Rubber grip

learner. Specific forms of touch cues are not standardized and therefore are often used inconsistently. Often teachers and parents use different touch cues to convey a similar message. Examples of touch cues that have been found to be effective and their corresponding contexts are provided in Table 4. The specific cue that is used is not critical. However, the consistency of a cue across persons, time, and settings is critical if the learner is to derive meaning from those cues and demonstrate appropriate responses. Remember: never act on a person with sensory impairments without first giving him/her information about what is about to happen.

Table 4. Receptive touch cues

Meaning	Touch cue
"Hi"—approach cue	Lightly rub learner's hand
"Bye"—termination cue	Lightly rub or tap lower shoulder
"Out/Down"—change in placement cue	Lightly pat bottom or pull on arm
"Change" or "bathroom" cue	Gently tug at waistband
"Up"	Gently tug on hand and arm
"No"	Tap firmly twice on outer wrist
"Name" or possession cue	Touch chest
"Want more?" cue	"M" fingers stroke from learner's knuckles to fingertips
"Give me"	"M" fingers stroke inside of learner's fingertips
"Take it"	Tap twice (with one finger) at mid–hand
"Let go"	Shake learner's wrist with thumb and forefinger
"Look for"	Put your hand over learner's flat outer hand and move from side to side
"Go"	Gently guide elbow
"Stop"	Take both hands and firmly put them down
"Finished"	Gently guide learner's hand to push away the object (at forefinger)
"Sit"	Gently push twice at shoulder
"Stand"	Gently stroke upward on both arms
"Play-interaction"	Gently rub rib area with both hands
"Bed/sleep"	Gently rub both eye lids
"Bath"	Gently rub between the breast bone
"Clothes on"	With your fist stroke or tap location of clothes on body

Gesture Cues Gesture cues include both conventional gestures and pantomimes that mimic an action or the shape of an object. For learners who have even limited vision, gesture cues may eventually replace object or touch cues. For example, the caregiver might gesture "up." If the learner does not respond, the teacher would know that there had been a breakdown in the communication exchange. He or she could then present an object or a touch cue paired with the gesture cue in a stimulus shift procedure (Tawney & Gast, 1985). In this way, the gesture cue would begin to take on meaning as it is paired with an already meaningful cue. Gradually, the touch or object cue would be distanced from the gesture cue in a temporal fading procedure (Touchette, 1971). During the early phases of intervention, gesture cues (and other receptive cues) should be used within motivating interactions and not simply as directives. For example, cues such as "give me," "take," "look for," "let's go," and "here" may be more motivational and interaction-oriented than "sit down," in that the learner gets something in exchange. A learner who responds to touch or object cues may learn to respond to equivalent gesture cues if they are paired consistently with the existing cues.

Abstract Receptive Forms Once the learner is responding to more complex touch cues or to conventional gesture cues, abstract symbolic forms of receptive input should be introduced systematically within functional routines in which the learner is focused on specific activities, persons, or events. Symbolic forms might include hand-in-hand (tactile) signing. Early training for tactile signing might involve teaching the learner to anticipate a message from an addressor by holding out his or her hands so that the signs may be signed into them. A learner must demonstrate good tactile discrimination skills and fairly high cognitive skills to be able to receive the subtle tactile cues in two-handed (or one-handed) tactile signing. For learners with some vision, gesture and/or object cues can be gradually faded and replaced by manual signs (Stremel-Campbell, Cantrell, & Halle, 1977) so that the learner begins to understand more abstract forms of input. Other abstract symbolic forms are speech, print, pictographic systems and braille.

Selecting a Receptive Form Even though teachers use forms of visual and gestural cues as well as speech, the use of these cues with sensory impaired learners has not been systematically examined. The primary considerations must be the selection of forms in relation to the responsivity of the learner. The "bottom line" in choosing receptive forms is not the learner's sensory abilities, but whether the learner *responds*. As with expressive communication, more than one form is often used at once. Most teachers speak to their students, even if the learners have limited hearing acuity. Not to speak may deprive the learner of any intonation cues or facial gestures that the learner may perceive. Although two- and three-dimensional symbol systems are often thought of as forms for the learner to use, teachers and parents should consider them as potential receptive modes as well. A learner should not be expected to use an expressive mode spontaneously if he or she does not perceive that it is used communicatively by other persons; in other words, it should be shared. It is important, however, not to go overboard in the use of different receptive forms. Too many forms of input may be confusing for some learners. Once a learner is responding at one level, a higher form should be systematically targeted.

The importance of consistent use of cues cannot be overstressed. Communication in the natural stream of events is inconsistent enough for nondisabled persons. For the learner with vision and hearing impairments, consistency in the forms of receptive communication is essential. Home and school environments must use identical literal markers, touch cues, and object cues to communicate identical meanings. Without such consistencies, the learner with dual sensory impairments cannot be expected to make "sense" of receptive input.

Functions of Receptive Communication

The function or intent of a message to the learner is a critical aspect of receptive communication. There are two major areas of concern regarding the functions of receptive communication. The first is the provision of cues to enable the learner with sensory impairments to correctly interpret the function of messages directed to him or her. Learners with intact sensory systems interpret the functions of communication before they comprehend the meaning of specific words. They learn that questions, commands and comments have different functions signaled by the various vocal intonation patterns, facial expressions, and gestures that accompany speech. The learner with impaired hearing may be able to derive function cues from vocal intonation, even if he or she cannot discriminate specific words. The learner with a total hearing loss who has some vision may be able to interpret function from facial expressions and general "body language" and gestures. The learner without vision or hearing, however, is deprived of any of the naturally occurring function cues. If the teacher signs "cup" into the hand of such a learner, the learner may have trouble understanding if the teacher is requesting an action, making a comment, requesting that the learner imitate the word, or expecting a yes/no response. The learner with dual sensory impairments needs more information to interpret the function of receptive input. Receptive communication should include additional gesture/tactile or object cues that serve as discriminative function cues to inform the learner of the intent or function of the speaker's message ("do what I did," "do what I said," "give me an answer," or "I'm just commenting/no response is necessary").

The second major area of concern regarding the functions of receptive communication is the provision of a wide range of functions in messages to learners with sensory impairments. Studies of mother-child interactions suggest that the mothers of learners with hearing impairments (Goss, 1970; Henggeler & Cooper, 1983; Wendell-Monnig & Lumley, 1980) and with vision impairments (Kekelis & Anderson, 1984; Rowland, 1984) may interact in ways that are not always facilitative to prelinguistic and linguistic growth. Recent studies of the functions of mothers' speech to their handicapped children (Cunningham, Reuler, Blackwell, & Deck, 1981; Eheart, 1982; Kekelis & Anderson, 1984) show that these mothers are more directive and give more commands to their children, often not providing positive feedback for cooperative interactions (Cunningham et al., 1981). There is a large body of data indicating that the maternal use of a high proportion of directives may have a negative influence on language acquisition (Cross, 1978; Field, 1977, 1980; McDonald & Pien, 1982) by decreasing the frequency and complexity of spontaneous speech (Hubbel, 1977) and by causing a slower rate of vocabulary acquisition (Nelson, 1973; Snow, 1979). It is important that teachers provide ample opportunities for communication and decrease the high frequency of directives that are often provided.

Content

A number of studies (Cross, 1978; Mueller, 1972; Phillips, 1970) indicate that caregivers focus their speech on what the learner is visually attending to or interacting with. It is clear that the mother's speech is highly synchronized with the learner's ongoing behavior in routine social interactions (Collis, 1977; Collis & Schaffer, 1975; Murphy, 1978). Schaffer et al. (1983) also suggest that mothers may actually adapt a task to increase the chance that the child can comply with the mother's directive or respond to the message. Thus, children may understand a message based on the environmental variables (person, place, context) rather than relying on lexical or syntactic variables. For learners who have sensory impairments, it may be difficult to determine what they are focused on or interacting with, since their interactions may be extremely limited. Teachers and parents may need to carefully determine what the learner attends to tactually. It may be necessary to provide the learner with numerous routine interactions so that the learner has a content/context to focus upon before attempting to add nonlanguage and language cues for receptive input.

Mervis (1983) contends that for a child to comprehend words to acquire a vocabulary, there must be a transparent relationship between the word and referent. Therefore, the content selected for receptive communication training must be based on: a) what the learner is focusing on/interacting with; and b) words for which there is a transparent relationship. Miller, Chapman, Branston and Reichle (1980) found that children comprehend words referring to objects and people before they comprehend action words. Children also comprehend words for objects that are visibly (and possibly tactually) present prior to words for objects outside the "here and now." These data suggest that learners with sensory impairments may learn the specific names of objects that are focused on before verbs, such as "eat, sit, go." Receptive content or meaning should be chosen as carefully as expressive content. It is critical that teachers and parents be consistent in the manner in which the targeted gestures or symbols are presented, in order for the learner to derive meaning and learn the one-to-one correspondence between the gesture/word and the referent.

DYADIC INTERACTION: A NATURAL CONTEXT FOR COMMUNICATION TRAINING

Dyadic interactions transcend the use of specific receptive or expressive communication systems, requiring effective execution of a communication exchange. Dyadic skills are those skills necessary to initiate, respond to, and sustain communication between two partners. Dyadic skills are social-interactive skills that allow the synthesis of isolated receptive and expressive skills into successful communication. Some of the most basic dyadic skills include: a) attracting a person's attention before communicating a message; b) directing a person's attention to the topic of the communication; c) providing the partner with opportunities to take turns; and d) filling one's own turn in the exchange. Without dyadic skills, isolated receptive and expressive skills are not effective. In other words, a learner may be able to produce correct expressive responses in specific settings and correct responses to specific receptive input, but be unable to communicate effectively. The effectiveness of communication skills cannot be judged outside of a functional dyadic interaction. Dyadic interaction thus becomes the logical context for intervention.

Bruner (1974, 1975a, 1975b) indicates that the social functions of communication are an outgrowth of early dyadic interactions between parents and infants that include "joint action" and "joint attention." For some learners with more severe sensory impairments who do not attend to objects, the early joint action and joint attention interactions with caregivers or teachers may be purely social, not involving objects. One of the first steps in initiating a social interaction with a learner who has sensory impairments is establishing mutual attention (attention between social partners). For many learners with low vision and hearing abilities, tactile and olfactory cues may need to be used in order to establish mutual attention. The learner needs to know that someone is there before initiating an interaction. The context of these early communicative exchanges may need to include both reciprocal game contexts (Rich, 1986) and personal-need contexts, such as eating, bathing, dressing (Rowland, Stremel-Campbell, Schweigert, Thorkildsen, & Hansen, 1985). Objects may be introduced later as mediators for joint actions in social exchanges, and as functional tools within personal-need routines. As routines are carried out repeatedly and consistently, objects begin to take on meaning. At this point, the learner with sensory impairments is more likely to attend to the objects, not for themselves, but because they serve a functional purpose within a routine activity. The learner begins to anticipate what objects/actions are needed within the communicative exchange of the routine and is more likely to establish joint attention or to attend to the object through a joint action. Once the learner can request continuation of object interactions (through physically manipulating the partner, for example, to request more drink), a temporal fading or distancing can be used to teach the learner to request further interaction through manipulating an object rather than acting directly on the partner. It becomes critical that the caregiver or partner provide opportunities for expanding the learner's communicative form so that the object (e.g., cup and pitcher) and social agent are more physically distanced from the learner. As the learner learns to act on objects (e.g., holding the cup while drinking), learns to anticipate the partner's actions (e.g., pouring the drink), and learns to sustain joint interactions with objects, the intervention may include having the learner extend the cup to the person as a process of physically distancing the learner himself or herself from the social agent. The object itself (not the partner's hand) becomes the medium or the tool to affect the environment (getting more drink).

One of the most important features of intervention at this point is allowing and encouraging the learner to fill his or her turn within the interaction. The communication partner must be prepared to allow extra time (wait) for the learner to fill his or her turn in the interaction and may also need to include additional contextual cues (as repair cues) if the learner does not fill his or her turn. The learner must also learn to reciprocate, by waiting—stopping the activity and allowing someone else to take a turn. Teachers must view themselves, not as trainers, but as "partners" within a shared exchange. If an effective exchange does not occur, it is the responsibility of the teacher to repair the exchange so that it is successful. Rieke and Lewis (1984) describe a useful strategy for conceptualizing the communicative interaction, suggesting that the teacher keep in mind the number "three," the number of turns necessary to complete a communicative interaction. Teacher initiates—learner responds—teacher reciprocates or expands; or learner initiates—teacher responds (prompting for further response)—learner responds. Teachers may want to analyze their own interactions with learners to ensure that they are targeting three-turn interactions.

Routines that include sequential or repetitive actions in which each partner assumes a role in a turn-taking manner are the types of functional interactive routines suggested for intervention. The dyadic interaction sequences that are utilized should be age appropriate and should be conducted, to the extent possible, in living, community, educational, vocational, and leisure environments. Early interactive routines for very young learners may be confined to specific locations (play in family room, dressing in bedroom) so that the learner receives redundant environmental cues. However, since many learners with sensory handicaps do not generalize readily across persons and settings, these routines should gradually be extended to other natural settings.

SUMMARY

This chapter blends an analysis of the foundations of communication with practical suggestions for applying this knowledge to communication intervention for learners with dual sensory impairments. There is presently a serious gap between the knowledge currently disseminated within the academic and research communities and the practices currently being applied in classrooms and clinics. Training programs for teachers of students with severe communication impairments should provide thorough groundwork in the basic processes of communication development as they are currently understood. Thorough grounding in this knowledge base will provide the tools for farsighted intervention planning. Communication is such a complex skill, and the population in question manifests such diverse cognitive, sensory and motor skills, that remediation must be highly individualized. No one sequence of communication programs or objectives is widely applicable—only the thorough understanding of basic communication processes will allow the educator to tailor form, function and content (both expressive and receptive) appropriately for individual learners.

As important as what is taught, however, is the context within which teaching occurs. Communication without function is meaningless. Communication intervention must occur within functional natural environments and must involve reciprocal interaction between at least two people, as discussed in the final section of this chapter. Finally, it is essential that educators validate successful intervention techniques through systematic data collection. Without proper data systems, it may be difficult to assess whether or not a very slowly developing learner is in fact acquiring new skills. For the more rapid learner, frequent modifications of communication systems and targets will be necessary to ensure steady development—these modifications should be based upon and judged by a systematic data base.

REFERENCES

Allen, R., & Shatz, M. (1983). What says meow? The role of context and linguistic experience in very young children's responses to what questions. *Journal of Child Language, 10*, 321–335.

Austin, J.L. (1962). *How to do things with words*. London: Oxford University Press.
Bates, E. (1976). *Language and context: The acquisition of pragmatics*. New York: Academic Press.
Bates, E., Benigni, L, Bretherton, I., Camaioni, L., & Volterra, V. (1977). From gesture to the first word: On cognitive and social prerequisites. In M. Lewis & L.A. Rosenblum (Eds.), *Interaction, conversation and the development of language* (pp. 247–307). New York: John Wiley.
Bates, E., Camaioni, L., & Volterra, V. (1975). The acquisition of performatives prior to speech. *Merrill-Palmer Quarterly, 21*, 205–226.
Bateson, M.C. (1975). Mother-infant exchanges: The epigenesis of conversational interaction. *Annals of the New York Academy of Sciences, 263*, 101–113.
Bloom, L. (1973). *One word at a time: The use of single-word utterances before syntax*. The Hague: Mouton.
Brinker, R.P., & Lewis, M. (1982). Discovering the competent handicapped infant: A process approach to assessment and intervention. *Topics in Early Childhood Special Education, 2*, 1–16.
Bruner, J.S. (1974). The organization of early skilled action. In M.P. Richards (Ed.), *The integration of the child into a social world*. London: Cambridge University Press.
Bruner, J.S. (1975a). The ontogenesis of speech acts. *Journal of Child Language, 2*, 1–19.
Bruner, J.S. (1975b). From communication to language: A psychological perspective. *Cognition, 3*, 255–287.
Carlson, F., & James, C.A. (1980). *Picsyms System and Symbol Systems*. Unpublished paper.
Carpenter, R.L., Mastergeorge, A.M., & Coggins, T.E. (1983). The acquisition of communicative intentions in infants eight to fifteen months of age. *Language and Speech, 26*(2), 101–116.
Carrier, J.K., & Peak, T. (1975). Non-speech language initiation program (Non-SLIP). Lawrence, KS: H & H Enterprises.
Chapman, R. (1981). Exploring children's communicative intents. In J. Miller (Ed.), *Assessing language production in children*. Baltimore: University Park Press.
Collis, G.M. (1977). Visual co-orientation and maternal speech. In H.R. Schaffer (Ed.), *Studies in mother-infant interaction*. London: Academic Press.
Collis, G.M., & Schaffer, H.R. (1975). Synchronization of visual attention in mother-infant pairs. *Journal of Child Psychiatry, 4*, 315–320.
Condon, W.S., & Sander, L.W. (1974). Synchrony demonstrated between movements of the neonate and adult speech. *Child Development, 45*, 456–462.
Craighead, N.A. (1984). Strategies for evaluating and targeting pragmatic behaviors in young children. *Seminars in Speech and Language, 5*(3), 241–252.
Cross, T. (1978). Motherese: Its association with rate of syntactic acquisition in young children. In N. Waterson & C. Snow (Eds.), *The development of communication: Social and pragmatic factors in language acquisition*. New York: Wiley & Sons.
Cunningham, C.E., Reuler, E., Blackwell, J., & Deck, J. (1981). Behavioral and linguistic developments in the interactions of normal and retarded children and their mothers. *Child Development, 52*, 62–70.
Curcio, F. (1978). Sensorimotor functioning and communication in mute autistic children. *Journal of Autism and Childhood Schizophrenia, 3*, 281–292.
Donnellan, A., Mirenda, P.L., Mesaros, R.A., & Fassbender, L.L. (1984). Analyzing the communication functions of aberrant behavior. *Journal of The Association for Persons with Severe Handicaps, 9*(3), 201–212.
Dore, J. (1974). A pragmatic description of early language development. *Journal of Psycholinguistic Research, 4*, 343–351.
Eheart, B.K. (1982). Mother-child interaction with non-retarded preschoolers. *American Journal of Mental Deficiency, 87*(1), 20–25.

Field, T. (1977). Effects of early separation, interactive deficits and experimental manipulations on infant-mother face-to-face interaction. *Child Development, 48*, 766–771.

Field, T. (1980). Interactions of high-risk infants: Quantitative and qualitative differences. In D. Savin, R. Hawkins, L. Walker, J. Penticuff (Eds.), *Exceptional infant: Psychosocial risks in infant-environment transactions* (Vol. 4, pp. 120–143). New York: Brunner/Mazel.

Folger, J.P., & Chapman, R.S. (1978). A pragmatic analysis of spontaneous imitations. *Journal of Child Language, 5*, 25–38.

Foster, S. (1985). The development of discourse topic skills by infants and young children. *Topics in Language Disorders, 5*(2), 31–45.

Fristoe, M., & Lloyd, L.L. (1979). Nonspeech communication. In N.R. Ellis (Ed.), *Handbook of mental deficiency: Psychological theory and research* (2nd ed.), (pp. 401–430). New York: Lawrence Erlbaum.

Goss, R.M. (1970). Language used by mothers of deaf children and mothers of hearing children. *American Annals of the Deaf, 115*, 93–96.

Griffith, P.L., Robinson, J.H., & Panagos, J.H. (1983). Tactile iconicity: Signs rated for use with deaf-blind children. *Journal of The Association for Persons with Severe Handicaps, 8*, 26–38.

Guillaume, P. (1978). First stages of sentence formation in children's speech. Translated by E. Clark in C.A. Ferguson & D.L. Slobin (Eds.), *Studies of child language development*, (pp. 240–251). NY: Holt, Rinehart & Winston.

Halle, J.W. (1984). Arranging the natural environment to occasion language: Giving severely language-delayed children reasons to communicate. *Seminars in Speech and Language, 5*(3), 185–198.

Halliday, M. (1975). Learning how to mean. In E. Lenneberg & E. Lenneberg (Eds.), *Foundations of language development: A multidisciplinary approach* (Vol. 1, pp. 239–265). New York: Academic Press.

Henggeler, S.W., & Cooper, P.F. (1983). Deaf child–hearing mother interaction: Extensiveness and reciprocity. *Journal of Pediatric Psychology, 8*(1), 83–95.

Hubbel, R.D. (1977). On facilitating spontaneous talking in your children. *Journal of Speech and Hearing Disorders, 42*, 216–231.

Johnson, R. (1981). *The Picture Communication Symbols*. Stillwater, MN: Mayer Johnson Co.

Karlan, G.R., & Lloyd, L.L. (1983). Considerations in the planning of communication intervention: Selecting a lexicon. *Journal of The Association for Persons with Severe Handicaps, 8*(2), 13–25.

Kekelis, L.S., & Anderson, E.S. (1984). Family communication styles and language development. *Journal of Vision Impairment and Blindness*, February, 54–65.

Kiernan, C. (1983). The use of nonvocal communication techniques with autistic individuals. *Journal of Child Psychology and Psychiatry, 24*(3), 334–375.

Lewis, M., & Rosenblum, L.A. (Eds.), (1977). *Interaction, conversation and the development of language*. New York: John Wiley.

Lloyd, L.L., & Karlan, G.R. (1984). Non-speech communication symbols and systems: Where have we been and where are we going? *Journal of Mental Deficiency Research, 28*, 3–20.

Luftig, R.L. (1984). An analysis of initial sign lexicons as a function of eight learnability variables. *Journal of The Association for Persons with Severe Handicaps, 9*(3), 193–200.

Mahoney, G. (1975). Ethological approach to delayed language acquisition. *American Journal of Mental Deficiency, 80*(2), 138–148.

McDonald, L., & Pien, D. (1982). Mother conversational behavior as a function of interactional intent. *Journal of Child Language, 9*, 337–358.

McInnes, J.M., & Treffrey, J.A. (1982). *Deaf-blind infants and children: A developmental guide*. Buffalo, NY: University of Toronto Press.

McNaughton, S., & Kates, B. (1980). The application of Blissymbolics. In R.L. Schiefelbusch

(Ed.), *Nonspeech Language and Communication*, (pp. 303–322). Baltimore: University Park Press.

McNeill, D. (1985). So you think gestures are nonverbal? *Psychological Review, 92*(3), 350–371.

Mervis, C.B. (1983). Acquisition of a lexicon. *Contemporary Educational Psychology, 8*, 210–236.

Miller, J.F., Chapman, R., Branston, M., & Reichle, J. (1980). Language comprehension in sensorimotor stages 5 and 6. *Journal of Speech and Hearing Research, 23*, 243–260.

Moerk, E. (1975). Verbal interactions between children and their mothers during the preschool years. *Developmental Psychology, 11*, 788–794.

Moerk, E. (1977). *Pragmatic and semantic aspects of early language development*. Baltimore: University Park Press.

Mueller, E. (1972). The maintenance of verbal exchanges between young children. *Child Development, 43*, 930–938.

Murphy, C.M. (1978). Pointing in the context of a shared activity. *Child Development, 49*, 371–380.

Murphy, C.M., & Messer, D.J. (1977). Mothers, infants, and pointing: A study of gesture. In H.R. Schaffer (Ed.), *Studies in mother-infant interaction* (pp. 325–354). London: Academic Press.

Musselwhite, C.R., & St. Louis, K.W. (1982). *Communication programming for the severely handicapped*. San Diego: College-Hill Press.

Nelson, K. (1973). Structure and strategy in learning to talk. *Monograph of the Society for Research in Child Development, 38*(1–2, Serial No. 149).

Phillips, J. (1970). Formal characteristics of speech which mothers address to their children. Unpublished doctoral dissertation, The Johns Hopkins University.

Reichle, J., Rogers, N., & Barrett, C. (1984). Establishing pragmatic discrimination among the communicative functions of requesting, rejecting, and commenting in an adolescent. *Journal of The Association for Persons with Severe Handicaps, 9*(1), 31–36.

Rich, J. (1986). Play, cognition, and communication. In M. Bullis (Ed.), *Communication development in children with deaf-blindness: Literature review II*, (pp. 107–120). Monmouth, OR: Teaching Research.

Rieke, J.A., & Lewis, J. (1984). Preschool intervention strategies: The communication base. *Topics in Language Disorders, 5*(1), 29–40.

Romski, M.A., Sevcik, R.A., & Joyner, S.E. (1984). Nonspeech communication systems: Implications for language intervention with mentally retarded children. *Topics in Language Disorders, 5*(1) 66–81.

Rondal, J. (1978). Maternal speech to normal and Down syndrome children matched for mean length of utterance. In C. Meyers (Ed.), *Quality of life in severely and profoundly retarded people: Research foundations for improvement*. Washington, DC: American Association on Mental Deficiency.

Rowland, C. (1984). Preverbal communication of blind infants and their mothers. *Journal of Visual Impairment and Blindness, 78*(7), 297–302.

Rowland, C., Stremel-Campbell, K., Schweigert, P., Thorkildsen, R., & Hansen, P. (1985). *The New CONCEPT: Communication training interactive videodisc*. Monmouth, OR: Teaching Research.

Schaffer, H.R. (1977). *Studies in mother-infant interaction*. London: Academic Press.

Schaffer, H.R., & Crook, C.K. (1979). Maternal control techniques in a directed play situation. *Child Development*, 989–998.

Schaffer, H.R., & Crook, C.K. (1980). Child compliance and maternal control techniques. *Developmental Psychology, 6*, 54–61

Schaffer, H.R., Hepburn, A., & Collis, G.M. (1983). Verbal and nonverbal aspects of mother's directives. *Child Language, 10*, 337–355.

Schiefelbusch, R.L. (1980). *Nonspeech language and communication: Analysis and intervention*. Baltimore: University Park Press.

Schweigert, P. (1986). Contingency intervention. In M. Bullis (Ed.), *Communication development in young children with deaf-blindness: Literature review II* (pp. 167–182). Monmouth, OR: Teaching Research.

Silverman, F.H. (1980). *Communication for the speechless*. Englewood Cliffs, NJ: Prentice Hall.

Snow, C.E. (1979). The role of social interaction in language acquisition. In W.A. Collins (Ed.), *Children's language and communication*. Hillside, NJ: Erlbaum.

Snyder-McLean, L.K., Solomonson, B., McLean, J.E., & Sack, S. (1984). Structuring joint action routines: A strategy for facilitating communication and language development in the classroom. *Seminars in Speech and Language, 5*(3), 213–228.

Stillman, R., & Battle, C.W. (1984). Developing prelanguage communication in the severely handicapped: An interpretation of the van Dijk method. *Seminars in Speech and Language, 5*(3), 159–170.

Stremel-Campbell, K., Cantrell, D., & Halle, J. (1977). Manual signing as a language system and as a speed initiator for the nonverbal severely handicapped student. In E. Sontag (Ed.), *Educational programming for the severely and profoundly handicapped* (pp. 335–347). Reston, VA: Council for Exceptional Children, Division on Mental Retardation.

Stremel-Campbell, K., Rowland, C., Schweigert, P., Bullis, M., & Hansen, P. (1985). *New CONCEPT Videodisc Training Manual*. Monmouth, OR: Teaching Research.

Sugarman-Bell, S. (1978). Some organizational aspects of pre-verbal communication. In I. Markova (Ed.), *Social context of language* (pp. 49–66). New York: John Wiley.

Tawney, J.W., & Gast, D.L. (1985). *Single subject research in special education*. Columbus, OH: Charles G. Merrill.

Touchette, P.E. (1971). Transfer of stimulus control: Measuring the moment of transfer. *Journal of Experimental Analysis of Behavior, 15*, 347–354.

van Dijk, J. (1964–67). *The non-verbal deaf-blind child and his world: His outgrowth towards the world of symbols*. Jaarverslag: Institut voor Doven.

van Dijk, J. (1966). The first steps of the deaf-blind child toward language. *International Journal for the Education of the Blind, 15*(4), 112–114.

Wendell-Monnig, J., & Lumley, J.M. (1980). Child deafness and mother-child interaction. *Child Development, 43*, 930–938.

Werner, H., & Kaplan, B. (1963). *Symbol formation*. New York: John Wiley and Sons.

Wilson, K.D. (1980). Selection of a core lexicon for use with graphic communicative systems. *Journal of Childhood Communication Disorders, 4*(2), 111–123.

Woodcock, R.W., Clark, C.R., & Danes, C.O. (1969). The Peabody Rebus Reading Program. Circle Pine, MN: American Guidance Service.

CHAPTER 4

Functional Vision Programming

A Model for Teaching Visual Behaviors in Natural Contexts

Lori Goetz and Kathleen Gee

CURRENT CURRICULUM MODELS for persons with multiple severe handicaps suggest a growing emphasis upon the context in which instruction occurs. The functional life skills curriculum model (Brown et al., 1980) derives curriculum content through systematic analysis of activities that regularly occur in a student's home, community, recreational and vocational environments (see Nietupski & Hamre-Nietupski, Chapter 9, this volume). The community intensive curriculum model (Sailor et al., 1986) shares an emphasis upon teaching functional activities in natural contexts and, in addition, stresses integration and interaction with nondisabled persons in both school and community environments. The individualized curriculum sequencing model (Guess & Helmstetter, 1986) focuses upon teaching skill clusters, or sets of skills that are functionally and/or environmentally interrelated (see Helmstetter & Guess, Chapter 10, this volume). While differences exist among and within these models, a major commonality is a shift away from artificial, highly controlled classroom instructional environments, and toward the use of multiple integrated environments and natural cues and consequences (Falvey, Brown, Lyon, Baumgart & Schroeder, 1980) as the basis for instructional activities.

Successful applications of these models have been reported with increasing frequency; individual students have learned such skills as grocery shopping (Wheeler, Ford, Nietupski, Loomis, & Brown, 1980), eating in public restaurants (van den Pol et al., 1981), and playing pool in a public recreation facility (Hill, Wehman, & Horst, 1982; see Snell & Browder, 1986, for review). However, relatively little literature is available for the educator specifically concerned with enhancing or improving sensory functioning within the context of a community-based, functional life skills curriculum model. With a few notable exceptions (Hamre-Nietupski, Nietupski, Sandvig, & Ayres, 1984; Helmstetter, Murphy-Herd, Roberts, & Guess, 1984), current curriculum and instructional procedures have overlooked specific visual and auditory functioning. While there is agreement that persons with visual impairments can learn to see better (Lundervold, Lewin, & Irvin, 1987), few models integrate naturally oc-

The work reported in this chapter was supported in part by the U.S. Office of Education Grant #G008300032; however, no official endorsement should be inferred.

curring cues, consequences, and contexts into effective instructional procedures to teach or improve a student's use of residual vision.

The instructional model presented in this chapter is an initial effort to provide such integration. It is based upon four years of field testing and formal research in educational programs serving students with multiple severe handicaps and dual sensory impairments (Goetz & Gee, 1987; Sailor & Goetz, 1981).

HISTORICAL OVERVIEW

Lundervold et al. (1987) reviewed and evaluated four methods traditionally used to enhance residual vision: 1) optical aids, 2) contrast effects, 3) vision stimulation, and 4) vision training. Based upon careful analysis of the available scientific evidence, Lundervold concluded that successful utilization of optical aids (e.g., spectacles, magnifiers, telescopes) had been documented primarily with persons who had only visual handicaps, and that effective applications with children having multiple handicaps remained to be demonstrated. Lundervold further concluded that the effectiveness of contrast effects, including manipulating figure-ground contrasts through changing the luminance (the comparative darkness of the foreground figure) or colors of the figure-ground relationship, was unsupported by current empirical data and did not merit further investigation as a low vision enhancement strategy.

Vision stimulation, the third method for enhancing residual vision, has been the most common traditional curricular approach to teaching students with severe disabilities functional vision use, as indicated by such visual behaviors as fixation, refixation, tracking, and scanning. Vision stimulation refers to the noncontingent presentation of visually interesting stimulus items such as blinking lights or colored mobiles (Barraga, 1970; Ficociello, 1974): The underlying assumption is that visual displays will elicit a visual response and thus motivate the student to become visually attentive, thereby increasing visual efficiency. Despite widespread popularity, the vision stimulation model is unsupported by research data (Hatlen & Goetz, 1981). Lundervold et al. (1987) further note that the research cited in support of this model is not available in scientific or educational journals.

In contrast to vision stimulation, more recent data suggest that visual behaviors can be taught using the same principles of systematic instruction that have characterized instructional programming for students with severe disabilities in more typical curricular domains such as domestic, recreational, or vocational skills (see Brown et al., 1979; Sailor & Guess, 1983). Utley, Duncan, Strain, and Scanlon (1983), working with infants with profound multiple handicaps, have demonstrated the operant nature of visual fixation through contingent reinforcement procedures. Mosk and Bucher (1984) successfully taught visual motor task performance to students with severe retardation using specific prompting and stimulus shaping procedures. In a series of investigations, Gee and Goetz (1985) and Goetz and Gee (1987) worked with six students who had low vision and/or specific vision impairments in addition to severe or profound retardation and motor disabilities. They established visual attention to motor tasks using specific prompting and reinforcement contingencies and functional, age-appropriate tasks.

Data such as those cited above led Lundervold to conclude that structured vision training was the most effective vision enhancement method for students with multiple handicaps. In light of these data, the vision programming strategy recommended in this chapter is based upon careful application of operant principles and data-based instruction (Haring, Liberty, & White, 1980; Snell, 1978). In addition, structured vision training occurs in the context of a community referenced, functional life skills curriculum model (Brown et al., 1980; Sailor et al., 1986). Teaching visual behaviors is presumed to involve more than just vision stimulation, or the provision of opportunities to receive input through the visual mode. Instead, effective strategies for teaching visual behaviors entail arranging the instructional environment so that use of vision results in specific natural, desirable, and functional consequences for the student. Visual skills are not taught in an isolated skill, massed trial format (see Mulligan, Guess, Holvoet, & Brown, 1980), but rather in the context of learning other age-appropriate tasks and activities. The student always has a functional and reinforcing reason to use his or her residual vision, and this consequence is contingent upon occurrence of the visual behavior.

FUNCTIONAL CONTEXT VISION TRAINING

Functional context vision training involves two major components. First, training of visual attention behaviors (i.e., fixation) occurs in the context of other skills and tasks which require visual attention for successful task completion. Training contexts are selected only for those visual motor tasks in which visual attention to the task items is genuinely necessary for effective performance. Additionally, the visual motor training contexts are also selected from the criteria of functionality and age-appropriateness of the task for the learner (Brown et al., 1980). Thus, the package is designed specifically to be a visual skill training procedure, rather than a compliance training procedure (cf. Striefel, 1974). The goal is not to teach eye contact upon request to students who have adequate visual acuity. The goal is to teach students with low or residual vision to use their vision to accomplish successful task performance.

The second component of the training package is the use of a repeated prompting (Koegel & Egel, 1979) or continuous correction (Utley, 1979) procedure. While engaging in the visual motor tasks, the student is repeatedly prompted until visual attention is established. Until visual attention to the relevant stimulus occurs, the student is not allowed to attempt to complete the task. Instead, the task response is interrupted, and the student is prompted again until visual attention occurs. Once visual attention does occur, the student may continue with task performance. No extrinsic, arbitrary reinforcers (e.g., edibles) for visual attention are utilized.

A schematic diagram of the model is presented in Figure 1. The model involves five steps:

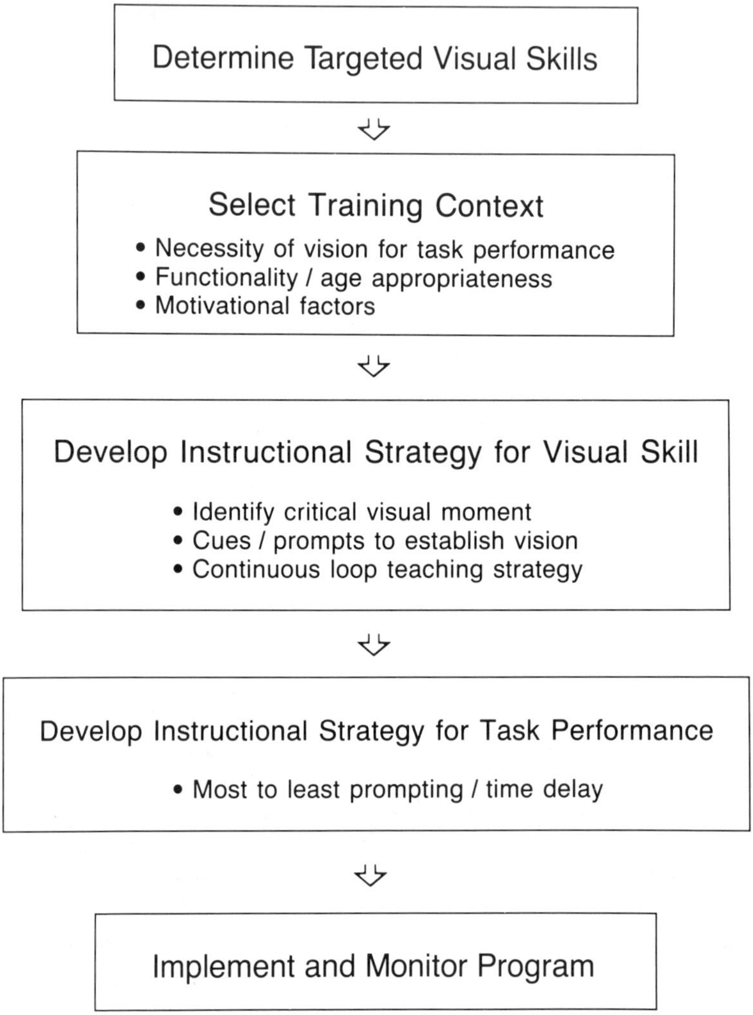

Figure 1. Lattice of steps involved in developing a functional vision program.

1. Determine the targeted visual skill
2. Select a training context
3. Develop an instructional strategy for the visual skill
4. Develop an instructional strategy for the other skills or tasks used as the training context for the visual skill
5. Implement the instructional programs and monitor skill acquisition through daily performance data

Each step has several subcomponents which are discussed in detail below. The chapter then concludes with a discussion of the model in terms of competence and motivational factors, and a brief summary of future research needs and directions.

DETERMINING RESIDUAL VISION SKILLS FOR INSTRUCTION

Determination of appropriate vision skills for instruction is a complex task dependent upon multiple data sources. Extensive variability exists among students with severe multiple disabilities in terms of visual functioning. A variety of vision impairments, including cataracts, glaucoma, optic atrophy, strabismus, and numerous other impairments, may be associated with retardation and cerebral palsy (cf. Donlon, 1966; Wolf & Anderson, 1973). All of these impairments influence a student's functional vision status.

A first step in determining the need for professional vision care is vision screening using a subjective visual acuity test. Cress et al. (1981) have pointed out the critical need for effective vision screening for persons with severe handicaps, and have reviewed numerous appropriate screening tools. If an appropriate screening procedure is not available, several acuity tests now exist which can be applied in the classroom by teachers who are knowledgeable about the principles of operant conditioning and individualized training techniques; such tests include, for example, the Parsons Visual Acuity Test (PVAT) (Spellman, DeBriere, & Cress, 1979). These tests have been designed specifically using principles of errorless learning (Terrace, 1963) to facilitate participation by persons often labeled "untestable."

For students who cannot participate in formal vision screening, numerous functional vision assessments are now available for use in a classroom context by the classroom teacher and/or vision resource teacher. Langley and Dubose's (1980) Functional Vision Inventory includes structured observations in seven major areas of visual functioning. Smith and Cote (1982) have adapted this inventory into a 12-item scale representing samples of visual sensation and visual motor skills. Utley et al. (1981) provide detailed information on measurement procedures for informal assessment of reflexive measures, ocular coordination, peripheral vision, and tracking and gaze shift in students who may have little voluntary movement, no effective communication systems, and undetermined vision status. Data from these assessment procedures can then be shared with a professional vision specialist.

Other sources of information are members of the transdisciplinary assessment team (Lyon & Lyon, 1980), including information from physical and occupational therapists concerning positioning and handling techniques which can enhance the student's visual functioning. Vision specialists, such as a vision resource teacher or consultant, can also provide valuable information about environmental modifications and optical aids that might enhance a student's visual functioning.

The aim of the assessment process is to obtain an understanding of what the student's current visual status is, and an understanding of what visual behaviors the student lacks. Table 1 presents a brief list of different visual functions, vision re-

Table 1. Visual functions and responses

Visual function	Possible response forms
Orient to presence of stimulus	Head turn, gaze shift, brief fixation (less than 1 second)
Fixation (bifoveal or monofoveal)	Sustained eye contact, presence of corneal light reflection
Accommodative convergence	Continuous fixation on object as it approaches nose; typically, fixation is broken as object moves within 4 inches of nose
Gaze shift	Fixation on one object, then on second object, without smooth tracking
Tracking	Smooth eye movement to follow object, both eyes aligned, head typically follows eyes
Scanning	Systematic search of visual display
Peripheral vision	Gaze shift to find object located on periphery of visual field

sponses and possible measures of these responses that the teacher may want to consider in determining appropriate vision objectives.

Unfortunately, there are no data available on the effects of using specific skill sequences in training residual vision (e.g., training convergence before tracking), and little evidence to suggest that training one specific skill, such as fixation, will improve performance of other visual skills, such as tracking (Lundervold et al., 1987). Without such data, the appropriateness of visual skill hierarchies based exclusively upon the developmental model (e.g., Barraga & Collins, 1979; Bernstein, 1979; Robinson & Robinson, 1978) for persons with multiple severe disabilities remains uncertain.

SELECTION OF A FUNCTIONAL SKILL CONTEXT

Once a specific vision objective has been selected (e.g., increasing frequency or duration of visual fixation), the second step is to select the functional context in which the vision skill will be trained. Three criteria are critical in selecting an effective training context.

Necessity of the Visual Response for Successful Task/Skill Performance

The first criterion is selection of a task or skill context in which the visual behavior being taught is genuinely required for accurate and efficient task performance (Goetz & Gee, 1987). For example, visual scanning might be taught in the context of a domestic task in which the student must match a sock to its mate and then fold the pair as part of an instructional program at the local laundromat. The student must scan the clothing items if he or she is to make a correct matching response. In contrast, it is not necessary for a student to visually scan the closet for a broom if the broom is always the only item hanging in a fixed place on the back of the closet door. Careful evaluation of the need for the visual behavior in a skill context can help to avoid purposeless demands to "look," "watch," and so on, when in fact the skill context does not really require looking behavior.

Functionality and Age Appropriateness of the Paired Skill/Context

Functional skills are skills which increase a student's level of independent functioning in his or her home, school, vocational and community environments (Brown et al., 1980). Selecting paired skills that are functional means selecting skills that will increase independence, and then teaching these skills with materials and contexts that are age appropriate and natural to the student's interaction with the environment. Thus, it is functional to use a pail and shovel in a sand box to teach visual attention in the context of a visual motor task such as pouring, if the student is of preschool age. If the student is an adolescent, visual attention during the act of pouring can be made more functional if the paired skill involves pouring laundry soap into a washing machine or pouring cake mix into a measuring cup.

Use of age-appropriate materials and contexts does not require overlooking developmental data concerning preferences for different types of visual stimuli at different stages of visual development. Familiarity with developmental sequences of pattern preferences (e.g., Fantz, Ordy, & Udelf, 1962; Kagan, 1973) may suggest guidelines in the selection of age-appropriate and functional materials. For example, a student who is to fixate on an object and then reach toward the object may learn this skill in the functional context of reaching toward a comb or hairbrush in order to partially participate (Baumgart et al., 1982) in personal hygiene activities at the local YMCA. Data on color and pattern preference suggest that red and orange are among the first colors for which preferences are shown. Thus, use of a red comb within this context may facilitate acquisition of the visual behavior without compromising a functional approach to instruction.

The use of a functional life skills curriculum generated through ecological inventories of individual students' current and future domestic, recreational, vocational and community environments (Brown et al., 1979; Nietupski & Hamre-Nietupski, Chapter 9, this volume) will automatically result in a wide range of age-appropriate, functional activities that can be considered as natural contexts for vision training.

Motivational Factors

Awareness of an individual student's choice and preference when determining curricular content may play an important role in enhancing motivation to learn new skills (see Datillo & Rusch, 1985; Helmstetter & Guess, Chapter 10, this volume). The process of selecting a visual skill and a context for teaching that skill also involves careful examination of whether the student *ever* performs the visual skill in any context. If a student does already perform the target visual skill in specific situations where it is a genuine necessity, instruction may not be needed. Presumably, the student is using the skill in contexts that are sufficiently motivating from the student's perspective.

The importance of gathering extensive baseline information about a student's use of the target visual skill across various contexts is illustrated by the data from Archie in Figure 2. Archie was a 6-year-old boy with hemiplegia and severe developmental delay whose visual status included hemianopsia. These data were gathered as part of subject selection screening procedures for an experimental validation of functional context vision training procedures (Gee & Goetz, 1985).

The data in Figure 2 represent Archie's visual attention (defined as fixation on the materials while manipulating them) during two different tasks: completing a puzzle by inserting one piece into the available spot, and inserting a toothbrush into a plastic tubular toothbrush case. Each baseline session consisted of five trials or opportunities to perform the task, with no reinforcers or instructional procedures in effect. While the data show some variability within each task, overall level differences indicate that Archie did already visually fixate on specific tasks such as inserting a toothbrush into its case, though not on other, presumably less motivating, tasks such as completing a puzzle. Replication of the data patterns in Figure 2 across several additional pairs of tasks led to the decision not to develop a training package for visual attention for Archie, as he already used his vision if the contexts were sufficiently motivating to him.

The selection of age-appropriate, functional activities through ecological inventories has already been identified as an initial step in developing a functional vision program. Informal observation of the students as they participate in these activities

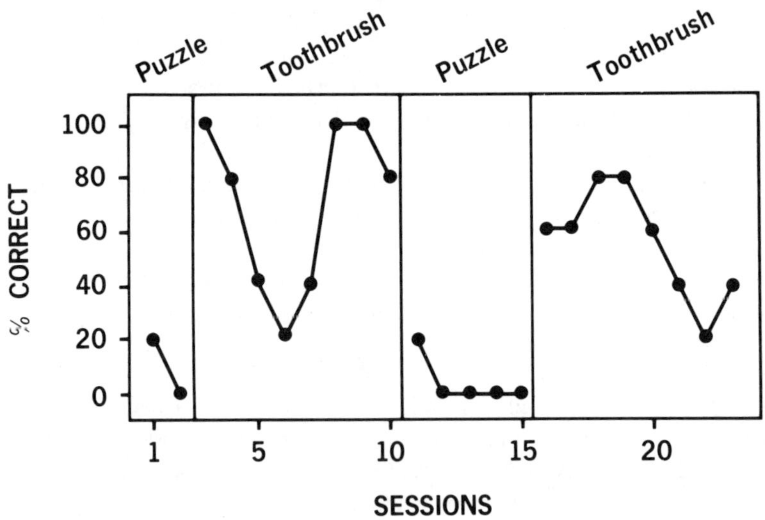

Figure 2. Archie's visual attention (defined as fixation on materials while manipulating them toward successful task performances) during baseline on two different tasks as indicated by ·______·.

will provide opportunities to assess whether or not they appear to use the target visual skill at those times when it is needed within these activity contexts. More formal baseline procedures, such as those described above, can then be carried out.

Table 2 presents five functional skill contexts selected for teaching a 5-year-old girl, Maria, sustained visual fixation skills (Gee & Goetz, 1985).

Selection of these tasks for Maria was based on consideration of all of the above factors. A total of eight possible tasks were originally selected that fell into either the leisure or vocational domain. These tasks were derived from parental requests during a home interview and/or the teacher's ecological inventory of appropriate environments. In addition, the teacher's knowledge of Maria's preferred objects (based upon classroom observation) was also a factor in selecting the initial activities. All tasks were analyzed to ensure that vision use was necessary for competent task performance (see "Critical Moment" section below). Lastly, a baseline assessment was conducted on each task to ensure that Maria did not already use the target visual skill to accomplish these tasks. Baselines indicated that Maria did not use her vision when interacting with these materials; however, for three of the selected tasks, Maria did not attempt to interact with them at all. These tasks were dropped, leaving the five tasks presented in Table 2.

Table 2. Maria's functional skill contexts for visual fixation

Skill context	Vision necessary	Activity source	Motivation
1. Stacking rings on spinning top toy	yes	Teacher observation/inventory of pre-school/first grade classrooms	Preferred toy
2. Stacking cups while clearing table	yes	Parent request for her to learn household chores	Dumping dirty dishes into water at end of task
3. Insert blocks into post office toy	yes	Teacher observations/inventory of pre-school/first grade classroom	Enjoys auditory feedback from this activity
4. Coins into purse before going into community	yes	Teacher inventory of shopping as community activity	No evidence other than baseline analysis
5. Caps on pens as part of classroom clean up job.	yes	Parental request to learn chores; teacher inventory of classroom activities	Often handles/chooses pens during leisure choice activity

INSTRUCTIONAL STRATEGIES FOR VISION SKILLS

Once a vision skill has been targeted for instruction and several contexts have been selected for instruction, a specific instructional program for teaching the visual behavior must be developed. Developing an effective program for the vision skill requires three steps: identifying the critical visual moment, selecting appropriate cues and prompts, and utilizing a continuous loop training procedure.

Identifying the Critical Moment

Deciding on a criterion which will designate correct or incorrect visual responses will depend, for the most part, on the choice of the paired functional skill and the student's functioning level. The decision involves identifying the critical moment at which the student must be fixating, tracking, scanning, and so forth, in order to accomplish the paired skill. When and for how long is the visual behavior required in order to correctly perform the task?

For example, when must a student be fixating in order to stack one glass into another? The critical moment might be stated as follows: The student must be fixating from the time one glass touches the other glass until insertion is completed. For putting a coin into a piggy bank, the critical moment to fixate might be designated as from the time the coin is within one inch of the slot until completion of insertion.

Important considerations in choosing a critical moment include the student's motoric ability and overall ability to perform the functional activity. Consider the visual behavior of fixation during a task involving controlled release of grasp. For a student with severe spasticity who has no independent feeding skills, fixation on his or her hand may be required for a 2-second duration as the student is prompted to begin releasing a bowl into the sink. Fixation is not required, however, for the duration of the time needed to complete the release. In contrast, a student who has numerous independent self-help skills may be required to fixate upon the toothbrush from the time he or she takes it out of his mouth until it is accurately released into a cup.

Few empirical data are available to assist a teacher in designating critical moments at which vision appears necessary for successful task completion. One suggestion is to physically go through the paired skill activity and note the times at which vision is needed to task completion. Establish from what starting to ending points the targeted visual behavior is actually needed to carry out the task, and then observe the speed and proficiency with which the student actually does the paired skill. Based on this information, a specific critical moment can be defined. This is the time during which the visual behavior will be measured during instruction.

For Maria's paired skill contexts shown in Table 2, for example, the critical moment during which she had to fixate on the materials while putting coins into a coin purse was defined as starting when the coin was within an inch of the opened purse and ending when the coin was released into the purse. Maria was not required to fixate on her hand as she picked up the coin and brought it within proximity of the purse, nor was she required to continue to fixate on the materials once the coin had been released.

Selecting Cues and Prompts

After a teacher has designed a vision objective, picked a paired skill, and designated the critical moment, the next step is to ensure that the student actually performs the desired visual behavior. Teaching strategies for establishing visual behaviors include two phases: selection of a prompting technique and, if needed, use of a correction procedure.

Utley et al. (1981) identified four prompting techniques for visual behaviors: 1) use of physical and tactile prompts; 2) use of auditory cues; 3) use of augmentative visual cues; and 4) use of "time-out" techniques.

Physical and tactile prompts refer to strategies that involve motorically assisting the student to fixate, track, or scan by moving his or her head, tapping a cheek, taking the student's hand and placing it where the student should be looking, and so on. Physical assistance is then faded until the student can do the visual behavior without prompting. For example, a teacher may use a physical prompt by manually orienting the student's face toward an item that he or she must fixate on and use or activate in some way.

Auditory prompts involve the use of supplemental speech or other sound cues different from the initial verbal cue or instruction. As an example, consider a student who is being taught to fixate while putting a cup on a hook. The final vision objective might be that he or she fixate while putting cups on hooks without any prompt or cue other than the instruction, "Put the cup on the hook." Any added verbal cues, such as "look" or "keep looking," would be considered part of the training strategy, and would ultimately need to be faded out.

Other types of auditory prompts include: tapping the item with a finger while pointing to it, tapping the item itself (such as a cup on a table), or calling the student's name. Auditory cues can be paired easily with other visual and tactile cues. For example, to get the student above to look at the hooks, the teacher might first point to the hook and then tap it as the student maintains fixation.

Any added visual stimulus which helps to call attention to the item the student should fixate on, track, scan, and so on, is considered an augmentative visual cue. Pointing to the item or shining a flashlight on it are two common visual prompts. Augmentative visual cues should be differentiated from visual aids. Some students may benefit from the use of low vision aids. These aids will remain stable throughout a vision training program. Vision or resource teachers may be a resource of information on ways to adapt materials for low vision students, although the data supporting the use of contrast effects is equivocal (Lundervold et al.,1987).

All of the prompting techniques described above operate by adding an additional cue to the instructional situation—a cue that is intended to prompt or facilitate performance of the visual behavior. As with any prompting strategy, systematic procedures for fading out these prompts must also be planned. Prompts can be faded using a time delay strategy (Touchette, 1971) or an intensity fading procedure in which the intensity of the added auditory or visual prompt is gradually diminished (cf. Goetz, Gee, Baldwin, & Sailor, 1982).

A fourth set of prompting strategies are time-out techniques. These strategies refer to various way of stopping the instructional activity when the student does not perform the visual behavior. One method is simply to remove all the task materials from the setting whenever the student looks away from the task. Materials are returned only when the student re-establishes visual attention (or demonstrates the targeted visual behavior). For example, a student who is working on fixating while performing the fine motor skill of stacking cups may begin to look and then look away while groping for the place to stack the cup. At that point the teacher using this technique would pull the stack of cups away. When the student re-establishes visual attention, the teacher can replace the materials and try again.

Selection of appropriate prompts is, of course, dependent on individual learner characteristics. While an auditory prompt would not be effective for a low vision student who in addition had a profound hearing loss, manual prompting would be appropriate.

Use of a specific prompting procedure is only one component of establishing visual behaviors. In addition, a systematic error correction procedure is also recommended as part of functional context vision instruction. If an auditory prompt such as tapping the object has been selected to establish visual tracking, and the student still fails to track the object, the error correction procedure described below may be appropriate.

Continuous Loop Training Procedures

The error correction procedure used as part of functional context vision instruction is one of repeated prompting (Koegel & Egel, 1979) or continuous correction (Utley, 1979). In using this procedure, students must make a correct visual response before they are able to continue with performance of the paired skill activity.

If a student reaches the critical visual moment and fails to do the targeted visual behavior, the teacher interrupts the trial, and visual performance is scored as (−). The trial is then repeated, providing the same cues, prompts, and assistance as before. If the student responds correctly this time, he or she is allowed to continue with the performance of the functional activity. A (−1) is scored to show that the initial response was incorrect and one additional trial was needed to achieve a correct response. The teacher continues to represent the trial with the designated assistance and prompting until a correct response is achieved. When the correct response is made, the student can continue his or her attempt to perform the paired skill, and the teacher records the number of times he repeated the trial next to the (−). The scores might look like this: (−5); (−3); (−1) for three separate trials. If the student responds correctly on the very first presentation of the trial, he or she receive a (+).

The advantage to using this system with visual behaviors is that the student always has to make a correct visual response before going on to the next behavior. In addition to using a paired skill that by its very nature required the visual behavior, the teacher using this correction procedure does not let the student try to do the paired skill without first exhibiting the desired visual behavior. Thus, the student consistently experiences a contingent relationship between vision use and competent skill performance.

For example, a student working on scanning paired with a three-choice object-picture matching task might receive the initial cue, "Look and find the (object)," while the teacher gives him or her a sample object. The student might begin to scan but look away before putting down the item. The teacher would stop the student and re-present the trial using whatever strategy (e.g., auditory cue, physical prompt, etc.) was designated. The student would not be allowed to make the discrimination response until he or she correctly scanned.

Use of this procedure requires care in structuring the task analysis and strategies for the visual behavior in a way which will ensure the likelihood of success. The teacher must be reasonably sure that the student *can* perform the visual behavior, or the repeated trials may be highly aversive. The data from the trials will assist the teacher in making decisions about the effectiveness of the continuous loop procedure.

The data are recorded in two ways. One graph depicts the percentage of correct responses on the very first presentation of the trial (+). If a student had to scan and match object to picture in a grocery store for ten items on a picture card shopping list, and scanned correctly (on the *first* presentation of trial) three times, the data would indicate 30% correct.

The other graph depicts the average number of times the trial had to be repeated during that session. The number is computed by adding up the number of re-presentations and dividing it by the total number of trials per session. In the same example above, there were 7 trials out of 10 in the grocery store in which an incorrect response was given on the first try. If those scores were as follows: (−3), (−5), (−2), (−1), (−3), (−2), the total number of re-presentation is 17. Computing the average number of corrections per trial, the score would be 17 corrections/10 trials = 1.7.

The average number of corrections will go down as the percentage of correct responses goes up. The correction data can show progress when the percentage correct data do not. If a student has just begun a program and rarely gets the response correct on the first trial, the data may show improvement in the average number of corrections. A decrease from 3.5 corrections per trial to .5 in the first five sessions indicates that the response is becoming less difficult, even though correct responses on the first trial have not yet improved.

The appropriateness of this procedure for use in community settings must be carefully considered. As Sailor et al. (1986) have noted, evaluation of instructional procedures for use in natural settings remains a major research need. Common sense, however, suggests that a continuous loop or repeated prompting procedure would not be practical in, for example, a crowded grocery store check-out line, while it might be effectively used for scanning the grocery shelves. As with all teaching procedures, application of this strategy in the community should be as unobtrusive as possible.

INSTRUCTIONAL STRATEGIES FOR THE FUNCTIONAL SKILL CONTEXT

Training visual attention within a functional skill context should be designed so that the student experiences a contingent relationship between visual attention and successful task performance; once the visual behavior is established at the critical moment (using the continuous loop if needed), competence in performing the task should be ensured through the instructional program that is developed for the functional or paired skill.

The functional paired skill may range from a complex fine motor task such as hanging cups on storage hooks in the dish cupboard, to a single motor action such as opening one's mouth to designate readiness to receive food, to a complex visual discrimination task such as selecting the correct coin from a wallet full of change. Student performance levels for the paired skill may also vary: one student may require only minimal assistance to perform the skill of putting pencils in a sharpener, while another student may require extensive training to learn to insert a wand successfully into a jar, withdraw it, and blow bubbles.

Regardless of the nature of the paired skill and the student's level of proficiency at the skill, it is crucial that a teaching strategy is specified that will allow the student to experience immediate competence at the skill when he or she performs the targeted visual behavior (Gee & Goetz, 1985). Thus, most to least prompt fading and shaping procedures (e.g., Sidman & Stoddard, 1967) are recommended rather than least to most prompting procedures (e.g., Correa, Poulson, & Salzberg, 1984).

For example, Gee & Goetz (1985) used a variation of time delay procedures to teach sustained visual attention during visual motor tasks such as those shown for Maria in Table 2 (stacking plastic cups, placing caps on marking pens, etc.). The first step of the paired skill instructional program specified immediate, hand-over-hand assistance to perform the motor task as soon as visual attention occurred. Assistance was withdrawn if at any point Maria discontinued visual attention. Assistance continued when visual attention was re-established through the continuous loop procedure. These procedures ensured that Maria was successful at completing the task *while* she was visually attending to it.

When the average number of performance loops per session decreased to .60, the instructor introduced a gradual, systematic increase in the amount of time Maria was required to visually attend while attempting task completion before she was assisted to be successful on the motor component. The delay interval (during which Maria had to continuously look while attempting task performance) was increased to 3 seconds, then 5, then 10, and finally 30 seconds. During the final delay steps, Maria frequently "anticipated" (Snell & Gast, 1981) and completed the motor task before any assistance was required.

SAMPLE DATA AND INSTRUCTIONAL PROGRAM

Table 3 presents a summary of the instructional program developed to teach Maria, a 5-year-old student, to attend visually in the context of functional motor tasks.

Table 3. Instructional program for visual fixation

Student's name: Maria Age: 5 Vision difficulty: reduced acuity/low vision

Targeted vision objective: Maria will sustain visual fixation long enough to successfully complete 5 targeted visual motor tasks with complete independence, 4/5 consecutive days.

Paired skills/ critical moment	Vision prompt	"Continuous loop" strategy	Paired skill steps
Play activities/leisure domain 1. Stack ring on spin toy 2. Block into post office toy **Chores/vocational and community domain** 1. Stack cups while clearing table 2. Coins into purse for community 3. Caps on pens when clearing teacher's desk **Critical moments:** From when items are within 1 inch of another until task is completed.	Point at item(s) and tap	Give student cue to "look and do" Wait 3 seconds for looking to begin At the critical moment assist student as designated under paired skill step Correct response: student looks at critical moment while teacher gives as much assistance as stated under skill step If student does not look or fails to continue to look, stop the assistance on the task, re-establish looking prior to continuing assistance Count the number of cues needed to establish or re-establish looking while doing. Score as (−3), (−5), etc. At the end of the session take the average number of continuous loops out of the number of trials.	1. Immediate hand over hand assistance to fully complete task. 2. 5 second delay before giving hand over hand assistance. 3. 10 second delay. 4. Independent task performance while looking. Score visual motor skill performance as (+) correct prompted response at designated level of physical assistance, (−) incorrect response at designated level of assistance, or (⊕) correct anticipated response with no physical assistance needed.

The objective, to increase visual fixation, is stated at the top of the table. The first column of the table lists the five skill contexts used to teach the visual attention skill. These contexts were selected based on criteria discussed earlier (see Table 2). The second column lists the prompt selected to teach visual attention. Since Maria did not have a hearing impairment, a combined auditory and visual prompt was selected.

The "continuous loop" strategy for the visual behavior is described in column 4, while the teaching steps for the paired skill are described in column 5. Maria required four time-delay steps. During Step 1, full physical assistance to complete the task was provided as soon as Maria demonstrated visual attention. During Step 2, Maria had to visually attend to the task for 5 seconds before full physical assistance was provided. Step 3 required 10 seconds of looking and attempting task completion before assistance was provided. By Step 4, no assistance to complete the task was provided. Throughout these steps, visual attention was prompted as needed, following the continuous loop correction procedure.

Figure 3 presents Maria's performance data for independent "looking and doing" while stacking cups, one of the five tasks selected for her vision training program. (These data are a subset of the experimental data reported in Gee & Goetz, 1985). During baseline, when no training procedures were in effect, Maria rarely attended visually and successfully completed the task on her first attempt, as indicated by the ________ line.

In session 12, Step 1 of functional vision training was introduced. As soon as Maria looked, she received complete hand-over-hand assistance to complete the task. Initially, she required numerous "loops" to establish looking at the critical moment (session 12, 13, and 14). By session 16, however, she independently looked and performed the task (with full assistance) 60% of the time, with no loops required to establish visual attention. Steps 2 and 3 show Maria's performance as she was required to look and do for increasing amounts of time (5 seconds and 10 seconds respectively) before assistance was provided to complete the task. During these steps, Maria did not require any "loops" to re-establish visual attention. By Step 4, Maria was required to independently look on the first cue and remain looking for as long as it took for her to successfully complete the task independently; i.e., no hand-over-hand assistance was provided.

CONCLUSION AND FUTURE RESEARCH DIRECTIONS

The assumption that efficient residual vision use is critical to all learning (cf. Barraga, 1970) remains a cornerstone in curriculum development for students with vision impairments. The assumption that persons with vision impairments can improve their visual function has also been a cornerstone in educational practices with these persons (cf. Lundervold, Lewin, & Irvin, 1987). This chapter has presented a procedure for teaching students to be visually efficient that is based upon both empirical data and theoretical models of learning.

The teaching procedures outlined here are acknowledged as complex and highly individualized. Developing a functional vision training program may require more

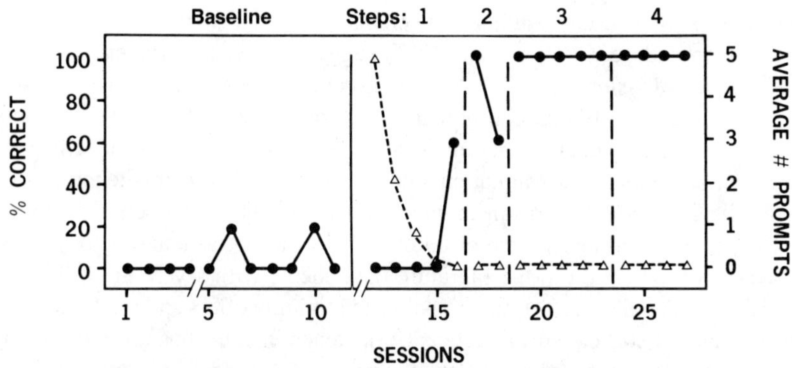

Figure 3. Maria's data for the stacking cups activity during the program described in Table 3. ______. Indicates Maria's successful looking and task completion on the first attempt. During Steps 1–3, successful looking and doing was scored even if a full physical prompt was provided, so long as Maria looked and attempted the task for the specified time interval. During Step 4, physical assistance was completely faded out. ▲______▲ indicates average number of correction loops per session for the visual behavior.

effort than is typically required for instructional programs in other domains. However, empirical evaluations of this model (Gee & Goetz, 1985; Goetz & Gee, 1987) suggest several critical benefits of this model. This training package resulted in *generalized* performance of visual attention across a variety of functional activity contexts. After experiencing the contingent relationship between visual attention and successful task performance (established through use of the continuous loop correction procedure) in two to three training contexts, all students generalized their visual attention to other, untrained functional activities.

Visual efficiency may also be a "target" skill that has multiple treatment effects (Rincover, 1981). Students who learned to use their residual vision with this procedure also demonstrated acquisition of the tasks used as the vision training contexts, *without* any direct teaching intervention on these tasks. Thus, teaching a basic sensory functioning skill within functional contexts may yield numerous unanticipated benefits to students with sensory impairments.

Functional vision training is consistent with a number of recommended "promising practices" curriculum models for students with multiple severe handicaps, including individual curriculum sequencing (ICS) (Helmstetter & Guess, Chapter 10, this volume; Mulligan et al., 1980), which stresses the clustering of behaviors into natural, common sense instructional sequences (e.g., look at an object, reach for it, and manipulate it), and distributed rather than massed trial practice. Functional vision training also utilizes recommendations that instructional content focus on activities that are age appropriate for the learner (Brown et al., 1980).

Utilization of natural cues and consequences is another frequent recommendation for learners with severe handicaps (Falvey et al., 1980). One of the natural consequences of using available vision is improved competence at tasks and activities that have a visual motor component. This is also the contingency in effect in functional vision training. Data documenting generalized visual attention as a function of this training procedure (Goetz & Gee, 1987) suggest that visual efficiency, or effective use of residual vision, may be a "self-reinforcing" behavior that is used independently of external or artificial consequences. Through use of the continuous loop, students experience a contingent relationship between "looking" and competent "doing." For students in our validation studies, this improved competence was evidently motivating enough to result in generalization of the visual behaviors to new, untrained contexts. While the role of competence as a motivational factor has only recently received attention in the literature on students with severe disabilities (cf. Goetz, Schuler, & Sailor, 1983), functional vision training offers an initial example of how to use natural consequences such as competence in educational programming.

Lastly, the procedure acknowledges the role of the students' task preference, or motivation to engage in the task, as part of the curriculum development process (Guess, Benson, & Siegel-Causey, 1985). As with the role of competence, choice and preference may suggest new models of motivation that go beyond traditional extrinsic reinforcers.

Developing effective curriculum model and instructional procedures for teaching basic sensory (e.g., visual efficiency) and basic motor skills (e.g., reach and grasp) within a community-referenced, functional life skills educational model will continue to be a pressing research priority. As individuals with the most severe multiple disabilities, including those who have combined motor and sensory impairments, and those who are medically fragile, are increasingly integrated into the community at large, educators face new questions about effective curriculum development and instructional strategies. Functional vision programming is an initial attempt to identify and synthesize some factors that might be of value to investigators and educators who are providing services to these individuals.

REFERENCES

Barraga, N. (1970). *Teacher's guide for the development of visual learning abilities and utilization of low vision.* American Printing House for the Blind.

Barraga, N., & Collins, M. (1979). Development of efficiency in visual functioning: Rationale for a comprehensive program. *Journal of Visual Impairment and Blindness, 73*, 121–126.

Baumgart, D., Brown, L., Pumpian, I., Nisbet, J., Ford, A., Sweet, M., Messina, R., & Schroeder, J. (1982). Principle of partial participation and individualized adaptations in educational programs for severely handicapped students. *Journal of The Association for Persons with Severe Handicaps, 7* , 17–27.

Bernstein, G.B. (1979). Integration of vision stimulation in the classroom II: Group programming. *Education of Visually Handicapped, 2*, 39–49.

Brown, L., Branston, M., Baumgart, D., Vincent, L., Falvey, M., & Schroeder, J. (1980). Utilizing characteristics of a variety of current and subsequent least restrictive environments as factors in development of curricular content for severely handicapped students. In L. Brown, M. Falvey, D. Baumgart, I. Pumpian, J. Schroeder, & L. Gruenewald (Eds.), *Strategies for teaching chronological age-appropriate functional skills to adolescent and young adult severely handicapped students* (Vol. IX, Part 1). Madison, WI: University of Wisconsin and Madison Metropolitan School District.

Brown, L., Branston, M., Hamre-Nietupski, S., Pumpian, I., Certo, N., & Gruenewald, L. (1979). A strategy for developing chronological age appropriate and functional curricular content for severely handicapped adolescents and young adults. *Journal of Special Education*, 13, 81–90.

Correa, V., Poulson, C., & Salzberg, C. (1984). Training and generalization of reach-group behavior in blind retarded young children. *Journal of Applied Behavioral Analysis, 17*, 56–69.

Cress, P., Spellman, C., DeBriere, T., Sizemore, A., Northam, J., & Johnson, J. (1981). Vision screening for persons with severe handicaps. *Journal of The Association for Persons with Severe Handicaps, 6*, 41–49.

Datillo, J., & Rusch, F. (1985). Effects of choice on behavior: Leisure participation for persons with severe handicaps. *Journal of The Association for Persons with Severe Handicaps, 10*, 194–199.

Donlon, E.T. (1966). Implications of visual disorders. In W.M. Cruickshank (ed.), *Cerebral Palsy: Its individual and community problems* (2nd ed.). Syracuse, NY: Syracuse University Press.

Falvey, M., Brown, L., Lyon, S., Baumgart, D., & Schroeder, J. (1980). Strategies for using cues and correction procedures. In W. Sailor, B. Wilcox, & L. Brown (Eds.), *Methods of instruction for severely handicapped students* (pp. 109–133). Baltimore: Paul H. Brookes Publishing Co.

Fantz, R.L., Ordy, J.M. & Udelf, M.S. (1962). Maturation of pattern vision in infants during the first six months. *Journal of Comparative and Physiological Psychology, 55*, 907–917.

Ficociello, C. (1974). *Observing visual functioning in deaf-blind children.* Visual Assessment Kit. South Central Regional Center for Deaf-Blind, Dallas, Texas.

Gee, K., & Goetz, L. (1985). *Establishing generalized use of residual vision through instruction in natural contexts.* San Francisco: Department of Special Education, San Francisco State University.

Goetz, L., & Gee, K. (1987). Teaching visual attention in functional contexts: Acquisition, generalization, and maintenance. *Journal of Visual Impairment and Blindness, 81*, 115–117.

Goetz, L., Gee, K., Baldwin, M., & Sailor, W. (1982). Classroom based sensory assessment procedures for severely handicapped students: Case studies of a stimulus transfer paradigm. *Analysis and Intervention in Developmental Disabilities, 2*, 171–185.

Goetz, L., Schuler, A., & Sailor, W. (1983). Motivational considerations in teaching language to severely handicapped students. In M. Hersen, V. Van Hasselt, & J. Matson (Eds.), *Behavior Therapy for the Developmentally and Physically Disabled* (pp. 57–77). New York: Academic Press.

Guess, D., Benson, H., & Siegel-Causey, E. (1985). Concepts and issues related to choice making and autonomy among persons with severe disabilities. *Journal of The Association for Persons with Severe Handicaps, 10*, 79–88.

Guess, D., & Helmstetter, E. (1986). Skill cluster instruction and the individualized curriculum sequencing model. In R. Horner, L. Meyer, & H.D.B. Fredericks (Eds.), *Education of learners with severe handicaps: Exemplary service strategies* (pp. 221–248). Baltimore: Paul H. Brookes Publishing Co.

Hamre-Nietupski, S., Nietupski, J., Sandvig, M., & Ayres, B. (1984). Leisure skills introduction in a community residential setting with young adults who are deaf/blind severely handicapped. *Journal of The Association for Persons with Severe Handicaps, 9*, 49–54.

Haring, N., Liberty, K., & White, O. (1980). Rules for data-based strategy decisions in instructional programs: Current research and instructional implications. In W. Sailor, B. Wilcox, L. Brown (Eds.), *Methods of instruction with severely handicapped students* (pp. 159–192). Baltimore: Paul H. Brookes Publishing Co.

Hatlen, P., & Goetz, L. (1981). Establishing generalized visual functioning in severely handicapped students (USOE Grant #G00830032). Field initiated research proposal.

Helmstetter, E., Murphy-Herd, M., Roberts, S., & Guess, D. (1984). *Individualized curriculum sequences and extended classroom models for learners who are deaf and blind.* Unpublished manuscript, Dept. of Special Education, University of Kansas, Lawrence, Kansas.

Hill, J., Wehman, P., & Horst, G. (1982). Toward generalization of appropriate leisure and social behavior in severely handicapped youth: Pinball machine use. *Journal of The Association for Persons with Severe Handicaps, 6*(4), 38–44.

Kagan, J. (1973). The determinants of attention in the infant. In L. Stone, H. Smith, & L. Murphy (Eds.), *The competent infant: research and commentary*. New York: Basic Books.

Koegel, R., & Egel, A. (1979). Motivating autistic children. *Journal of Abnormal Psychology, 88*, 418–426.

Langley, B., & DuBose, R. (1980). *Functional vision inventory for the multiply and severely handicapped*. Chicago: Stoelting.

Lovaas, O.I., Berberich, J., Perloff, B., & Schaeffer, B. (1966). Acquisition of imitative speech of schizophrenic children. *Science, 151*, 705–707.

Lundervold, D., Lewin, L., & Irvin, L. (1987). Rehabilitation of visual impairments: A critical review. *Clinical Psychology Review, 7*, 169–185.

Lyon, S., & Lyon, G. (1980). Team functioning and staff development: A role release approach to providing integrated services for severely handicapped students. *Journal of The Association for Persons with Severe Handicaps, 5*, 250–263.

Mosk, M., & Bucher, B. (1984). Prompting and stimulus shaping procedures for teaching visual motor skills to retarded children. *Journal of The Association for Persons with Severe Handicaps, 17*, 23–34.

Mulligan, M., Guess, D., Holvoet, J., & Brown, F. (1980). The individualized curriculum sequencing model I: Implications from research on massed, distributed to spaced trial training. *Journal of The Association for Persons with Severe Handicaps, 5*, 325–336.

Rincover, A. (1981). Some directions for analysis and intervention in developmental disabilities: An editorial. *Analysis and Intervention in Developmental Disabilities, 1*, 109–115.

Robinson, C., & Robinson, J. (1978). Sensorimotor functions and cognitive development. In M. Snell (Ed.), *Systematic instruction of the moderately and severely handicapped*. Columbus, Ohio: Charles Merrill.

Sailor, W., & Goetz, L. (1981). *Bay Area Severely Handicapped Deaf Blind Project: Final Report*. ERIC Document Reproduction #ED 250 841. Reston, VA: Council for Exceptional Children.

Sailor, W., & Guess, D. (1983). *Severely handicapped students: An instructional design*. Boston: Houghton Mifflin.

Sailor, W., Halvorsen, A., Anderson, J., Goetz, L. Gee, K., Doering, K., & Hunt, P. (1986). Community intensive instruction. In R. Horner, L. Meyer, & H.D.B. Fredericks (Eds.), *Education of learners with severe handicaps: Exemplary service strategies* (pp. 251–288). Baltimore: Paul H. Brookes Publishing Co.

Sidman, M., & Stoddard, L. (1967). The effectiveness of fading in programming a simultaneous form discrimination for retarded children. *Journal of the Experimental Analysis of Behavior, 10*, 3–15.

Smith, A., & Cote, K. (1982). *Look at me*. Philadelphia: The Pennsylvania College of Optometry.

Snell, M. (1978). *Systematic Instruction of the moderately and severely handicapped*. Columbus, OH: Charles E. Merrill.

Snell, M., & Browder, D. (1986). Community referenced instruction: Research and issues. *Journal of The Association for Persons with Severe Handicaps, 11*, 1–11.

Snell, J., & Gast, D. (1981). Applying time delay procedure to the instruction of the severely handicapped. *Journal of The Association for Persons with Severe Handicaps, 6*, 3–14.

Spellman, C., DeBriere, T., & Cress, P. (1979). *Person's visual acuity test.* South Bend, IN: The Bernell Corp.

Striefel, S. (1974). *Teaching a child to imitate.* Lawrence, KS: H and H Enterprises.

Terrace, H.S. (1963). Discrimination learning with and without "errors." *Journal of Experimental Analysis of Behavior, 6*, 1–27.

Touchette, P. (1971). Transfer of stimulus control: Measuring the moment of transfer. *Journal of the Experimental Analysis of Behavior, 15*, 347–354.

Utley, B. (1979). *Annual report: The Bay Area severely handicapped deaf-blind project* (USOE contract #300-78-0338). San Francisco: Department of Special Education, San Francisco State University.

Utley, B., Duncan, D., Strain, P., & Scanlon, K. (1983). Effects of contingent and noncontingent vision stimulation on visual fixation in multiply handicapped children. *Journal of The Association for Persons with Severe Handicaps, 8*, 29–42.

Utley, B., Goetz, L., Gee, K., Baldwin, M., & Sailor, W. (1981). *Vision assessment and program manual for severely handicapped and/or deaf-blind students* [(ERIC Document Reproduction Service No. ED 250 840).] Reston, VA: Council for Exceptional Children.

van den Pol, R. Iwata, B., Ivancic, I., Page, T., Neef, N., & Whitley, F. (1981). Teaching the handicapped to eat in public places. *Journal of Applied Behavioral Analysis, 14*, 61–69.

Wheeler, J., Ford, A., Nietupski, J., Loomis, R., & Brown, L. (1980). Teaching moderately and severely handicapped adolescents to shop in supermarkets using pocket calculators. *Education and Training of the Mentally Retarded, 15*, 105–112.

Wolf, J.M., & Anderson, R.M. (1973). *The multiply handicapped child.* Springfield, IL: Charles C Thomas.

CHAPTER 5

Audiometric Assessment and Management

Paul S. Niswander

AUDIOMETRIC ASSESSMENT AND management of the child with both visual and auditory impairments can present the audiologist with a very difficult challenge. Currently the term "difficult-to-test" seems to be in vogue for describing any client who seems to present more than a normal assessment challenge. However, there probably is no client who is more appropriately described by this label than the young child with severe impairments of both vision and hearing. Standard auditory assessment procedures that utilize behavioral responses rely heavily on vision, either to guide the client in the testing task or as an input for whatever reinforcer might be in use. With the child who is visually impaired, not only are the routine procedures of questionable value but even those techniques that have been developed for the difficult-to-test client may be miserable failures.

Habilitation of the hearing impaired child with severe visual impairment likewise presents a serious challenge. Auditory prosthetic devices such as hearing aids and cochlear implants are meant to supplement visual input. If vision is limited, the use of such devices may be of minimal value. Traditional habilitation that uses speechreading (lipreading) or manual signing to supplement input from auditory prosthetic devices may be of limited value for the child with significant vision impairment. In general, practically every current auditory device and/or habilitation strategy presumes vision in order to provide maximum benefit. Achievements with the hearing impaired–visual impaired child have been extremely limited. Nevertheless, growing attention to the child with multihandicaps in general and the child with deafblindness in particular has led to recent progress in both assessment and habilitation.

The purpose of the present chapter is to provide teachers, who may have limited knowledge of audiology, some background in the current status of both diagnostics and habilitation involving the child with the dual handicaps of hearing loss and vision impairment. Teachers need to have an understanding of assessment so that they can interpret the results of testing, and need to have some knowledge of auditory devices so that they understand the strength and limitations of such devices.

This chapter includes a brief discussion of the anatomy of the ear and of the types of hearing loss (including some etiologies of hearing loss); considerations of some of the newer assessment techniques for determining type and extent of hearing loss; and finally an overview of current auditory prosthetics, such as hearing aids, cochlear implants, and vibrotactile devices.

ANATOMY OF THE EAR

The peripheral portion of the ear is composed of three parts that have separate embryological derivation and functional significance (Martin, 1981). Reference to Figure 1 will be helpful in following this discussion.

Outer Ear

The portion of the ear that includes the pinna and external auditory meatus (ear canal) up to the tympanic membrane (ear drum) is referred to as the outer ear. A hearing loss that involves the outer ear is termed a conductive hearing loss.

Middle Ear

Central to the tympanic membrane is a cavity that contains the ossicular chain (malleus, incus and stapes), two muscles (tensor tympani and stapedius) and numerous suspensory ligaments. This cavity and its contents comprise the middle ear. The purpose of the middle ear is to transform the airborne vibrations that impinge on the tympanic membrane into mechanical vibrations that can set into motion the fluids of the inner ear. Hearing loss associated with the middle ear, like that involving the outer ear, is known as a conductive hearing loss.

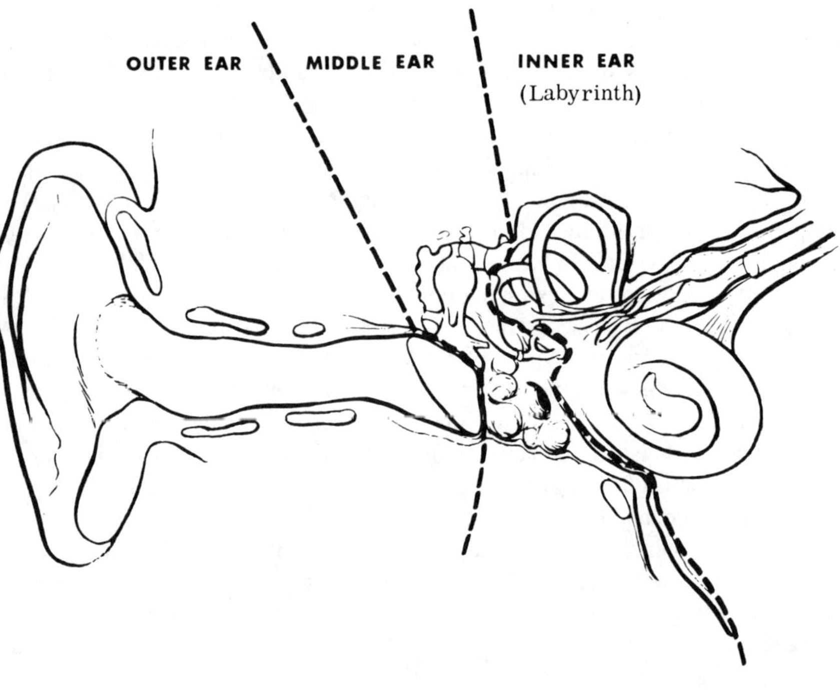

Figure 1. A cross-section of the human ear (Illustration courtesy of Zenetron, Inc.).

Inner Ear

The cochlea (inner ear) is the complex organ that transforms vibratory movements into electric nerve impulses. The "in and out" movements of the footplate of the stapes in the oval window set into motion the fluid (perilymph) contained in the inner ear. These hydrodynamic disturbances cause the basilar membrane to move, which, in turn, causes bending of the thousands of hair cells that rest on the basilar membrane. This bending of the hair cells initiates the nerve impulses that are transmitted to the central nervous system via the cochlear portion of the auditory nerve.

Hearing loss that involves the inner ear is termed a sensorineural hearing loss. Sensorineural hearing loss typically is due either to loss of hair cells, and/or to anatomical deformations of the structures that support the hair cells.

Central Auditory Pathways

The eighth cranial nerve, which originates in the inner ear, conducts nerve impulses from the cochlea to the brainstem. From the brainstem the impulses are conveyed to the centers of hearing in the temporal lobes. These central pathways are quite complex, and include connections to many parts of the brain.

Retrocochlear pathologies that involve the central auditory pathways are relatively rare in childhood deafness; these pathologies are more likely to be found in adults in association with such conditions as multiple sclerosis and auditory nerve tumors.

THE NATURE AND CAUSES OF HEARING LOSS

Conductive Hearing Loss

Conductive hearing loss may involve the outer and/or middle ear. There are several malformations that can involve the external auditory meatus and thereby cause such conductive hearing loss. With atresia (or congenital atresia), the failure of the external auditory canal to open during prenatal development, a plug or block of cartilage completely occludes the external auditory canal and thereby causes the hearing loss. Congenital atresia frequently is accompanied by additional abnormalities of the head and face. Both Treacher Collins syndrome and Goldenhaar syndrome may combine congenital atresia with additional craniofacial anomalies (Martin, 1981; Northern & Downs, 1984).

Stenosis, an external auditory canal more narrow than is normal, will not by itself cause a hearing loss, but it does make it easier for the canal to become occluded with cerumen (ear wax) and thereby cause a hearing loss. Stenosis may occur in isolation but, like atresia, is more likely to appear in conjunction with other craniofacial anomalies. Stenosis of the external auditory canal is quite common in individuals with Down syndrome, and may be accompanied by additional malformations of the middle ear.

When the pinna is malformed, the condition is known as microtia. The impact of microtia on hearing is likely to be minimal. However, the presence of microtia may signal the presence of other more important but less visible problems in the outer and middle ear, since abnormalities of the outer and middle ear are frequently found in association with each other.

Of the various problems that cause conductive hearing loss in children, by far the most common is the condition of otitis media, which may include both inflamation of tissue lining the middle ear cavity and accumulation of either thin serous or thick mucoid fluid in the middle ear cavity. If this fluid surrounds and immerses the individual bones of the ossicular chain, it will interfere with their normal ease of movement and thereby cause a conductive hearing loss. Otitis media commonly arises as a result of upper respiratory infections or allergies, and normally is treated successfully with antibiotics and decongestants.

A far more serious but less common problem involving the middle ear occurs when one or more of the bones comprising the ossicular chain is not formed properly, or when the bones are fused and, therefore, prevented from vibrating in a normal fashion. Such conditions, which often are of genetic origin, may occur alone or in conjunction with atresia or stenosis as in Treacher Collins and Goldenhaar syndromes. Abnormalities involving the structure of the ossicular chain cause a conductive hearing loss. This, like all conductive losses, may be medically treated.

In general, conductive hearing loss is less severe than that resulting from sensorineural pathology. Additionally, in contrast with sensorineural hearing loss, the hearing loss associated with conductive factors tends to be more serious at the low frequencies. High frequency thresholds may be near or within normal limits. This type of hearing loss makes sounds softer but does not appreciably affect their quality.

Sensorineural Hearing Loss

Many cases of sensorineural hearing loss are congenital; that is, they were present at birth. Some of these are genetically related and others are acquired as the result of medications used or illness suffered by the mother during the prenatal period. It is generally assumed that approximately half the cases of congenital hearing loss result from genetic factors. Approximately 25 genetic syndromes involving hearing loss in conjunction with eye disease have been documented. Usher's syndrome, one of the more common of these, combines congenital hearing loss, often severe to profound in degree, with progressive retinitis pigmentosa.

Acquired congenital deafness can result from numerous causes during the prenatal period. Rubella is a virus that, if contracted by the mother during pregnancy, can cause a variety of handicaps that include both severe hearing loss and visual deficits. The development of the rubella vaccine has greatly decreased the incidence of handicaps associated with prenatal rubella. Cytomegalovirus (CMV) is a virus that may infect the infant either *in utero* prior to birth or during the birth process. Likewise, herpes may be contracted by an infant during a normal vaginal delivery. Both CMV and herpes can cause hearing loss in conjunction with a variety of other handicaps, including visual deficits and mental retardation. In the case of CMV, it appears that the hearing loss may have progressive aspects, increasing in severity during the infant's first year of life.

Other causes of hearing loss dating from the neonatal period include anoxia, apnea and jaundice associated with elevated bilirubin levels. In addition, hearing loss is associated with the use of certain antibiotics (aminoglycosides), which are used frequently to treat severe infections in neonates.

Many children have sensorineural hearing loss that has been acquired during early childhood from illness or infection. Whereas most of these losses undoubtedly are caused by the illness itself, it is possible that some of the losses may be attributable to medications used to treat the illness. Meningitis (especially that associated with bacterial causes) can result in particularly severe sensorineural hearing loss. Viral infections, such as those associated with chicken pox and unspecified upper respiratory infection, have also been implicated in producing sensorineural hearing loss in children.

In contrast to conductive hearing loss, sensorineural hearing loss can be quite severe and the hearing loss normally is more severe for the high frequencies than for low frequencies. This, in turn, causes a sort of "filtering" effect in the cochlea. Therefore, not only do the sounds seem softer, but their quality is also changed. In fact, it frequently happens that the sounds of speech can be heard but not understood. Perhaps the most important concern with sensorineural hearing loss is that the use of hearing aids to simply increase the loudness of sounds does not solve the problem, for the filtering effect still remains. Hearing aids typically are not successful for children who are profoundly hearing impaired, not because these hearing aids cannot amplify sound sufficiently, but because they cannot restore the clarity to sounds that the filtering effect of the hearing loss has affected.

Additional problems caused by cochlear hearing loss may include decreased ability to discriminate both intensity and pitch differences, and decreased tolerance for loud sounds (a very great problem if use of a hearing aid is under consideration). In reality, there are many dimensions of auditory experience that may be affected by hearing loss. Since most hearing aids only make sounds louder, they do not remediate other abnormalities of auditory function that may be associated with hearing loss. The failure of hearing aids to effectively ameliorate hearing loss due to most of these other abnormalities only reflects the current limited understanding of the complex problems associated with hearing loss.

AUDIOMETRIC ASSESSMENT

Purpose of Audiometric Assessment

Audiometric assessment serves to identify the presence of a hearing loss, quantify its magnitude and determine whether it is conductive or sensorineural in nature. Determination of type of hearing loss is important because treatment options are different for conductive and for sensorineural loss. Many types of conductive hearing loss can be alleviated by means of appropriate medical management, whereas sensorineural hearing loss typically is permanent. If a hearing loss can be medically corrected, this certainly is preferable to having to compensate for its effects by means of hearing aid amplification.

In general, audiometric tests are known as *behavioral* if they use voluntary, behavioral responses. They are known as *physiological* if they monitor some physiological response of the auditory mechanism. Tangible-reinforcer operant-conditioning audiometry (TROCA) is an example of a behavioral procedure; measurement of auditory brainstem response (ABR) is an example of a physiological method. This general classification scheme will be utilized for the remainder of this chapter.

At the outset it should be noted that physiological tests are not necessarily better or more accurate than behavioral tests. They simply provide a different means for viewing the same system. Strictly speaking, physiological assessments are not hearing tests at all, and therefore do not provide "audiograms." They only assess the general functional status of the auditory system. This distinction becomes very important as one attempts to reconcile differences that may appear to exist between the results of behavioral and physiological tests. The primary value of physiological tests is that they assess the auditory system without any need to involve behavioral responses. This is particularly useful for assessing hearing in individuals who are severely delayed. The general status of the auditory system can be assessed and, if a hearing loss is found, some estimate of the relative contributions of conductive and sensorineural components is available.

With an individual who is severely delayed, if behavioral testing can be completed and if normal hearing is indicated, then no further testing is normally necessary. However, if responses to sounds are inconsistent or non-existent, then the use of physiological methods is indicated. Behavioral methods should always receive first consideration, for they provide the only means to define quantitatively the magnitude of hearing loss. Some individuals will demonstrate no behavioral responses to sounds, yet physiological testing will reveal normal responses. Since most physiological tests currently in use examine physiological activity at the brainstem level, normal responses mean that the system is functionally intact at this level. One is forced to conclude that the lack of behavioral responses is related to impaired cortical processing, and perhaps is part of an overall nonresponsiveness to environmental stimuli. The ability to determine whether lack of responsiveness to sound is due to hearing loss or to impaired cortical functioning is quite important, for hearing aids typically are not effective for an individual who receives sounds perfectly well but has difficulty bringing the stimulus to the cognitive level. An intervention option for such an individual, to be tried on an experimental basis, is the use of some sort of augmentative device that utilizes another sensory modality, such as the visual modality or, if the visual handicap precludes this, the tactile modality.

The Audiogram

The audiogram is the graph that summarizes hearing sensitivity at various frequencies within the audible range. Figure 2 shows a typical audiogram form. The x-axis

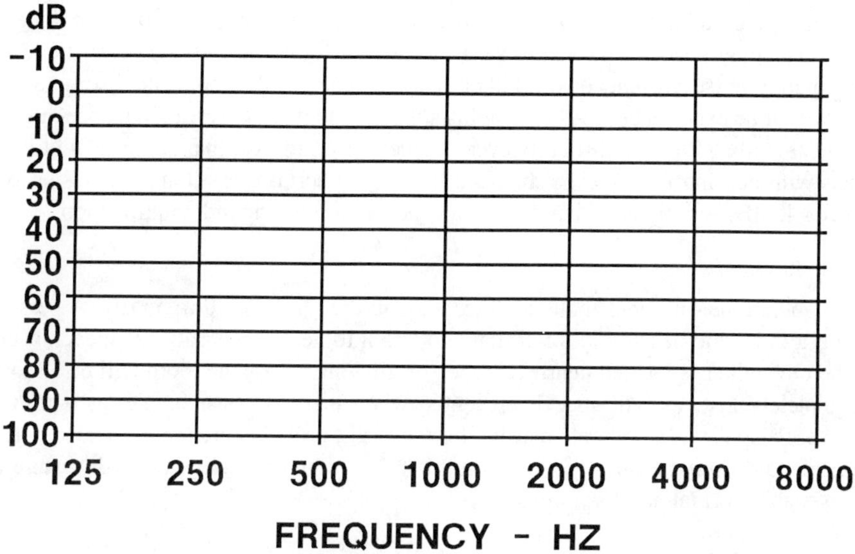

Figure 2. A sample audiogram form.

(abscissa) summarizes the frequency of the test tone expressed in Hertz (Hz). The lowest frequency normally tested is 250 Hz and the highest is 8,000 Hz. In reality, the human ear can hear frequencies down to about 20 Hz and up to about 18,000 Hz. Audiometric testing normally is limited to frequencies from 250 Hz to 8,000 Hz. However, frequencies higher and lower than this contribute very little to our ability to hear and understand environmental and speech sounds. In fact, most information in the speech signal is contained in the frequencies between 500 Hz and 2,000 Hz. For this reason, these are often designated as the "speech frequencies."

The y-axis (ordinate) summarizes loudness of the test tone in units termed decibels or dB. Decibels are units derived empirically from how the human ear operates. The human ear can detect intensity differences between sounds as small as about 1 dB. The decibel scale has been adjusted so that a young adult with normal hearing can hear tones of about 0 dB.

CLASSIFICATION OF HEARING LOSS

Sounds of −10 to 0 dB are very faint and can be heard only by those with the best hearing acuity who are listening in a very quiet room. Most people with normal hearing acuity can hear tones of 10 to 20 dB in a room that is reasonably quiet. A person is considered to have normal hearing if the hearing threshold is no poorer than 25 dB.

Mild Loss

Hearing sensitivity falling in the 25 to 40 dB range comprises a mild hearing loss. Since conversational speech is about 40 to 45 dB when one is face to face with a talker about 1 meter distant, a person with a hearing threshold of 30 to 35 dB will still hear conversational speech reasonably well in quiet surroundings. If, however, there is competing noise present, or if a talker is situated across the room, then some difficulty will be experienced. As thresholds approach 40 dB, conversational speech will be heard only with great difficulty even in quiet surroundings. In most cases, individuals with hearing loss in even the mild range (and certainly as it approaches or exceeds 40 dB) will be good candidates for the use of hearing aid amplification.

Moderate Loss

A moderate hearing loss includes thresholds in the range of 40 to 55 dB. A person with a moderate hearing loss will have to strain to hear conversational speech even when the talker is located nearby. Speech originating across the room will be almost completely lost, as will speech presented when there is considerable background noise. Persons with moderate hearing loss, overall, probably are the most successful hearing aid users because the loss is not too severe and a hearing aid will restore a reasonably normal auditory signal.

Moderately Severe Loss

Moderately severe hearing loss comprises the range of thresholds between 55 and 70 dB. A person with hearing loss in this range will not hear normal conversational speech, but may be able to hear some individual speech sounds if the speaker is adjacent and shouting. For most purposes, an individual with moderately severe hearing loss has quite limited functional hearing without the use of a hearing aid.

Severe Loss

Hearing thresholds in the 70 to 90 dB range comprise a severe hearing loss. Individuals with hearing loss in this range are deprived of all but the most intense sounds (e.g., the honk of a car horn heard from just in front of the car). Individuals with severe hearing loss certainly can be expected to benefit from the use of a hearing aid, but even the most powerful aid will not restore the ability to hear all sounds.

Profound Loss

Hearing thresholds that exceed about 90 dB are considered to constitute profound loss or deafness. Individuals with profound hearing loss can never expect to develop functional hearing for speech, even with a powerful body-style hearing aid. A hearing aid might be used, however, to provide supplemental environmental cues such as the blare of a car horn or the wail of an emergency vehicle siren. This information could help an individual function more independently by providing environmental cues that would help to avoid injury in dangerous situations.

These comments regarding the functional limitations associated with differing degrees of hearing loss assume that some degree of vision is present to help compensate for, or at least supplement, residual hearing. If a severe visual deficit accompanies the hearing loss, then the overall handicap associated with the combined impairments will be much more serious. The seriousness of the dual handicaps of vision of hearing impairment can hardly be overestimated.

ASSESSMENT METHODS

Behavioral Tests

Behavioral Observation Audiometry (BOA) Methods The most simple—and least accurate—means of screening for hearing loss is to examine changes in ongoing behavior produced by various noisemakers in a very unstructured test situation. This technique most often is used for very young infants or those with severe developmental handicaps. Although the auditory stimuli for behavioral observation testing can be produced by an audiometer, noisemakers work best.

In general, a response for this type of test is any behavior change that is noted between the prestimulus and post-stimulus periods. Therefore, a response could be a startle, cessation of activity (stilling), searching movement with the eyes, localization involving head turn, and so on. The specific behavior change noted will depend on the activity of the infant at the precise time of stimulation and the developmental level of the infant.

Two principal problems are associated with the use of behavioral observation methods. First, when using environmental noisemakers as the source of sound, it usually is impossible to control either the intensity of the noisemaker or its frequency characteristics. When responses are observed, therefore, it generally is impossible to know to what stimulus frequencies these responses may be attributed, nor is it normally possible to change the intensity of the noisemaker to determine where the "threshold" for the response lies. Moreover, responses in such a testing situation usually occur only when the sounds are of a supra-threshold intensity (generally around a "comfortable" loudness level). This further complicates attempts to specify exact threshold levels. Although behavioral observation methods provide little more than gross indications of hearing sensitivity, this information may be of considerable value.

Visual Reinforcer Audiometry (VRA) Procedures The VRA procedures incorporate more strict control of the stimuli and responses, yet require only relatively primitive localization (head turn) responses, which normally are present at 3–4 months in the infant who demonstrates apparently normal development. Thus, these procedures can be useful for the infant who is very young either chronologically or developmentally.

Although it may seem strange to discuss visual reinforcer methods as viable test procedures for visually impaired infants, in many situations the VRA procedures may be quite successful. In particular, those infants who display some interest in bright lights are candidates for this type of testing. Actual visual acuity is of lesser importance. In some cases, a plain light bulb is used as the visual reinforcer. A typical VRA reinforcer unit may consist of a mechanical toy housed in a plexiglass box. When the unit is activated, the mechanical toy and the lights within the box are turned on simultaneously so that the movement of the toy and the illumination provided by the lights are presented together. For a child who is visually impaired, it might be that just the illumination and not the movement of the toy will provide adequate reinforcement.

The VRA procedure utilizes an association between a sound and activation of the visual reinforcer so that a head turn or localization response will occur. Normally this is done by initially pairing presentation of a sound with activation of the visual reinforcement unit. Most infants will, upon hearing the sound, anticipate the appearance of the lighted and moving toy after a few of these paired presentations. Thereafter, the procedure is to present a sound and observe whether an anticipatory head turn towards the reinforcer occurs. If it does, then it can be assumed that the sound was heard. Next, the intensity of the sound is decreased on successive presentations until responses no longer occur. By examining responses for tones of different frequency and for speech, an idea of the full range of auditory sensitivity can be obtained.

The minimum stimulus intensity levels at which responses can be expected using the VRA procedure will depend on the developmental level of the infant or child. Most infants of 5–6 months of age who have no significant developmental delay will respond to speech and tones at levels of 25 dB–30 dB, which is borderline normal in the hearing loss classification scheme noted earlier. If an infant shows significant developmental delay, then such localization responses may not take place until much later than 5 to 6 months. As with all testing procedures, the mental level of the child must be considered so that response failures resulting from delayed development can be differentiated from those attributed to hearing loss. Sometimes this differentiation is most difficult to make.

The infant with severe visual impairment lacks the means to develop an association between sound and sight and, therefore, may be significantly delayed in developing localization responses. It is important in such a case not to immediately assume that a lack of localization is the result of a hearing loss. If the cognitive level of the child and/or the precise degree of visual impairment is not known, the VRA procedures are a reasonable place to begin testing. They normally provide more objective information than the behavioral observation methods noted earlier, yet are easier for the child to understand than the tangible reinforcer methods discussed below.

Tangible-Reinforcer Operant Conditioning Audiometry (TROCA) Methods The TROCA procedure provides an example of the application of strict behavior modification methods to audiometric assessment (Martin, 1978). TROCA originally was developed to assess the hearing of adult clients with severe and profound retardation, but this method also works very well both with children having less severe cognitive delay and with children who have visual handicaps.

Briefly, TROCA utilizes an operant discrimination paradigm for assessing hearing sensitivity. By means of suitable reinforcers, a button-push response is brought under auditory stimulus control. When a correct response is made, the client is reinforced by means of a tangible reinforcer, which is dispensed into a small plastic tray located on the front of the TROCA unit. Responses made not in conjunction with a stimulus presentation (random responses) are not reinforced and may, in fact, be consequated by a time-out. Once responses have been trained, the intensity and frequency of the stimulus can be changed and the pure tone audiogram can be obtained.

TROCA testing is an invaluable assessment tool in a number of clinics and it is utilized frequently for children (older than 20 to 24 months) as well as adults who are lower functioning. The procedure allows determination of pure tone thresholds for both air-conducted and bone-conducted tones, speech awareness and speech reception threshold. Testing can be with earphones if the client will tolerate them. If not, soundfield testing with the stimuli presented through loudspeakers in the test room can be used. For children with severe developmental delay, or those with motor problems where the required button-press responses may be difficult, TROCA has little value. Likewise, TROCA procedures are infrequently used with deaf-blind children who are younger than 20–24 months.

Acoustic Immittance Measurements

Acoustic immittance (impedance) measurements should not be considered hearing tests. Rather, they provide a means to assess the mechanical resistance encountered by sound waves as they impinge on the tympanic membrane. This mechanical resistance, in turn, is dependent primarily on conditions in the middle ear. As a result, acoustic immittance measurements are useful for identifying such middle ear pathologies as otitis media, otosclerosis and ossicular disarticulation. Hearing tests can identify a hearing loss and indicate that the source of the problem lies in the middle ear, but they normally cannot provide any more precise information than this. Acoustic immittance measurements can supplement hearing tests since they can indicate with greater precision the actual type of pathology within the middle ear that is responsible for the hearing loss.

Because acoustic immittance measurements assess resistance to sound flow resulting from middle ear conditions, they are affected by and provide an indicator of acoustic reflex (stapedius) muscle activity in the middle ear. Because the level at which the acoustic reflex (AR) is activated depends on the hearing status of the individual, this portion of the acoustic immittance battery can be used to "predict" hearing levels. Although this test certainly is only a gross indicator of possible hearing loss, it is quickly administered and may even eliminate the need to resort to more complicated procedures such as auditory brainstem response measurements.

Basic Measurement Procedure Figure 3 provides a schematic representation of the components of acoustic immittance measurements. A small probe tip is inserted into the ear canal, and this serves to direct a low frequency probe tone (typically about 220 Hz) into the external auditory meatus and hence to the tympanic membrane. When this tone impinges on the tympanic membrane, part of the tone is transmitted through to the middle ear and part is reflected back into the external auditory meatus. The reflected sound is detected by a microphone connected to the probe tip. The electronic circuitry within the immittance bridge compares the magnitude of the reflected sound

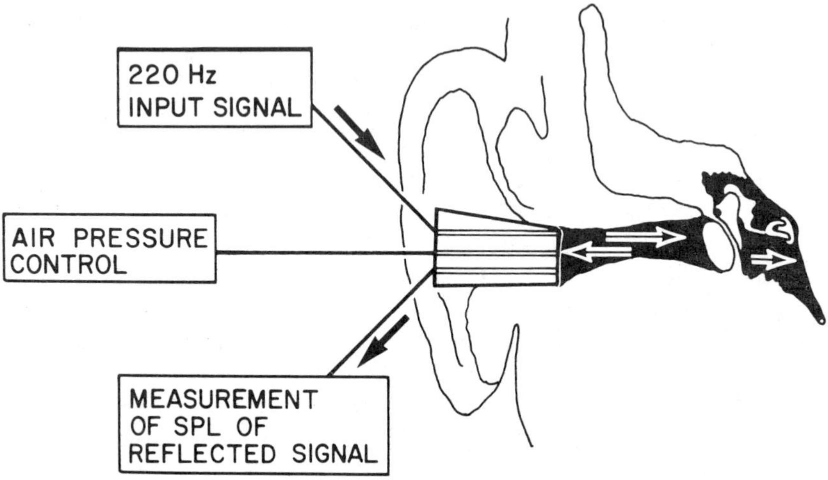

Figure 3. A schematic of acoustic immittance measurement system. (SPL = sound pressure levels.)

(measured in sound pressure level or SPL) to that which is delivered originally via the probe tip. If the magnitude of the reflected tone is either too high or too low, middle ear pathology is indicated. Too much reflected tone indicates a middle ear mechanism that is too stiff, as is found, for example, with otitis media, in which the middle ear cavity is filled with fluid. Too little reflected tone indicates a lack of proper coupling in the middle ear mechanism, such as might result from ossicular discontinuity.

If these acoustic immittance measurements are conducted while air pressure in the external ear canal is varied, the procedure is termed "tympanometry" and the graphs that are plotted are known as tympanograms. Tympanometry provides an ideal follow-up to pure tone threshold measurements, especially if a conductive hearing loss is indicated, for it can indicate more precisely the likely site of the conductive loss.

Acoustic Reflex Measurement and Prediction of Hearing Sensitivity Like any child, the deaf-blind child/youth may have middle ear infections that require detection and treatment. Tympanometry may be extremely useful in these cases. However, it is in the area of prediction of hearing sensitivity in the difficult-to-test child that acoustic immittance measurement can be of immense value to the audiologist. When the ear is stimulated with sounds moderately loud in intensity, contractions of the stapedius muscle in the middle ear occur. These contractions cause a tightening of the ossicular chain that in turn causes measured immittance at the eardrum to change. These reflex-related immittance changes can be detected by acoustic immittance measurements. By determining the minimum stimulus intensities that cause these reflex changes to occur and comparing these to norm values obtained from subjects without hearing loss, some estimate of hearing sensitivity can be made. Since this can be done with only the passive cooperation of the patient, it provides a very useful estimate of hearing in difficult-to-test clients.

One strength of acoustic reflex methods is that they are very accurate when they identify normal hearing. They almost never identify normal hearing in an individual who has a hearing loss. However, they do tend to overestimate hearing loss. On the average, they will identify a hearing loss in about one-third of clients who actually have normal hearing. Nonetheless, these methods do provide a useful screening function; if they predict normal hearing, there is no need to conduct further testing, but if a hearing loss is identified, additional testing must be completed to determine whether this hearing loss really exists and, if so, its magnitude.

Another problem associated with acoustic reflex measurements is that many mentally retarded clients unexplicably have no detectable reflexes in response to any level of eliciting stimulus. This absence may be related to minor middle ear pathology, to certain drugs (e.g., tranquilizers) used by the individuals, or to gross neurological abnormalities associated with the mental retardation. In the absence of such reflexes, of course, acoustic reflex-based hearing prediction methods cannot be used and other techniques need to be employed.

Auditory Brainstem Response Measurement

Without question, auditory brainstem response (ABR) measurement provides the audiologist with one of the most powerful assessment techniques available for assessing the hearing of the difficult-to-test client. Nevertheless, ABR procedures can provide information that can be vague and even misleading. It is wise to be aware of both the power and the limitations of this technique.

At the outset, it should be noted that measurements of brainstem electrical activity elicited by auditory stimulation are labeled by various names. *Auditory brainstem responses* (ABR) is the term favored by most audiologists; *evoked response audiometry* (ERA), and *brainstem auditory evoked responses* (BAER) tend to be terms more favored by neurologists and physiologists. The labels are different, but the procedure is the same.

General Nature Of Auditory Evoked Responses When the ear is stimulated by sounds, electrical potentials are generated in the auditory nerve that traverse the central auditory pathways and ultimately reach the cortex (Jacobson, 1985). Surface reflections of these potentials can be recorded by means of small electrodes attached to the skin of the head. In hearing assessment, the early component of this response, the auditory brainstem response, is of primary concern. This component is used for assessment purposes because it is not significantly affected by state of the subject (sleeping or awake), cognitive level, presence of medications, general neural integrity, and so on. On the other hand, it is greatly affected by the presence of hearing loss. Therefore, this component is ideal for use in assessing the hearing sensitivity of an individual who might be difficult to test by any other means.

Characteristics of ABR Responses Figure 4 illustrates normal ABR responses at several stimulus intensity levels. The x–axis is the time axis and the total duration of the graph (from left to right) is approximately 10 milliseconds. The reference point at 0 milliseconds represents the time when the auditory stimulus is delivered to the ear.

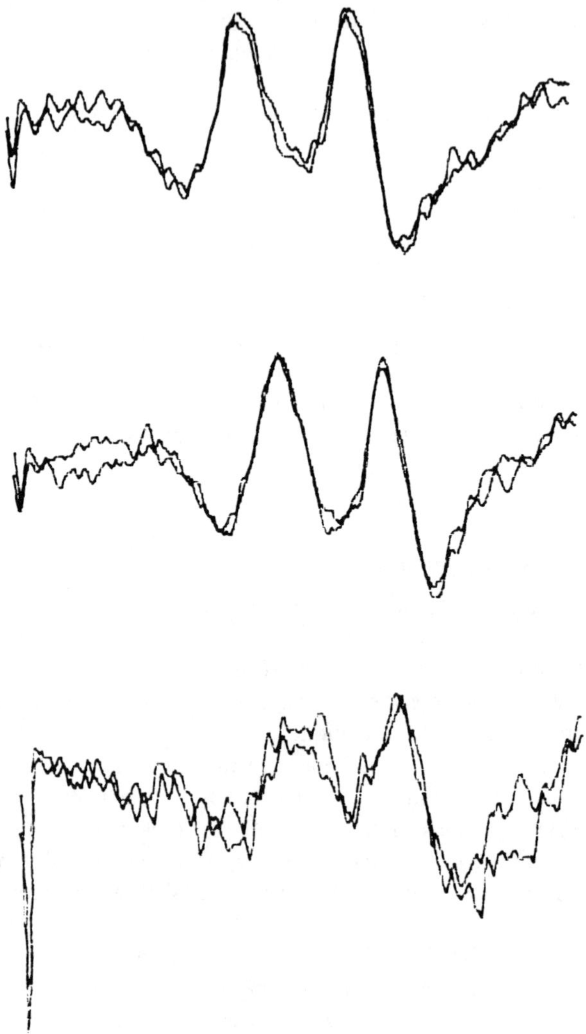

Figure 4. Auditory brainstem responses (ABR) for varying stimulus intensity levels. Stimulus intensity for top trace was 70 dB; 50 dB for middle trace; and 30 dB for bottom trace. The peak furthest to the right is Wave V.

The y–axis represents the intensity of the response in microvolts—the peaks of a good healthy response typically are on the order of 0.2–0.4 microvolts. It can be seen that the responses (at least for the louder stimuli) are characterized by a series of peaks from left to right. These are the hallmarks of an ABR response; response interpretation is a matter of identifying these components.

The peaks are labeled in Roman numerals in the manner proposed by Jewett (Jewett, Romano, & Williston, 1970), who was one of the original discoverers of the

ABR response; these peaks are sometimes referred to as Jewett Wave I, Jewett Wave II, and so on. The various waves represent sequential activation of the auditory system as the auditory-evoked nerve potential proceeds from the auditory nerve to the upper region of the brainstem. In the typical response, Waves I, II, and V normally are quite easy to identify with Waves II and IV often being nearly impossible to determine. Of these, Wave V tends to be easiest to locate, particularly for the softest levels of stimulation. For this reason, Wave V is the component of the response that is most useful for assessment purposes.

Two aspects of the response are used for assessment purposes: (a) whether the response can be identified at all, and (b) if so, the "latency" of the Wave V component. *Latency* refers to the time interval from delivery of the stimulus to the ear (zero time on the response illustrated above) to the peak of the Wave V component. These time intervals, which are expressed in milliseconds, are compared to normative values to examine for a possible hearing loss.

It is clear from Figure 4 that the entire response tends to move to the right as the stimulus intensity is decreased. This, in turn, causes the latency of Wave V to increase with decreasing stimulus intensity. The relationship between stimulus intensity and latency of Wave V forms the basis for the latency-intensity functions illustrated in Figure 5. The latency-intensity function forms the basis for providing a quantitative analysis of ABR responses. Figure 5 contains three separate functions that are typical of those found in normal hearing, conductive hearing loss, and sensorineural hearing loss. Note that with conductive hearing loss, the shape of the latency-intensity function is similar to that of the normal but is displaced from it. With sensorineural hearing loss, the slope of the latency-intensity function is quite different from normal.

In summary then, analysis of ABR responses is a two-stage process. One examines first the presence of responses and, if they cannot be demonstrated, it is assumed that a hearing loss exists. In general, research has indicated that responses tend to be absent when hearing loss exceeds about 70 dB. Therefore, the best statement that can be made on the basis of no responses is that a hearing loss seems to exist that appears to be at least 70 dB in magnitude. If responses can be identified, then one stimulates at several different intensity levels in order to generate a latency-intensity function as illustrated above. One uses these data to estimate magnitude of hearing loss and guess its type (it frequently is the case that "real" data are not so easily classified as are those illustrated in Figure 5).

Measurement Technique The ABR responses are detected by means of three small electrodes pasted onto the skin. One of these normally is attached to each earlobe (or to the mastoid prominence behind the ear) and the other to the forehead. Electrical activity is detected by these electrodes and fed to a sophisticated electronic instrument that filters and averages the responses, displays them on a screen so that latency times can be determined, and outputs them to a plotter so that permanent records of the responses can be obtained.

One slightly technical aspect of the ABR analysis procedure should be discussed

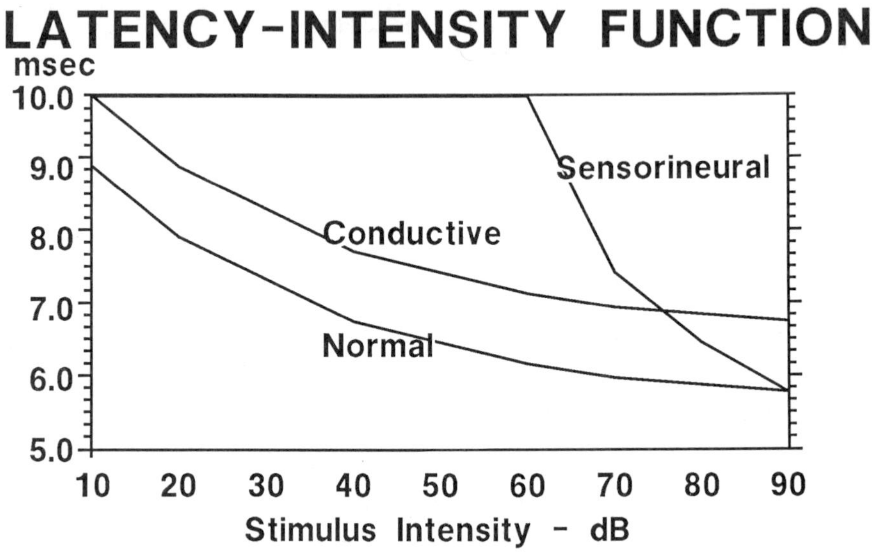

Figure 5. Typical wave V latency-intensity functions.

at this point since it is of importance for interpreting responses. Referring back to Figure 4, the responses illustrated can be thought of as those that result from a single stimulus presentation. In reality, the magnitude of evoked responses is so small and the level of physiological background electrical activity so high that it is nearly impossible to observe a response for a single stimulus presentation. In order to make responses observable, a relatively large number of stimulus presentations (1000 or so) are delivered to the ear and the responses are averaged by the ABR equipment over the total number of stimuli. Therefore, the responses portrayed in Figure 4 are actually averaged responses resulting from a relatively large number of stimulus presentations. If an individual response could be detected, it would look like these responses.

An important characteristic of responses that need to be averaged is that they be "time-locked" with the stimulus. That is, they need always to appear at exactly the same interval of time following the presentation of the stimulus. If they do not, then the ABR equipment will assume that they are random noise patterns and will attempt to eliminate them from the response record. This averaging function of the ABR equipment allows responses to be enhanced and irrelevant background activity to be eliminated. In most cases, ABR responses are time-locked with the eliciting stimulus and therefore this averaging type of analysis works quite well.

Although time-locking occurs in the normal auditory system, it may not occur completely in certain neurological pathologies such as multiple sclerosis. In addition, there is some current controversy over the degree to which mental retardation might affect time-locking to auditory stimuli. Where time-locking does not occur, responses will not be identified in the response trace. In this situation, therefore, the lack of responses is not due to hearing loss but to more subtle dysfunction in the auditory system. In fact, hearing sensitivity may be perfectly normal. It is apparent, therefore, that ABR responses might be absent in situations where hearing sensitivity is not depressed, and that in these situations, the use of a hearing aid certainly would not be appropriate. This particular interpretive pitfall confronts an audiologist each and every time a client is tested and no identifiable responses are demonstrated. Does this mean severe to profound hearing loss or does it indicate only subtle timing abnormalities in the auditory pathway? One hopes to avoid diagnostic errors by examining both ABR and behavioral responses (to whatever extent they exist) in order to find some sort of agreement between the two.

A final comment on ABR measurement should be made. In all cases, permanent records of *all* responses should be made on a plotter (or by photographing response traces on the viewing screen) so that these can be available for later analysis and possibly for later comparison with the results obtained from separate testing sessions.

Use of ABR in Audiometric Assessment The use of some behavioral-based procedures (such as TROCA, VRA, or even gross responses to noisemakers) should always be given first consideration in the assessment of any client, no matter how severe the handicaps or how depressed the cognitive functioning. Behavioral methods, based on some overt and voluntary response to sound, are the only way that the entire auditory system from ear to brain can be assessed.

In addition, behavioral techniques offer the only means to obtain an audiogram in which sensitivity can be specified for each test frequency. The normal ABR stimulus, the click, contains a mixture of many frequencies and so it is impossible to know for sure what frequencies are contributing to any responses that are observed. This is perhaps one of the most important limitations of ABR measurements. To be sure, different clinics use various combinations of tone bursts and filtered noise in an attempt to provide more frequency-specific responses. However, none of these methods has come close to providing the frequency specificity that is obtained from the audiogram.

Another serious limitation of ABR measurements is that the relationship between ABR responses and "real" threshold is quite variable from individual to individual. If one looks at group data, then the averaged relationship between ABR threshold and behavioral threshold may be quite good, with the two varying by only a few decibels. However, if one examines the variation between ABR and behavioral thresholds for individuals within the group, it will be seen that these individual differences frequently can exceed 15 dB–20 dB. This means that when one uses ABR thresholds to estimate behavioral thresholds, threshold estimation errors of 15 dB–20 dB will occur. Usually the magnitude of hearing loss is overestimated, but not always. This lack of accuracy makes hearing aid fitting based solely on ABR results somewhat risky. Sometimes it has to be done, however.

With these limitations in mind, perhaps a few positive statements in support of ABR measurements should be made. As a start, it should be noted that ABR procedures may provide the only quantitative information that can be obtained regarding hearing level in clients who are low-functioning. The suspicion of hearing loss certainly may exist from informal observations of the individual's response (or lack of them) and from delayed or nonexistent speech. On the other hand, it may be difficult to separate hearing loss from depressed cognitive ability as the major underlying etiology. Auditory brainstem measurement can provide a great deal of help in sorting out these factors. ABR is at its sterling best when the responses are normal. In this case, there can be little doubt that hearing sensitivity is normal. False negatives are not a problem with ABR.

Abnormal ABR findings present a problem, however, particularly if no responses are observed at all. In this case, it is entirely reasonable to assume, as noted earlier, that hearing loss must exceed at least 70 dB within that range of frequencies that is assessed by ABR procedures. However, alternate explanations may exist. In particular, one must eliminate the possibility of technical errors. Are the headphones connected and working properly? Are the electrodes connected and is interelectrode impedance sufficiently low? Are all connections secure between the client and the ABR instrumentation? Is the client sufficiently quiet so that movement artifact is not likely? Are the proper settings being used on the ABR instrumentation? Any of these could result in an unidentifiable response pattern. The audiologist must eliminate the possibility of technical error before judgments regarding hearing loss can be made.

Other explanations for abnormal or absent responses exist that are more difficult to evaluate. For example, it was noted earlier that time-locking between stimulus and response must occur if ABR signal processing is to work. A lack of time-locking does not mean that the auditory system is not conducting nerve impulses, but only that the averaging process utilized by ABR instrumentation will not work. Research has not clarified exactly when this problem might exist or how frequently it occurs, but its potential presence seems greater in the abnormal neural system. Hence, its possible presence must always be considered in the client with multiple handicaps. It seems likely that attempting to place hearing aids on such a person not only would not help but would probably produce a noise-induced hearing loss due to the excessive signal levels impressed on the normal peripheral hearing mechanism by the hearing aid.

A limitation of ABR information that many people do not understand is that it does not provide direct measures of stimulus processing at the cortical level. It does seem reasonable to assume that any procedure that attaches electrodes to the cortex should provide information about what is happening in the brain. In the case of the auditory brainstem, that is not the case. If an individual does not respond behaviorally to sounds or speech and ABR measurements demonstrate normal responses, then it is reasonable to assume that the lack of response is due to cortical processing factors. However, this conclusion is drawn only by inference; auditory brainstem responses do not provide direct information about cortical processing. Certain laboratories and clinics do look at such things as extended inter-wave latency intervals as a means of making statements about central auditory processing. However, such information is tentative at best and probably misleading at worst.

In summary, ABR remains one of the most powerful assessment techniques for the difficult-to-test client. However, like any test, it should be used as a component in a battery of tests to determine presence and magnitude of hearing loss.

PROSTHETIC DEVICES

Prosthetic devices used by persons with severe to profound hearing impairment fall generally into one of two classes: those that utilize residual hearing and those that provide input via some alternate sensory modality. Hearing aids and cochlear implants are examples of the former and devices that utilize vibrotactile stimulation typify the latter.

Hearing Aids

Hearing aids are certainly the most common prosthetic device used by persons who are hearing impaired. Depending generally on the degree of hearing loss, hearing aids can provide benefits that range from the ability to understand speech with reasonable clarity to a general awareness of loud sounds in the environment.

Types of Hearing Aids Hearing aids are of three different styles: in-the-ear, ear-level (or behind-the-ear), and body style (Hodgson, 1986). These types vary in size, placement, maximum gain, and frequency response capabilities. An additional difference between these three types of hearing aids is the location of the loudspeaker or receiver. Both in-the-ear hearing aids and ear-level aids utilize a receiver that is built into the case of the hearing aid. The receiver of the body style hearing aid is separate from the hearing aid case and is connected to it by means of a thin cord. The receiver itself is clipped onto the earmold.

In-the-Ear Hearing Aids A significant number of hearing aids in current use are of the in-the-ear variety. That is, the hearing aid and earmold are one integral unit, and both fit within the ear of the wearer. Because these hearing aids are not often used with children and normally are useful only with lesser degrees of hearing loss, they will not be considered further in this discussion.

Ear-Level Hearing Aids Although in-the-ear aids are becoming increasingly popular, the ear-level aid has been the most common style of hearing aid. The ear-level aid fits over the ear of the wearer and is coupled to the ear by means of a short length of plastic tubing that, in turn, is connected to an earmold. The earmold serves to channel amplified sound into the auditory canal and also helps to anchor the hearing aid in place.

Many individuals consider the ear-level hearing aid inferior to the body-style aid in terms of maximum gain, and therefore less appropriate for the individual with severe hearing impairment. However, there are quite a number of ear-level hearing aids that provide nearly as much gain as current body-style aids. The problem is not how much gain the aid is capable of providing, but rather how much of the potential gain is usable because of acoustic feedback considerations. Feedback is indicated by a high-pitched squealing sound. It is acoustic feedback, and not the basic power of the hearing aid, that limits its amplification potential in many cases and particularly with children. Ear-level hearing aids are physically located nearer to the ear than are body-style aids, and therefore are most susceptible to feedback problems.

In addition to having less usable amplification, ear-level hearing aids do have a more restricted frequency range than body-style hearing aids. In particular, body-style aids have better low-frequency responses. This is due primarily to the physical properties of the microphone and receiver. The more limited low-frequency response of an ear-level hearing aid may be extremely critical for an individual who demonstrates residual hearing only at quite low frequencies, and may render this type of aid unsuitable for such a hearing loss.

However, in situations where they can provide sufficient gain and frequency response, ear-level aids have many advantages over body-style hearing aids. First, they are easier to fit in pairs in a binaural configuration. Two ears allow binaural hearing and this is of immense value in many listening situations. It is quite difficult to hear speech in noise and nearly impossible to localize with only one ear. Ear-level hearing aids, when fit in pairs, allow normal binaural function of the ears to be more nearly restored. It is much more difficult to achieve true binaural amplification with body-style hearing aids, since two of them have to be used. The use of two relatively large body-style hearing aids on a small child presents obvious problems.

A second advantage of ear-level hearing aids is that the location of sound pick-up is in the vicinity of the ear. With a body-style hearing aid, the microphone is in the hearing aid case that is worn on the chest or perhaps, with a very young child who is not yet walking, on the back, thus making localization of sound more difficult.

Finally, an ear-level hearing aid tends to be smaller, and therefore seems to be more comfortable for many small children. The weight of the receiver of a body-style aid, which is attached to the mold, tends to pivot the earmold down and out of the ear (particularly in a small ear) and this may cause some discomfort or at least aggravation to the child (and the caregivers). Although earmold retention clips and wires are available, they seldom solve this problem.

Body-Style Hearing Aids If a hearing loss is very severe or if there is residual hearing only at quite low frequencies, then there may be no choice but to use a body-style hearing aid. However, this is a last resort, and most audiologists fit a body aid with some reluctance and trepidation.

The obvious advantages of a body-style hearing aid are high gain, wide frequency response, and low distortion. Some of the disadvantages have already been discussed. One other should be noted. Clothing noise resulting from the hearing aid rubbing on the child's clothing is a persistent problem with a body-style hearing aid, because this noise interferes with and tends to mask environmental and speech sounds.

Another source of problems with the body-style aid is the cord that connects the receiver to the aid. These cords are thin, in order to be flexible, and therefore are subject to frequent breakage either from normal flexing or due to chewing by the child. Finally, the cords frequently are a source of aggravation for the mother in her normal care of the child, for they get in the way of dressing and undressing, and serve as convenient "handles" for the child to either knowingly or accidentally pull out the attached earmolds. A final problem associated with the use of a body-style hearing aid by a young child is that food and liquid tend to dribble from the child's mouth directly into the microphone opening on the top of the hearing aid case. This situation results in many service problems.

Additional Hearing Aid Considerations Age is no real factor in deciding either whether a hearing aid should be fitted or what type should be used. It is recommended that a child be fitted with a hearing aid as soon as it is certain that a hearing loss exists and that there is some indication of its magnitude. In reality, body-style hearing aids are traditionally recommended for the child younger than 1 year of age simply because if a hearing loss has been detected at such an early age, it likely is more severe in degree. However, whenever possible it is preferable to fit with ear-level hearing aids, and this is done with increasing frequency even with children under the age of one year.

There are many factors to consider when attempting to decide between an ear-level and body-style hearing aid. If the client in question is an infant or a multiply handicapped child, there may be minimal information on which to base a specific hearing aid recommendation. As a rule of thumb, if there are responses apparent from ABR measurements, then it is often preferable to use an ear-level aid. If, however, there are no responses observed for any level of stimulation, then it may be preferable to start with a body-style instrument.

In general, there are very few individuals who cannot benefit in some way from the use of a high-gain hearing aid. That benefit may be considerably less than the ability to hear and understand speech, and in some cases it may be a matter of the individual being aware of the presence of environmental sounds and noises. Certainly the ability to hear sounds such as car horns, emergency sirens and various alarm or warning signals in the home can be of help in providing more information about the environment. The ultimate goal is to provide the individual the means to live a safer, more independent and fulfilling life, and appropriate amplification can help achieve this in many cases.

In order for a hearing aid to be of any value, it must be worn and it must be working. The simple presence of a hearing aid does not guarantee that it is operating. Either the parent or the teacher should ascertain by means of a listening check (at the beginning of the day at least) that the hearing aid is working. Teachers in particular frequently feel very uncomfortable with the technical complexity of hearing aids, and therefore may not check a child's hearing aid for days at a time. Dead batteries or wax in the earmold are easily remedied, yet make the difference between a functional hearing aid or an expensive but non-functional piece of ear ornamentation.

Cochlear Implants

Cochlear implant research provides hope that, for the first time, a useful prosthetic device is available to help the individual who is profoundly hearing impaired. Although research findings have been somewhat sensationalized by the popular press, it remains a fact that cochlear implants remain the only potential source of help for thousands of children and adults who are profoundly hearing impaired. Although great strides have been made in cochlear implant work in the past several years, at the present time these implants hardly deserve the billing that the term "artificial ear" connotes.

Components of the Cochlear Implant A cochlear implant is quite similar in many respects to a body-style hearing aid, except that some of its components are surgically implanted in the wearer. A microphone is worn in the vicinity of the ear to detect sounds and feed them to a processor unit that, in appearance, resembles a body-style hearing aid case. The processor unit converts the sound energy to electrical impulses that are, in turn, directed into the inner ear via a single electrode or a multiple electrode array. These electrical impulses stimulate the auditory nerve directly and provide a certain, albeit limited, auditory awareness. The auditory sensations resemble a series of buzzes and beeps rather than actual sound patterns. It is this series of buzzes and beeps that serve as a window to the world of sound.

Cochlear Implants with Children Implants developed by the 3M/House group and by the Nucleus Corporation have been granted FDA approval for use with children; in both cases, for clinical trial as investigational devices (Debout, 1986). Because of the limited data available from young children who have received a cochlear implant device, there is not complete unanimity of opinion regarding the advisibility of wholesale use of implants with this population (Simmons, 1985). The position can be taken that, given the limited available options for the prelingually deafened infant or child, there is not much to be lost and much to be gained from an implant. If this were an external aid, such as a hearing aid vibrotactile device, then this certainly would be a valid argument. However, the irreversible nature of the implant, along with associated uncertainties regarding the long-term effects of stimulation, tempers this argument somewhat. In addition, the fitting of an implant includes setting stimulation intensities based on behavioral responses of the client, not unlike fitting a hearing aid. Because of the different nature of auditory perceptual experiences with an implant, and due to the fact that direct electrical stimulation is involved, problems associated with adjusting these parameters have not been resolved for the young prelingual child.

If there remain questions regarding use of cochlear implants with young children whose "only" handicap is the presence of a profound hearing loss, with children having a severe visual handicap the problem is exacerbated. Since the implant is considered to be primarily a means to supplement vision in establishing a relationship with the environment and perhaps in facilitating communication skills, its potential benefit to those with severe visual impairment must be considered as questionable at best. Certainly the potential benefits would be expected to vary with the degree of visual impairment. House Ear Institute personnel report that ordinarily a person with a severe visual handicap would not be considered a suitable candidate for implant surgery (M. Thielemeir, personal communication, November, 1985).

General Benefits from Cochlear Implants Many of the subjects with postlingual-deafness describe sounds as having a "mechanical" or "static-like" quality. Speech frequently can be heard but not understood. Patients typically can distinguish between male and female voices. They also feel that they are helped to better control the volume and pitch of their own voices and this has been reported as one of the more important functional aspects of the implant. In addition, transplant users can hear such warning signals as sirens and fire alarms, and can hear doorbells, telephones and someone calling to get their attention. These subjects also report that the implants have helped their ability to speechread.

Problems and Risks Associated with Cochlear Implants To be sure, the implant operation and device are not without potential complications. Although relatively rare, the fact remains that complications can and do occur, and this possibility must be weighed when determining the benefit-risk ratio. As with any major surgical procedure, there are risks associated with the general anesthesia; these would not differ from the risks associated with any other surgical procedure of similar magnitude. As with any surgical procedure involving the mastoid, there are risks of facial nerve injury or paralysis, infection, or meningitis.

In conclusion, it appears that the cochlear implant is not yet the panacea that the popular press suggests. In the long term, it may represent the approach that has the most potential for restoring a usable sense of hearing for the individual who is profoundly hearing impaired, and perhaps may yet reach a level of functionality at which it can stand on its own, rather than just serving as an adjunct to visual input. If and when this time is reached, then the cochlear implant will offer powerful benefits for the individual who is deaf-blind. For the present, however, the client who is visually-impaired will receive very little benefit from such a device.

Vibrotactile Communication Aids

The purpose of vibrotactile stimulation is to help compensate for the loss of hearing by providing an alternate sensory input via vibrations on the skin. Vibrotactile units typically are used by individuals who receive very little or no benefit from the use of a hearing aid. Such units may be used by individuals who are profoundly hearing impaired, either to supplement hearing aids—or cochlear implants—or as a substitute for them.

Components Like hearing aids, vibrotactile devices incorporate a microphone to pick up sounds and an amplifier to amplify and filter them. In contrast with a hearing aid that delivers the amplified signal to a receiver and hence to the ear, the vibrotactile unit delivers the signal to a small vibrator that is attached to the arm or finger of the user. These vibratory signals provide temporal, pitch, and intensity information from the original sounds, and therefore provide some information about the nature of those sounds.

Most commercial vibrotactile systems utilize a single channel of stimulation; however, some newer ones use two channels and two vibrators. Experimental units utilizing multiple vibrator arrays are employed in devices called vocoders. Multiple vibrator arrays have the ability to retain and transmit more complex aspects of the original sounds. This will be discussed in a later section.

Single-Channel Vibrotactile Devices This device utilizes a single-channel amplifier that is connected to a single vibrator. The amplifier incorporates controls for adjusting the intensity of the signal and normally allows some frequency selectivity by means of bass and treble emphasis controls.

The vibrator itself is about the size of a pocket watch and may be held either in the palm of the hand or on the finger tips, or may be attached to either the front or back of the wrist by means of a strap. This latter position is more convenient because it allows the wearer more freedom of movement. As might be expected, the finger tip location is more sensitive to small changes in vibratory pattern than are either of the wrist locations (Cholewiak & Craig, 1984). Sensitivity also is related to vibrator size, with wearer sensitivity increased by the use of larger vibrators, and the greater sensitivity associated with finger tip placement may be more than offset by the larger physical vibrator size that can be utilized with a wrist attachment.

Because of the mechanical limitations of the vibrator, the full range of sound frequencies cannot be transmitted to the wearer. Most of the energy of the vibrator signal lies between about 200 and 2000 Hz. Although limited, this range certainly captures the most important speech frequencies and most environmental sounds. Because the entire sound spectrum is fed to a single vibrator that contacts a relatively small area of skin, only a limited amount of information about the sound can be discriminated by the wearer. Aspects of the sound that can be discriminated include sound frequency (at least to the extent that the vibrator can transmit it), intensity, and duration. These can be useful for providing information about the presence of an acoustic stimulus, its rhythm, stress, and duration. Single channel units, without supplemental auditory or visual stimulation, can provide some information about what specific environmental sounds are present, and can allow some discriminations to occur between selected speech sounds. In general, these finer discriminations are quite difficult to make from single-channel vibrotactile units.

Perhaps one of the best uses of single-channel vibrotactile cues is in the area of voice training for the person who is hearing impaired. Since vibrotactile units establish the awareness of sounds, they can be used to help the wearer learn to vocalize. Moreover, the device provides a means to allow a wearer to monitor vocal pitch, duration, loudness, inflection, and rhythm pattern, and can prove useful in training vocal skills. This may be helpful in attempting to eliminate some of the "deaf" vocal qualities typically found in those with severe hearing impairment.

Undoubtedly the best known commercial vibrotactile device is made by the Siemens Corporation and marketed under the name "Fonator." The Fonator Speech Trainer includes vibratory stimulation only; the Fonator Auditory Speech Trainer provides both vibratory and amplified auditory stimulation. Both of these are tabletop units.

The Mini-Fonator recently introduced by Siemens is a completely wearable vibrotactile device. The amplifier, which is battery powered, is about the size of two body-style hearing aids, and normally would be worn on a belt or placed in a pocket. Unlike a body-style hearing aid, the pick-up microphone is not built into the unit, but rather is separate, and is hand-held or attached to a lapel.

It is interesting that the Mini-Fonator is recommended by House Institute personnel to assist post-implant patients in the development of auditory perception skills. Because such individuals had already demonstrated no significant benefits from the use of a hearing aid, the vibrotactile stimulation is intended for use in place of amplification. Research indicates that single-channel implants and vibrotactile aids may both provide similar types of information. Units similar to the Fonator are marketed under the names of Tactaid, Minivib and Tactone. Except for minor differences, all operate in essentially the same manner.

Two-Channel Vibrotactile Devices The need to provide more information via tactile channels has led to the development of a two-channel system, built in Israel and marketed under the name of Kanievski Sound. The developer of this unit is himself deaf. The Kanievski Sound system makes use of two vibrators, both of which are worn together on a single wristband. The purpose of the two vibrators is to provide speech voicing information; voiced speech sounds activate one vibrator and voiceless speech sounds activate the other. Therefore, in addition to pitch, intensity and temporal cues, this system provides voicing information. Although this system has been developed with speech discrimination uses in mind, it is claimed to be useful for providing an awareness of environmental sounds. A domestic version of an earlier Kanievski Sound system has recently been developed by Telex Corporation.

Multiple-Channel Vibrotactile Devices Multiple-channel systems, or vocoders, have been developed in an attempt to incorporate more acoustic information into the vibratory signal (Green, Craig, Wilson, Pisoni, & Rhodes, 1983). As with a single-channel system, the sound is picked up with a microphone and fed to an amplifier. The amplifier unit incorporates a number of filters (the use of up to 24 is not uncommon) that divide the sound into separate channels based on the frequency spectrum. The output from each channel is fed to a separate vibrator pin. The vibrator pins from all channels are arranged in a tactile array or matrix.

Several means of delivering the vibrations to the user have been developed. Perhaps the most common is by means of a tactile array that may be contacted by one or two fingers. The sounds excite certain patterns of vibrations in the tactile array and these are picked up by the finger tips. An alternative type of tactile array arranges the vibrators in a linear fashion along the forearm, an arrangement that has the advantage of permitting a greater area of skin to be stimulated. Because of the larger number of stimulators involved, the multi-channel device can convey much more acoustic information. In fact, as many as 150 words have been discriminated by means of the linear forearm display noted above. Due to the complexity of signal processing involved, these multi-channel units are quite sophisticated, and most require the use of a computer to filter the sounds and drive the vibrator elements. As a result, those units that use more than about six to eight channels of stimulation are not portable.

Multi-channel systems are completely experimental at this time and no commercial units are yet available. Neither is much research data available regarding their benefits for persons who are deaf-blind. Development work has been carried out primarily on subjects who are hearing-seeing.

Since vibrotactile units provide the user with only a sample or abstract of speech and environmental sounds, the sensory information is limited and their potential benefits must be evaluated within this context. They can provide for the individual who is profoundly hearing impaired the means to be in better touch with the environment; the means to be aware, at least, of the presence of sounds. This could be valuable in learning to detect and discriminate important environmental sounds and warning signals such as approaching traffic. In general, these units can help provide an individual with a sense of contact with the environment.

At least one company (Siemens) notes that their vibrotactile unit was originally developed for use, in part, by persons who are deaf-blind. Currently these devices have no general use with this population. In fact, like hearing aids and cochlear implants, they seem to have gained their greatest application as a means of supplementing visual information, both in communication situations and situations in which a better sense of the environment is desirable. They have gained very little use as "stand-alone" devices. This is unfortunate, for they would appear to have significant potential for use by individuals who are deaf-blind. Perhaps as more attention is paid to this population, use of these vibrotactile devices will increase.

SUMMARY

A number of quite different assessment procedures have been discussed in this chapter. The availability of numerous tests increases the probability that at least one of the methods will be successful in assessing every client. Unfortunately, some clients prove so difficult to test that one ends with little more information than was available initially. However, the incidence of these situations decreases in direct proportion to the number of different assessment approaches available. Combined visual and hearing handicaps significantly reduce the repertoire of available behavioral responses for assessment purposes. In spite of its limitations, the fact of the matter is that ABR represents the single most powerful assessment tool currently available to the audiologist when working with these clients. ABR cannot provide the same degree of accuracy as can behavioral methods. It cannot identify precise degree of hearing loss as loss becomes greater than moderately severe in degree. Additionally, the absence of responses does not necessarily guarantee that peripheral hearing loss is present. Although ABR may not be the ultimate assessment tool for these children, it remains the single most useful test for many audiologists. Whatever else may be done, ABR testing is nearly always conducted for children with multiple sensory impairments.

The teacher can assume an important role in evaluating the hearing of difficult-to-test children. For example, the teacher probably has identified tangible objects or activities, such as vibrations or air movement, that are reinforcing for the child and that may already be in use in a classroom. If the audiologist is provided with this information, perhaps the use of these reinforcers can be incorporated into the audiological evaluation. Sometimes it is possible for the teacher to assist the audiologist by implementing a classroom-based training program that will prepare the child for audiological assessment. Extended training of a localization response by means of suitable noisemakers could assist in the use of VRA procedures. Once an effective reinforcer is identified, a large repertoire of responses can be developed, given enough time. The teacher and audiologist can work together to help prepare the "difficult-to-test" child for testing.

Once testing has been completed and a hearing loss has been identified, the next step is to determine the type of prosthetic device that should be utilized. Sometimes these children display such monumental delays that there is an inclination to ask whether it really makes any difference anyhow. As a professional whose primary concern is to identify hearing loss and assist in alleviating its effects, the audiologist has a responsibility to assist in the selection of whatever prosthetic device appears to have the greatest potential for increasing environmental input to the child. This selection task should be viewed as a process, with trial use of a device monitored and changes implemented as necessary in order to finally determine the best device.

A primary assumption is that very few hearing losses are so severe that some benefit will not be obtained from the use of a hearing aid. For this reason, it is usual to recommend the use of a hearing aid as a first step. Selection of the best type of aid will be based on the diagnostic information that is available, and this admittedly is very sketchy at times. There is no "minimum" age (cognitively or chronologically) that needs to be achieved in order for a hearing aid fitting to be made. The main criterion is to have established that a hearing loss does exist (or probably exists) and that a lack of responses to sounds is not due to general developmental delay.

Sometimes a trial fitting of a hearing aid will be helpful in determining how the child adapts to the feel of the hearing aid and how amplification changes general patterns of auditory awareness. If the hearing loss is severe, it may take months and even years to determine whether a hearing aid is really of any benefit, and for this reason a normal trial fitting period typically is of little value. If a hearing loss is indicated, then there must be commitment to the use of a hearing aid.

If a hearing loss is likely to be present, and cognitive level is significantly depressed, a hearing aid (or similar prosthetic device) might or might not provide beneficial sensory input. If a hearing aid is not used, however, then a decision has been made to withhold potentially useful input. A hearing aid may or may not help, but at least it provides for the possibility of benefits, even if these are not immediately obvious. All hearing aids provide at least a potential for benefit.

There are some young children who are so resistant to the use of a hearing aid that trying to keep the aid on actually interferes with important training activities in other areas. This occurs most commonly in the child with a high degree of tactile defensiveness, in which anything on or around the face is not tolerated. Children who display self-abusive behavior involving the ear (a common site, for some reason) will also not be good candidates for a hearing aid. In these cases, programming to reduce either the tactile defensiveness or self-abusive behavior must precede possible use of hearing aid amplification. Sometimes, when faced with such cases, it must with great reluctance be conceded that the use of a hearing aid just cannot occur. At this juncture, there should be a consideration of the use of other devices, such as vibrotactile units, to maximize sensory input.

Vibrotactile units have been used for children who are blind and deaf, but not extensively with individuals having both handicaps. Because these devices may provide some benefits as part of long-term training programs, it is unfortunate that they have not been used to a greater extent with this population. Currently, there seems to be an increased interest in vibrotactile units; perhaps this will lead to greater use of these units with individuals who are deaf-blind.

REFERENCES

Cholewiak, R., & Craig, J. (1984). Vibrotactile pattern recognition and discrimination at several body sites. *Perception and Psychophysics, 35*, 503–514.

Debout, J.M. (1986). Update: Cochlear implants. Beyond the first generation. *The Hearing Journal, 39*, 7–14.

Green, B., Craig, J., Wilson, A., Pisoni, D., & Rhodes, R. (1983). Vibrotactile identification of vowels. *Journal of the Acoustical Society of America, 73*, 1766–1778.

Hodgson, W. (1986). *Hearing aid assessment and use in audiologic habilitation*. Baltimore: Williams and Wilkins, (3rd Ed.).

Jacobson, J. (1985). *The auditory brainstem response*. San Diego: College-Hill Press.

Jewett, D., Romano, M., & Williston, J. (1970). Human auditory evoked potentials: Possible brainstem components detected on the scalp. *Science, 167*, 1517–1518.

Martin, F. (1978). *Pediatric audiology*. Englewood Cliffs, NJ: Prentice-Hall.

Martin, F. (1981). *Medical audiology*. Englewood Cliffs, NJ: Prentice-Hall.

Northern J., & Downs, M. (1984). *Hearing in children* (3rd ed.). Baltimore: Williams and Wilkins.

Simmons, F. (1985). Cochlear implants in young children: Some dilemmas. *Ear and Hearing, 6*, 61–63.

CHAPTER 6

Teaching Orientation and Mobility Skills within and across Natural Opportunities for Travel

A Model Designed for Learners with Multiple Severe Disabilities

Kathleen Gee, Rona Harrell, and Richard Rosenberg

RECENT LITERATURE DOCUMENTING the efficacy of teaching students with severe multiple handicaps in integrated, community settings (Brown et al., 1983; Sailor et al., 1986) has shifted the emphasis from the instruction of functional skills in classroom simulated environments to an emphasis on the instruction of functional skills within the natural environments in which their performance is necessary (Brown et al., 1979). Educators have placed additional emphasis on the student's natural motivation to perform an activity (Goetz, Schuler, & Sailor, 1983) and the importance of participation in activities that are age appropriate and future oriented (Baumgart et al., 1982; see Nietupski & Hamre-Nietupski, Chapter 9, this volume). Current curriculum models stress the development of instructional goals and programs that increase the student's ability to participate to the fullest extent possible in domestic, recreational, community, and work activities that are critical for a normalized life-style.

While there has been a significant number of studies documenting the success of instruction within multiple environments (see Snell & Browder, 1986), educators have recently noted the need for more research into instructional techniques that teach students to take advantage of the cues and stimulus arrays available in the natural environment (Ford & Mirenda, 1984; Sailor et al., 1986). Educators have also begun to direct their efforts toward the development of techniques that facilitate the instruction of basic skills (i.e., motor, auditory, vision and communication skills) within the context of ongoing sequences of behavior (see Helmstetter & Guess, Chapter 10, this volume).

The work reported in this chapter was supported in part by U.S. Office of Education Grant #G008300032; however, no official endorsement should be inferred.

Participation in multiple environments makes safe, efficient mobility an important goal for many students. Despite the instructional technology now available to educators (Sailor & Guess, 1983; Snell, 1983), the literature shows very few systematic applications of experimentally validated strategies to teach orientation and mobility to students having vision disabilities in addition to other severe handicaps.

Advances in orientation and mobility techniques (Eisenberg, 1979; Hill & Ponder, 1976), as well as an understanding of some of the underlying processes of independent travel (Welsh & Blasch, 1980) have been developed primarily by professionals focusing on persons whose only disability is visual impairment. The field of orientation and mobility has rapidly expanded since the 1940s. Following World War II the long cane and the touch technique method of travel were developed. It was not until 1953, at the first conference on mobility (Welsh & Blasch, 1980) that an expansion of orientation and mobility services to children and adults other than war veterans who were blind was considered. Professional licensing for instructors began in 1959, and the 1960s brought the introduction of specific training strategies and sequences. Services were still primarily limited to persons whose only disability was blindness. For these individuals, orientation and mobility instruction has been community based and functional in nature. Instruction of travel skills is provided in the person's home, school, community, or work environment. Instruction is also provided on conceptual and discrimination skills, and on other aspects of orientation considered necessary for successful and purposeful travel.

Since the 1960s there has been an expanding application of orientation and mobility sequences and techniques with a wider, more varied population, including individuals with low vision, elderly persons with acquired visual impairments, infants, preschoolers, and individuals with multiple handicaps. Direct applications of orientation and mobility assessments and curricula to persons with severe multiple handicaps have been known to exclude these individuals from the opportunity to increase their mobility. Being developmental and sequential in nature, instruction typically stresses the acquisition of certain presumed, prerequisite abilities—conceptual, psychomotor, and affective—on a step-by-step basis prior to the introduction of travel skills. Many persons with severe multiple handicaps may never acquire the "prerequisites" to begin instruction in travel skills. The heavy reliance on the use of verbal instruction and verbal feedback (Lolli, 1980) that is also typical of traditional orientation and mobility instruction, may exclude young children, persons with severe handicaps, and persons with dual sensory impairments.

While it is recognized that the level of one's conceptual, motor, communicative, and social abilities will directly influence the speed and degree of acquisition of orientation and mobility skills, some professionals in the field of orientation and mobility have also recognized the importance of semi-independent travel and the positive effects of successful independent movement for students with more severe disabilities (Bryant & Jansen, 1980; Gamble, 1980). Specific techniques and training strategies to benefit this population are, however, extremely limited in the orientation and mobility literature.

The purpose of this chapter is to provide an initial model for the development of instructional programs designed to teach orientation and mobility skills to students with severe multiple handicaps and sensory impairments (see also Warren, Horn, and Hill, Chapter 11, this volume, for a discussion of advanced technologies to teach orientation and mobility skills). It is an attempt to utilize the techniques of safe, efficient travel developed by the field of orientation and mobility (O&M), in conjunction with current community-intensive curriculum practices for this population. The model is based on the premise that the contexts for instruction of orientation and mobility skills, from the most basic to the most advanced, should be natural situations that require movement or travel.

The chapter also provides a review of adaptations and instructional strategies that are particularly useful in community-based instruction. An additional effort has been made to delineate areas in which further research is needed.

RATIONALE AND THEORETICAL PERSPECTIVE

Literature from the field of O&M has focused on assessment and intervention programs which stress the development of prerequisite sensory, motor, and conceptual skills (Harley, Wood, & Merbler, 1975, 1980). A precise teaching approach to O&M skills that follows a developmental/sequential approach was developed by Harley, Wood, and Merbler in 1975, and later adapted by the same authors (1980). The resulting assessment and programmed instruction, known as the Peabody Mobility Scale (1980), was successful in teaching basic O&M skills to students with moderate multiple disabilities. In a more recent report, Merbler and Wood (1984) concluded that there was a moderate to high correlation between students' performance scores on the sensory, concept, and motor sub-scales and their performance on the mobility skills scale. Additional authors have outlined many developmental concepts believed to relate to O&M skills (Foulke, 1971; Hapeman, 1967; Kay, 1974, Welsh & Blasch, 1980). This body of literature is often used as the basis to support the use of certain sensory, motor and conceptual skills as prerequisites for instruction in independent travel and cane use.

Despite the increasing use of various O&M assessment tools and instructional techniques, authors have noted as problems the wide variability among learners and the lack of knowledge of the interactions between the processes of perception, spatial learning, and actual mobility (Shingledecker & Foulke, 1978; Welsh & Blasch, 1980). Conflicting reports regarding the processes involved in mobility and the complexity of travel within natural environments cast doubt on the ability to determine the specific cognitive, sensory, and motor skills necessary for successful mobility within various environments (Rieser, Gruth, & Hill, 1982; Miller, 1982; Strelow, 1985).

Miller (1982) concluded that there was little relationship between the level of mobility and the development of positional concepts; and that, in fact, they are two separate entities. Bachman (1961) and Singer (1966) demonstrated high task specificity among individual motor abilities, supporting Miller's conclusion that the development of conceptual skills and levels of mobility are highly specific, yet equally important, skills.

In a comprehensive discussion of cognitive and perceptual processes related to mobility, Strelow (1985) describes the ability to travel as involving no single principle; rather, any or all perceptual and conceptual strategies could be involved in any particular instance of travel. He discusses certain mobility tasks as being purely perceptual but other situations where concepts and memory play a more important role. Strelow states that the person's ability to take in information useful for travel and the ability to use this information based on previous experience will determine successful mobility. He proposes that the difference in travel without sight is found in the informational bases available to the traveler. Determining information sources and the actual information most useful to a student on each part of any particular route is a difficult task, made even more complex by the ever-changing stimulus field created as the student moves.

Although relatively little is understood about the relationship between mobility and discrete travel skills, many mobility programs still require successful performance on certain sensory discrimination tasks, as well as a demonstrated understanding of certain spatial and positional concepts *prior* to instruction in more advanced skills. Recommended instruction for students with severe handicaps has tended to follow the same basic sequences but at a slower pace (Bryant and Jansen, 1980). As a result, many students with severe handicaps may never receive the opportunity to learn independent or semi-independent travel because they lack these readiness skills.

Rather than continue with a readiness model, some authors have suggested that adaptations to the standard practice be made (Hill & Ponder, 1976) and that "splinter skills" or "route travel" be taught to these individuals in order to increase independence and participation in daily activities (Gamble, 1980). Drawing a distinction between "route travel" and independent travel skills, Gamble suggests that students can be taught specific routes to home, work, and recreational areas even if they are unable to learn skills which will make them successful independent travelers in unfamiliar environments. She also suggests that "splinter" skills—skills specific for a particular response, but often not transferable to another situation—be taught to assist the student to function in present and future environments. Careful evaluation of the student and his or her skills is recommended to ensure that the right decision is made when teaching splinter skills vs. generalizable mobility skills.

In a recent study, Gee and Goetz (1985) found that four students with severe disabilities, including blindness, were able to learn four specific O&M skills (i.e., a modified trailing technique; maneuvering around obstacles; trailing around corners, and crossing short open spaces with no trailing surface) taught within the context of several functional travel routes, despite their failure to pass the conceptual and sensory skills on the Peabody Mobility Scale. These same students were also able to generalize the use of these O&M skills to new and unfamiliar routes and environments. In addition, they demonstrated evidence of incidental learning of the landmarks, clues, and memory tasks specific to the training routes. The students acquired semi-independent travel—travel with supervision and occasional assistance—within designated environments to specific destinations and activities. They also gained valuable O&M skills that are basic to travel in almost any environment or route.

Based on this research, the proposed model suggests that students with severe handicaps can learn specific O&M skills which may generalize to many environments and situations. The model is designed to teach the interrelationships of the skills necessary for mobility through the direct application of systematic instruction within the actual contexts in which the student is expected to be mobile.

O&M Skills Definitions

Orientation and mobility has been defined by Welsh and Blasch (1980) as the task of teaching persons with visual impairments to move independently, safely and purposefully through the environment. *Orientation skills* refer to the processes of utilizing the remaining senses to establish one's position and relationships to all other significant objects in one's environment (Hill & Ponder, 1976). *Mobility skills* refer to the ability to navigate safely from one's present fixed position to a desired position in another part of the environment. Hill and Ponder (1976) state that

> . . . the ultimate goal of orientation and mobility is to enable the student to enter any environment, familiar or unfamiliar, and to function safely, efficiently, gracefully, and independently by utilizing a combination of these two skills. (p. 1)

A variety of assessment instruments have been developed for evaluating the current O&M skill levels of students with visual impairments (see Table 1). Most of these assessment tools are in the form of developmental sequences or checklists of skills. There are checklists for basic O&M skills, concept development, functional vision, and motor development. In addition, many informal checklists have been developed by various school districts, private agencies, and O&M specialists.

While these assessment tools can be useful in identifying potential curricular content areas for instruction, they should be used with careful scrutiny for the student with severe multiple disabilities. As discussed earlier, there is little empirical evidence that training of certain concept skills such as body image prior to the instruction of travel skills will indeed improve the student's performance on these travel skills (Strelow, 1985). A student's potential may be limited if he or she is required to pass tests of tactile discrimination of items at a table in the classroom prior to being allowed to learn to recognize tactile clues and landmarks on a mobility route.

Educators who work with the O&M specialist may gain a greater understanding of the potential services this specialist can provide to students if these educators are aware of the traditional scope and sequence of successful O&M training for students whose only disability is serious visual impairment. A basic outline of the O&M skills taught to an individual who is totally blind (Eisenberg, 1979) is shown in Table 2. It is utilized by students in, and graduates of, mobility training programs, as a reference

Table 1. O&M assessment scales

Peabody Mobility Scale—Designed for measuring O&M skills in multihandicapped, visually impaired children (Harley, Wood, & Merbler, 1980)

Functional Vision Inventory—Assessment of vision in children who have low-vision and mental retardation (Langley, 1980)

Body Image of Blind Children—Designed to assess the child's ability to identify body planes and body parts, laterality, and directionality (Cratty & Sams, 1968)

Hill Performance Test of Selected Positional Concepts—Developed to assess spatial concepts needed in O&M by children from ages six to ten who have visual impairments (Hill, 1981)

The Tactile Analog to the Boehm Test of Basic Concepts—designed to assess potential concepts of persons with visual impairments (Caton, 1977)

The Peabody Mobility Kit—Assesses sensory and motor function of children with mental handicaps, visual impairments, and low vision (Harley, Henderson, & Wood, 1975)

Peabody Developmental Motor Scales and Activity Cards—Assesses sensory and motor functions (Folio & Fewell, 1983)

AMMP—Assesses awareness, movement, manipulation of environment, posture, and locomotion (Webb, 1969)

Additional examples of informal assessment strategies have been delineated by Swallow, Mangold, and Mangold (1977). For more specific information contact a local O&M instructor, or write to:

> The National Office of the Association for Education and Rehabilitation of the Blind and Visually Impaired (AER)
> 206 North Washington Street, Suite 320
> Alexandria, VA 22314-2528
>
> or
>
> The American Foundation for the Blind
> Orientation and Mobility Consultant
> 15 West 16th Street
> New York, NY 10011

guide for sequencing skill instruction. It is developmental in nature, going from "simple skills related to basic mobility needs to advanced techniques for complex independent travel in the extended geographical outdoor world" (p. iv). Upon instruction, each skill area is expanded into many more steps.

This sequence assumes that the individual moves from the concrete to the abstract and that the goal is independent travel in any environment, whether familiar or unfamiliar. The skills of orienting oneself within an environment—i.e., knowing where one is in space, where the destination is in space, and a way of ordering what must be done to arrive at that destination (Hill & Ponder, 1976)—are taught in conjunction with movement skills.

Table 2. Traditional scope and sequence of O&M (Eisenberg, 1979)

Concept development

Basic techniques
- Sighted guide
- Protective and information gathering
- Forearm technique
- Trailing
- Lower body protective technique
- Independent room orientation

Introduction to cane techniques
- Touch technique
- Training with the touch technique
- Diagonal cane technique
- Touch and slide technique
- Stair travel
- Congested area cane technique
- Entering and exiting doorways, cars, and so on
- Touch and drag technique
- Three-point touch technique

Residential travel

Light business travel

Major metropolitan travel

Rural travel

Snow travel and other adverse conditions

A brief description of orientation and mobility skills follows. It is not intended to be a comprehensive discussion of all techniques available, but rather a summary useful for the educator with primary responsibility for the student with severe multiple handicaps. The reader is referred to the texts by Hill and Ponder (1976), Welsh and Blasch (1980), and the sequence by Eisenberg (1979) for a more detailed description of O&M techniques used with individuals who have only a visual impairment.

Concept Skills Generally, when O&M specialists refer to concept skills they are indicating three basic areas: body, spatial, and environmental concepts. Body concepts refer to the student's body image and body schema (Hill & Blasch, 1980). The sequence of instruction includes body parts, functions, surfaces, and relationships. Spatial concepts include positional and relational concepts of the body and the environment (such as beside, under, lateral, internal, external, etc.), concepts of measurement, and action concepts such as the terms for various movements (i.e., turn at 45 degrees, 90 degrees, right-angle turn; and move, scoot, creep, crawl, roll, walk, run).

The environmental concepts emphasized by Hill and Blasch (1980) are those related to travel. Their list is a series of terms such as *traffic light, city, business district, road, crosswalk,* and so on. In addition, they include topography concepts such as *side, border, flat,* and *straight*; and concepts of texture such as *pavement, stone, slick,* and *gravel*. Their list also includes temperature concepts important to the traveler, such as *hot, cold, muggy,* and *chilly*.

Orientation Skills Hill and Ponder (1976) refer to six components of orientation: landmarks, clues, indoor and outdoor numbering systems, measurement, compass directions, and self-familiarizations. Landmarks include "any familiar object, sound, odor, temperature, or tactile clue that is easily recognized, is constant, and that has a known permanent location in the environment" (p. 4). "Landmarks" are used to establish and maintain direction, to locate specific destinations, to use for perpendicular or parallel alignment for straightline travel, or to obtain information about an area such as a floor. Examples of landmarks are the drinking fountain next to the gymnasium entrance, or the bump in the hallway floor right before the turn to the locker room.

"Clues" are not necessarily permanent. They refer to tactile, auditory, visual, and olfactory stimuli which give the student information about his or her direction, position and orientation relative to specific landmarks or locations. For example, the student may smell the food in the cafeteria and use it as the clue that he or she must turn left and head toward the door.

"Indoor and outdoor numbering systems" refer to the arrangement of numbers of rooms in buildings and the addresses on streets within a town or city. "Compass directions" are transferable from one environment to another and, once understood, are a valuable aid to the person with a visual impairment. "Self-familiarization" is the ability to tie together all the orientation concepts as one becomes familiar with a strange environment. Hill and Ponder (1976) have outlined a specific process for self-familiarization in which the student enters a room or building and systematically explores and notes all the necessary landmarks, and positions of objects in relation to each other.

Basic Mobility Techniques and Cane Techniques A list of mobility skills and techniques, both basic and advanced, are depicted in Table 3. The definitions are taken from Hill and Ponder (1976). The reader can see that these skills follow a sequence from what are considered easier skills to those that are more advanced. Working with a sighted guide, the student is expected to learn many travel concepts that can be used later while trailing or using a cane. Similarly, the student is taken through a series of skill-building procedures while using a sighted guide, prior to the use of the cane.

Recently, many O&M specialists have begun to use the cane with preschool students and students with multiple disabilities, even though these students have not mastered many of the skills that precede the cane techniques on the list. For example, an 18-year-old student with dual sensory impairments and intellectual delay, who had never been independently mobile before, learned to trail, cross open doorways, and follow a straight line of travel, while also learning to use the cane in the diagonal position. A 6-year-old student with severe intellectual delay learned to move independently, trail, maneuver around obstacles and turn corners, also while learning to hold the cane in a diagonal position (Gee & Goetz, 1985).

When the student's severe handicaps suggest that the typical assessment instruments and instructional sequences may be inappropriate, it is suggested that assessment and instruction be carried out using the strategies identified in the remainder of the chapter. Caution should be taken, however, in making the decision for children with visual impairments and more mild handicaps, who may follow the traditional developmental sequence but at a slower rate.

Table 3. Mobility skills and purpose (the sequence is modified from Hill & Ponder, 1976)

Skill	Purpose
Sighted guide Basic Reversing Transferring Narrow passages Accept & refuse aid Stairways Doorways Seating	To travel safely and efficiently with a sighted person within different environments and under varying conditions
Self-protection Upper hand & forearm Lower hand & forearm Trailing Traversing open doorways Direction taking Search patterns Dropped objects	To enable the student to travel efficiently and independently, primarily in familiar indoor environments, affording the student maximum protection without the use of a mobility aid
Basic cane skills Walking with a guide Transferring sides with a guide Doorways with a guide Accept or refuse aid	To enable the student to travel safely, efficiently, and independently in familiar and unfamiliar environments
Placement of the cane	To enable the student to position his or her cane so that it is easily accessible and will not interfere with others
Diagonal technique Changing hands Objects/Obstacles Doorways Trailing Stairways Cane manipulation	To enable the student to travel independently, primarily in a familiar indoor environment with some degree of protection Cane is held at a diagonal across and in front of the student and pushed forward ahead of the student

(continued)

Table 3. *(continued)*

Skill	Purpose
Touch technique	To enable the student to detect drop-offs and objects in the vertical plane in familiar or unfamiliar environments
Basic	
Trailing	
Changing from diagonal to touch technique	
Examine objects	
Outdoors/residential	
Car familiarization	Enter and exit cars
Outdoor travel	
Shorelining	To establish and maintain a desired line of travel and to locate a specific object perpendicular to his line of travel
Sidewalk recovery	
Touch & slide	To detect textual changes, subtle drop-offs, etc.
Touch & drag	For use on curbs, expansion joints, elevated walkways and platforms
Residential street crossings	
Outdoors/commercial	
Street crossing at traffic light	
Pedestrian traffic control	
Soliciting aid	
Buses	
Primary commercial facilities	
Escalators, elevators	
Revolving doors	
Airports, etc.	

FUNCTIONAL ORIENTATION & MOBILITY PROGRAM DEVELOPMENT

The model of instructional development that follows has four main components. First, instruction of orientation and mobility skills—from the most basic to the most complex—takes place within and across the activities and environments that naturally require performance of the skills. The contexts for instruction are selected as part of a functional, community-based curriculum model (see Nietupski & Hamre-Nietupski, Chapter 9, this volume). Training of specific objectives occurs when travel is necessary and instructional trials of each objective are distributed across several travel routes used as training contexts (cf. Helmstetter & Guess, Chapter 10, this volume). Instruction is carried out in at least four contexts concurrently.

The second component of the model is the use of interspersed training trials (Gee & Goetz, 1985). The student learning basic O&M skills may not be initially required to perform all the skills necessary to get from one place to another in a given route. Rather, he or she may be taught two or three skills which are required within the route of travel. These skills are required at various points along the route, and thus are instructed when their performance is necessary. The instructor assists the student on all other parts of the route, stopping and giving instruction when the skills designated for training are required. As the student passes the initial objectives, more of each route can be added to his or her performance requirements.

The third component is the use of a "context instruction" phase in the program (Gee & Goetz, 1985). Because most students will not previously have been required to participate in their travel, other than to use a sighted guide, it cannot be assumed that they have an understanding of the natural cues for travel along the route, nor the expectation that a specific event will occur at the end of a particular path. During this phase the instructor completely assists the student to travel through the route from one destination to another (i.e., from the classroom to the bus stop; or the snack table to the play area) in the manner in which the student would eventually be expected to travel. The purpose is to establish a functional motivation for travel. By setting up an expectation that at the end of the route is an event or activity that the student regularly participates in, the teacher provides a context in which the student can perceive travel as necessary. Functionally motivating contexts have been used similarly in communication and vision instruction (Goetz & Gee, Chapter 4, this volume; Goetz et al., 1983) and in the interrupted chain training strategy outlined by Goetz, Gee, and Sailor (1985). Thus, the model attempts to provide intrinsic motivation for movement.

The fourth component is the use of systematic, operant training procedures. Antecedent fading procedures, or the systematic use of most-to-least assistance prompting, are used most often for initial instruction. Consequential procedures, or the use of least-to-most prompt hierarchies, are suggested for the student who has reached a "fluency" stage of performance (Ford, 1983). The use of time delay (Touchette, 1971) as a procedure for shifting stimulus control and avoiding prompt dependency is also recommended.

The model is a process with six phases (see Figure 1). Phase one involves planned observations of targeted O&M skills based upon team assessment information. The transdisciplinary team may consist of the student's primary caregiver(s), teacher, O&M specialist, vision specialist, and any other professionals involved in the student's educational program development. The reader is referred to Lyon and Lyon (1980) for further information on the transdisciplinary team. Phase two is the selection of the contexts for instruction. In phase three, the O&M specialist and the student's teacher conduct a baseline route analysis in which the route and the student's performance are both analyzed. Phase four involves context instruction and a second baseline, and phase five is the actual construction of the instructional program. In the final phase, the program is implemented and the data are continuously monitored.

Assessment of the Student's Current O&M Performance

Prior to the assessment process, the transdisciplinary team (Haynes et al., 1976) should review information from several sources. Among students with severe handi-

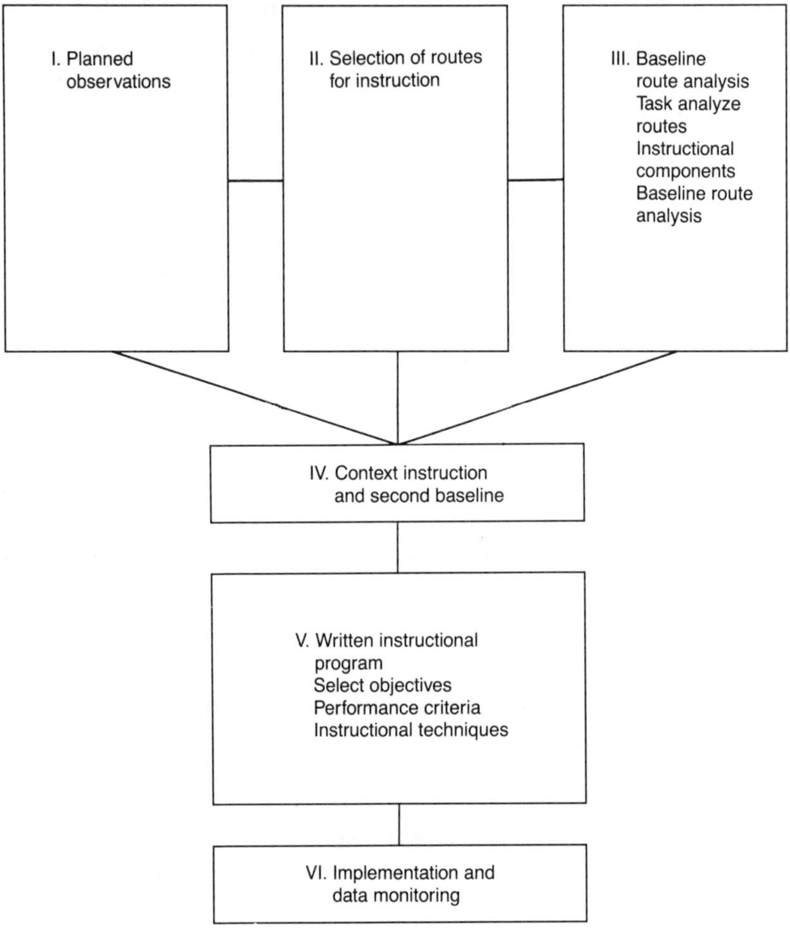

Figure 1. Model for the development of O&M instruction.

caps, a wide range of visual impairments occur in conjunction with varying levels of intellectual functioning and other physical disabilities. Each student's individual combination of disabilities will influence his or her ability to be mobile.

Understanding an individual's vision problem thoroughly will assist in developing appropriate O&M goals and objectives. If a field loss exists in the lower quadrants, for example, the use of a cane or special scanning procedure may be necessary even though the student has a great deal of functional vision. Based on the recommendation and/or prescription made by a qualified eye care specialist, low vision aids, contact lenses, sunglasses, and so forth may also be appropriate for students to maximize their remaining vision. Objectives should reflect strategies to teach the use of any residual vision within mobility routes. The reader is referred to Goetz and Gee (Chapter 4, this volume) for a review of vision assessment tools.

Just as the amount of vision is often difficult to assess by traditional means, the amount of hearing loss is equally uncertain in many individuals with multiply handicapping conditions. If a hearing loss is suspected, the O&M specialist should consult with the special education teacher, audiologist, speech and language specialist, and/or the teacher of students with hearing impairments, for these professionals may have relevant data to assist in programming. Programmatic assessment techniques to prepare students for an audiological evaluation can be found in Goetz et al. (1985). The amount of residual hearing students have and their ability to make use of hearing aid(s) will also have an impact on their mobility skills.

Information from physical and occupational therapists, regarding such concerns as the student's balance, reflexes, trunk control, and wheelchair guidelines, is also necessary in the development of an O&M program. The student's physical abilities will affect his or her ability to learn to travel. The speech therapist and teacher should also provide information to the team regarding the student's current system for communication.

Planned Observations

The initial step in conducting a functional assessment of O&M skills is to structure planned observations of the performance of each skill. The teacher observes the student using the skill at a time when there are natural cues for its performance. In order to adequately use this strategy the teacher and O&M specialist must review the skills they wish to assess, determine a functional, age-appropriate context in which the skill is necessary, and arrange for the opportunity to observe or gather baseline data on the student in that context. Examples of some O&M skills and contexts in which they might be assessed are shown in Table 4. The primary purpose of the planned observations is to provide the instructor with initial information about the student's performance of specific O&M skills.

Selection of Contexts for Instruction

While completing planned observations in order to become familiar with the student's performance levels of targeted O&M skills, instructional staff can concurrently begin to select contexts for instruction. It is recommended that instruction be given in as many contexts as possible, and in at least four contexts within the instructional day. The student's ecological assessment, involving the parents and other transdisciplinary team members, and the IEP process will identify the priority activities and environments in which the student will need to use his or her O&M skills (see Harrell & Rosenberg, 1986).

Based on this information, the teacher and O&M instructor together review the student's activities and regular destinations to select the contexts in which instruction will take place. Four main factors should be considered in route/context selection.

Table 4. Contexts in which O&M skills are essential

Category	Skill	Function	Age-appropriate contexts in which the student can demonstrate skill performance: 3–7 years	13–18 years
Underlying basic skill	Tactile discrimination	To determine differences between tactile stimuli	Stop or sit down on the mat with the group after noticing the difference in surface (in the school gym)	Stop or slow down and cautiously approach the swimming pool when students' bare feet touch the tile surrounding the edge of the pool
Underlying basic skill	Sound localization	To recognize the direction from which a sound came	Turn toward the sounds from other children on the playground	Turn toward the sounds coming from the bus arriving at the corner
Orientation skill	Utilize clues	Change movement or direction based on an environmental clue	Move or attempt to leave when the bell rings for recess	Stop and turn left down a hallway when the flow of air hits face
Orientation skill	Utilize landmarks	Change movement behavior or direction based on recognition of a landmark	Slow for the stairway when the railing is felt with the hand	After passing the drinking fountain, enter the next doorway
Mobility skill	Trailing	Move continuously using a guiding surface	Follow the hallway at home to the bathroom	Follow the classroom wall to the coat rack
Mobility skill	Crossing a defined open space 14–30 feet	Moving continuously across a defined space in a purposeful and relatively straight path	Cross the hallway leading to the school cafeteria	Bring dishes to the sink from the table in the kitchen

First, routes of travel should be chosen which will be used on a regular and continuing basis. For example, a kindergarten-age student may regularly travel from his or her classroom to the kindergarten classroom for one period a day. He or she may also regularly travel from the bathroom to the classroom, the snack table to the play area, the classroom to the cafeteria, and to the bus stop. On a daily basis, a 15-year-old student may use the school locker room; travel from the school to the laundromat, restaurants, and local services; and travel to a nearby vocational site.

Second, it is preferable to choose routes that can most practically be instructed, given teacher–student ratios. In addition to the instructional time provided by the O&M specialist, the student's teacher and other classroom staff will carry out the mutually agreed upon O&M programs across daily travel routes. There may be certain times during the instructional day when there are more classroom staff available, allowing the kind of close one-on-one assistance that is often necessary for mobility instruction. Particular groupings of students (i.e., one student who is blind with two students who are ambulatory and sighted) may also make O&M instruction more manageable.

The third factor is motivation. If the routes lead to some desirable activity that occurs regularly on arrival, the student's motivation for movement may increase. Thus, the teacher may choose to train O&M skills on the way to the swimming pool if the student enjoys swimming, to a worksite where the student interacts with a friend, or to the cafeteria or a restaurant if the student enjoys eating.

Lastly, consideration should be given to the variations in the skills required in the routes. The team may decide, for example, that certain routines require too many advanced skills, or that some routes are too short to allow enough practice. It is preferable to train across routes that allow several opportunities for practice on each skill. The information gathered from the route analysis will assist in this decision.

Baseline Route Analysis

Task Analysis of the Route After a route is chosen, the team determines the most efficient path for the student and the O&M skills which are required for traveling through the route. First, the entire route is analyzed. Every change in direction, change of hand or foot, turn, shift of cane, landmarks, and so on, is considered to be a separate component of the route. The educators (O&M specialist and teacher) write down each component, organizing the route for safety, efficiency, and appearance (see section on *performance criteria*).

The O&M specialist advises the teacher of the path that would be taken by a person with only a visual disability, and together they determine any adaptations that might be necessary. For example, on a route from the classroom to the front entrance of the school building, there may be a section where the independent blind traveler would cross a crowded, open area with no surface to continuously trail, in order to reach a series of steps. The teacher and O&M specialist may decide to have the student with severe handicaps take a different path at that point in the route, allowing the student to follow a wall which eventually leads to the steps. While less efficient, it may allow the student more independence.

Table 5 depicts two routes which have been task analyzed for two students with dual sensory impairments. The first is the route from the classroom to the bus stop for Tim, a 17-year-old high school student who is learning cane travel for parts of his routes. The second route is for Rebecca, a 5-year-old elementary school student who uses a walker to travel from her classroom to the kindergarten classroom daily.

Determine Instructional Components Unlike some activities in which one training

Table 5. Task-analyzed routes for Tim and Rebecca

Tim's route from classroom to corner bus stop	Rebecca's route from classroom to kindergarten room
1. Open door of classroom	1. Exit classroom
2. Trail around right corner	2. Follow short wall on left
3. Cane in left hand	3. Cross hallway
4. Trail the wall	4. At wall, turn right
5. Three obstacles: garbage can, chair, chair	5. Follow wall
6. Trail around right corner	6. At end of wall, go around corner
7. Down first set of stairs	7. When walker hits stairs, move walker to right
8. Trail wall	8. Grasp railing—both hands
9. Down second set of stairs	9. Upstairs—5
10. At bottom of stairs, turn left	10. At top of stairs, grasp walker
11. Follow bottom step with cane	11. Follow wall
12. At end of stair, walk straight	12. Cross open doorway
13. Cross open space	13. Follow wall
14. When cane hits short stairs, turn left	14. When reach children singing, stop and turn right
15. Find wall	15. Cross hallway
16. Down 3 steps	16. Find doorknob
17. Turn left	17. Open door of classroom
18. Cross open space	18. Enter kindergarten class
19. When cane hits stairs, find railing	
20. Down 3 steps	
21. Find doors	
22. Push open doors/exit	
23. Cross open space to outside steps	
24. Down four steps without railing	
25. At bottom, turn left, wait for guide	
26. Walk one block on sidewalk with sighted guide	
27. At curb, stop and wait for bus	

procedure can be used across the entire task analysis, each mobility route requires the use of many different skills. Each skill may require a different instructional approach. Instructional programs are written for each of the varied skills required within and across the routes.

The steps in each route can be divided into two general categories: steps representing skills that can be used across any travel route, and steps that are specific to one particular route. The first category includes basic movement skills, sighted guide techniques, and cane techniques. These are skills that can be practiced across many contexts and can be generalized to new and unfamiliar contexts (Gee & Goetz, 1985). Performance of these skills will be the same on any route. For example, the technique to travel up and down stairs with a railing will be the same across most routes. Similarly, trailing a wall, making turns, crossing doorways, and other movement skills can be used in many environments.

The second category includes the steps that are only necessary to the particular route being analyzed. Landmarks and clues are usually included in this category. While the ability to use landmarks and clues may be general for the more advanced student, each clue or landmark must be remembered and used in its specific location on the route. For example, the student may need to remember that the sound of the kindergarten children singing is his or her clue to turn left to cross the hallway and enter the kindergarten room. The clue is specific to that particular route.

A format for analyzing routes and collecting baseline data was developed by Gee and Goetz (1985). Figure 2 depicts a partial baseline route analysis for Tim's route from the class to the bus stop. At the top of the form the instructor notes any adaptations that have previously been made (see adaptations section), and the current status of the student's vision, hearing, and communication mode. In the vertical column on the right side of the form the steps of the route are listed in order. Several columns for data are available. The instructor uses the columns to the left of the route to indicate the required skills for each corresponding step. The specific skill is written in at the top of the column and the box that is parallel to the step is checked. (A complete route analysis would include all skills required for the entire training route.)

The columns on the right side of the form are used to collect baseline data (or posttest data) before or after instruction. On 6/7 and 6/8, Tim's teacher collected baseline data by going through the route with him and providing opportunities to perform each of the skills listed. Based on his performance, four skills were chosen for instruction: trailing walls, trailing corners, maneuvering around obstacles, and crossing over spaces. Baseline data on these skills were then taken on 6/20, after context instruction had occurred (see below).

Baseline With the baseline data collected, the teacher and O&M specialist can complete the analysis. The purpose of the baseline is to determine the present level of the student's performance, possible instructional techniques, and where instruction is necessary. The instructor uses a format of least–to–most assistance throughout the route, allowing the student to demonstrate any current ability to perform the step required.

Baseline Route Analysis
School site or other community site: ____________________
Student: Tim — 17
Route: Classroom to front entrance and bus stop on corner
Communication System: A few tactile signs and gestures
Vision Status: No vision Hearing Status: Profound Loss
* = Indicates that data from this step is to be combined with data on the same objective from other routes.

*Stairs without railing	*Open classroom door	Route memory	Open large front doors	*Turn, square off	*Sighted guide	*Shift cane	*Correct position on stairs — down	*Trail with cane only	*Cross defined open spaces	*Maneuver obstacles	*Continue to hand trail while turning corner	*Maintain trailing — diagonal and hand	Route description **by objective** Cane with marshmallow tip in use	Date of baseline/posttest (open squares indicate the objectives to be tested.) 6/7/84	6/8/84	6/20/84
	x												Open door of classroom	-	-	
		x									x		Trail around right corner	-	-	-
		x				x							Cane in left hand	-	-	
												x 23	Trail the wall (23 trials)	+1	+6	+7
										3 x			3 obstacles: garbage can, chair, chair	- - -	- - -	- - -
		x									x		Trail around right corner	-	-	+
							x						Down 1st set of stairs	-	+	
												x 2	Trail wall	- -	- +	+ -
													Down 2nd set of stairs	-	-	

. . . etc.

Goal: 4 routes within school building
Date: 6/21/86, steps chosen for instruction: trailing with hand cane at diagonal; trail around corners; maneuver around obstacles in trailing path; cross defined open spaces using diagonal techniques.

Figure 2. Baseline route analysis: Tim.

Changes in performance criteria or the route itself may be indicated. For example, it may be discovered that rather than trailing with the cane, the student can benefit from learning the more advanced touch technique; or, that rather than the diagonal technique, an adaptation should be made. Following baseline it was determined that Tim's method of travel in buildings would be trailing with the cane held in the diagonal position, rather than using open space travel techniques (see Table 6).

Table 6. Objectives and definitions

Goal: Tim will be able to travel at least 4 routes independently under supervision within the school building.

Objective #1: While traveling within the school building to specific destinations, Tim will be able to trail the walls using correct position for his hand and the diagonal cane position, continuously moving until encountering an obstacle or a route marker, with at least 90% accuracy maintained for 2 weeks.

Objective #2: While traveling within the school building to specific destinations, Tim will be able to maintain the diagonal trailing position with hand and cane while going around corners, with 100% accuracy, maintained for at least 2 weeks.

Objective	*Instructional trial definitions*
1. Trailing by hand with the cane	Approximately every 7 feet, using natural markers in the fence, wall, and so on, or masking tape and chalk to mark each trial
2. Corners	Each time the student has to turn a corner *while trailing*, and continue trailing

The route analysis will be different for each route, and each student will have an individualized set of movement skills depending on his or her ability level and specific disabilities. For example, a student using a walker to ambulate must travel without a cane. Thus, the skills represented by the steps which indicate traveling down hallways, across rooms, and along sidewalks will be different than the skills used by the student with a cane. A route analysis for a student using a walker is shown in Figure 3. This student will use a different method for getting up and down stairs (i.e., holding the railing with both hands) than will Tim, who is ambulatory and learning to use a cane (see Table 6). Figure 4 gives a route description by step for this student.

Context Instruction and Second Baseline

The "context instruction" phase is designed to establish the motivation for travel. The instructor uses this phase before he or she writes the instructional objectives. Before receiving O&M instruction, most students with severe handicaps either use a sighted guide or, unfortunately, are pushed or pulled through most environments. As a result they have not experienced the landmarks and clues, the surfaces, or any of the other steps in the route they will travel. It cannot be assumed that the student understands the natural cues for travel along the route, nor the presumed motivation of the activity at the end of a particular path.

During context instruction the student is assisted to travel through each route in the manner in which she or he will eventually be expected to travel it independently. This phase is an adaptation of the initial training used to develop independent travel in a frequently used indoor environment for a person who is blind. The instructor calls attention to tactile, auditory, and other situational cues, and manipulates the student's

Baseline Route Analysis
School site or other community site: ____________
Student: Rebecca — 4
Route: Classroom to kindergarten
Communication Status: Uses 3–5 tactile signs receptively
Vision Status: Residual peripheral vision and spots on right side.
Hearing Status: Severe loss in both ears.
* = Indicates that data from this step is to be combined with data on the same objective from other routes.

*Turn, square off	*Localize to sound	*Use one arm to balance	*Walk upstairs—no walker	*Move walker aside	*Corners	*Cross open space	Route memory	*Follow walls in walker		Route Description **by Step** Four legged rollator walker in use. Instructor carries walker upstairs and places in position	Date of baseline/posttest (open squares indicate the objectives to be tested).		
							x			Exit classroom.			
								x1		Follow short wall on left.			
						x				Cross hallway.			
							x			At wall, turn right.			
								x4		Follow wall (4 trials).			
					x					At end of wall, go around corner 24			
				x			x			When walker hits stairs, move walker to right.			
							x			Grasp railing—both hands.			
			x							Upstairs — 5.			

Figure 3. Baseline route analysis: Rebecca. *(continued)*

body through moving, turning, holding the cane, and any other components necessary to reach the destination. The one demand placed on the student is cooperation in participation. No data are collected during this phase. Rather, the purpose is to establish a level of expectation in the student of an event to take place at the end of movement through the environment. From five to ten days of context instruction are suggested, after which a second baseline is taken.

Data from the second baseline reflect the student's ability to perform the skills after some expectation of what should happen has presumably been established through the context training phase. These sessions are run identically to the first baseline. Baseline data on particular basic movement skills (e.g., taking steps independently, trailing, and moving up and down stairs) following context instruction have been shown to demonstrate a higher level of performance than the data on the initial

*Turn, square off	*Localize to sound	*Use one arm to balance	*Walk upstairs—no walker	*Move walker aside	*Corners	*Cross open space	Route memory	*Follow walls in walker	Route Description **by Step** Four-legged rollator walker in use. Instructor carries walker upstairs and places in position.	Date of baseline/ Posttest (open squares indicate the objectives to be tested.)		
		x					x		At top of stairs, grasp walker.			
								x2	Follow wall (2 trials).			
						x			Cross open doorway.			
								x2	Follow wall (2 trials).			
x	x								When reach children singing, stop and turn right.			
						x			Cross hallway.			
									Find doorknob.			
		x					x		Open door of classroom.			
							x		Enter kindergarten.			
	1	2			1			9	= #Trials Score =			

Goal: Four routes within building with minimal assistance.

Date: 1/86, steps chosen for instruction:
1) localize to sound;
2) use one arm to balance;
3) follow walls;
4) go around corners and continue to follow wall.

Figure 3. *(continued)*

baseline (Gee & Goetz, 1985). Presumably, the students may learn some of the skills by simply being put through the movements during the context instruction phase. The data may also reflect the student's knowledge or anticipation of the event at the end of the route. With an expectation of the events that will follow the route, the student may be more likely to continue to move along the route and at least attempt to continue travel.

Writing the Instructional Program

Selection and Ordering of Objectives Instructional objectives for students with severe multiple disabilities may range from very basic movement skills to more advanced cane skills. A few general guidelines follow.

Based on the data from Gee and Goetz (1985) indicating that many route memory steps (landmarks, clues, etc.) can be learned incidentally, it may be preferable to begin instruction on the basic motor movement skills (e.g., turning corners) and cane techniques which will get a student from place to place—the heart of the ability to be mobile. As the student meets the criteria on the initial movement objectives, more steps within the route can be added to the student's repertoire.

The number of opportunities for practice on the skill is another variable to consider. If the necessity to use a particular skill only arises once out of several trailing routes, it may not be a priority.

Age is another factor that will influence the objectives. The older student will travel to more environments in the community, requiring skills which are not necessary inside buildings. It may also be more advantageous to make adaptations for older students who have only a short amount of time left in school to receive instruction.

Table 6 presents a long-term goal and two short-term mobility objectives for Tim. Also included are definitions of the targeted skills for purposes of instruction and measurement. These objectives were taught in the context of four natural travel routes, including travel between the bus stop and classroom, the classroom and restroom, and from the classroom to a store in the community.

Setting the Performance Criteria Before setting the performance criteria on long- and short-term objectives, it is useful to consider the criteria which the O&M specialist would set for a person whose only disability is blindness. Based on the data from the baseline observations, the criteria can be adapted temporarily or permanently to suit the student with a severe handicap.

Safety, efficiency, and appearance are the three levels of competency which are considered within the traditional orientation and mobility paradigm. The same levels should be considered when defining goals and objectives for the student with severe multiple handicaps. Adaptations in the program and materials can be made accordingly.

The first priority in O&M instruction is the safety of the student. Insuring that the student has the necessary skills to move about safely in familiar and unfamiliar environments is essential before independent travel is considered. Protective techniques for low and overhanging obstacles are essential if the student with visual impairments is to move freely in various environments. It is often a disservice to the student to unnaturally modify his or her environment to make it safe. It is preferable to teach the student how to recognize hazards and how to safely maneuver around them. Since most O&M training occurs in the community, the safety of the student is of great importance (e.g., street crossings, avoiding overhanging tree branches).

The second area of emphasis in O&M instruction is efficiency. A variety of skills, strategies, and "tricks of the trade" make traveling easier for individuals who are visually impaired. Locating a door knob by rotating one's wrist and holding one's cane vertically an inch off the ground while moving it across the door is a much faster way to find the door knob than groping aimlessly all over the door with one's free hand.

A third area of emphasis in O&M instruction is appearance. If the student with severe multiple handicaps and a visual impairment is expected to assimilate into society and move about to the greatest extent possible, then consideration should be given to appearance. In order for normalization and integration to occur, students should be taught to look as unobtrusive as possible as they travel in the school and throughout their community. Teaching appropriate posture, gait, and coordinated movements will assist the student in presenting an acceptable appearance.

The need for training in each of these three areas of competency must be decided in relation to each student individually. Safety should always be given first consideration; however, efficiency and appearance should also be considered and prioritized. For example, the O&M specialist may choose to forgo efficiency and appearance criteria for a particular student who is able to safely travel to his or her after-school job, even though he or she is not always efficient and might appear awkward. Performance criteria must ultimately be based on the student's abilities.

Instructional Strategies A wide variety of instructional strategies are available to the teacher and O&M specialist (see Sailor & Guess, 1983; Snell, 1983). Shaping and gradual fading of physical assistance and reinforcement are commonly used. Since some O&M instructors have not received in-depth training in teaching strategies appropriate to persons with severe handicaps, the student's classroom teacher may have primary responsibility for developing the instructional strategies to be used in the O&M program. The O&M specialist will have primary responsibility, however, for the technique and adaptations; and will provide ongoing supervision and training for all staff implementing the instruction.

Physically assisting the students through the correct motions may be an effective means to let them know exactly how the correct movements feel. Students can easily become prompt dependent, however, from too much physical attention and verbal prompting, learning that if they stop moving someone will make contact with them or talk to them to initiate movement. Careful use of tactile and verbal feedback and praise can help avoid the problem. Another effective means to avoid prompt dependence is the use of time delay (Touchette, 1971). Time delay is an instructional technique that gradually increases the amount of time between the natural cue to use an O&M skill and the prompt which will initiate it.

An important component of the instructional program is placement of the instructional trials within route travel. This means that parts of the route (the components being systematically instructed) must be performed to the criteria designated in the program, but the teacher assists the student to perform the remaining components of the route. Using this method the teacher can begin with instruction on one, two, or three objectives and continue to gradually add more components of the route as components are mastered.

Periodically, it is advisable to run a *probe session*. During a probe session, the teacher requires performance on all steps of the route, thus providing a baseline for all the non-training steps in the route. The data will point out any steps which have been incidentally learned or partially trained.

Implementation and Data Monitoring

The model is data based—the instructor records the student's score on the performance of each component that is being instructed. Data may be collected daily or on a varied schedule basis (i.e., every third day). For practical purposes the instructor may choose only to collect data on one objective at a time, and periodically probe all objectives (components) across the route. The data from the skills used across more than one training route can be compiled into graphs that show overall performance on each skill. The teacher gathers the scores from all the routes for each skill and plots the student's performance. The number of trials per skill will depend on the performance criteria and the number of opportunities for practice across all the training routes.

Figure 4 shows a partial data sheet for teaching trailing on Tim's route from the classroom to the bus stop. Data from trailing trials (Steps 4 and 8) are combined with trailing data from other routes. On 7/5, trailing around corners, the next objective was probed. On 7/11, the entire route was probed. The data suggest that trailing around corners is being learned incidentally as part of the contextual training package.

In addition, the teacher can plot the student's performance on each individual route. This can be done simply by adding the number of components in the route that the student can perform correctly, and plotting the data on a graph. As mentioned earlier, periodic probes should be conducted to determine performance on steps not yet being instructed. The data sheets and graph also provide a means for the O&M specialist and the teacher to communicate about the student's progress, in order to make decisions about the program based on objective criteria.

Program and Material Adaptations

The intent of all mobility techniques is to provide protection and information for individuals with visual impairments to allow them to successfully and safely move within and between various environments. Basic instructional format and procedures may need to be adapted to accommodate the unique needs of each student.

If it is determined by the O&M specialist that the use of a long cane is necesary, modifications from the traditional touch technique may be needed. The cane serves as a bumper and probe, it protects the traveler from contacting low obstacles, and it provides tactile and auditory feedback. The long cane is traditionally thought of as an extension of the index finger as it explores the path in front of the person who is blind. The touch technique involves keeping the hand and arm centered as the cane is extended out from the midline of the body. As the cane tip moves slightly off the ground in an arc to the right, the left foot steps forward, alternating foot and cane as one walks. All cane movements are to emanate from the wrist, and a rhythmic movement is necessary to remain in step and keep a safe arc size. Significant coordination and integration of body movements are needed when utilizing the traditional touch technique.

Instruction on objective #1 only: Trailing
Student: Tim
Route: Classroom to bus stop

				Probe trailing corners			Probe entire route		
Route steps	Trials ↓ Date →	7/1	7/2	7/3	7/5	7/8	7/9	7/10	7/11
1. Open door of classroom									–
2. *Trail around right corner					+				+
3. Cane in left hand									–
4. *Trail the wall	23	+7	+11	+10	+15	+17	+19	+21	+20
5. *Obstacles	3								+ + –
6. *Trail corner to the right					+				+
7. Down first set of stairs									+
8. *Trail wall	2	+ –	+ +	+ +	+ +	+ –	+ +	+ +	+ +
9. Down second set of stairs									+
10. At bottom of stairs, turn left									–
11. Square off									–
12. Follow bottom steps with cane									–
13. At end of stair, walk straight									+
14. Cross open space	2								+ –
15. When cane hits stairs, turn left									–

. . . etc. for remainder of route

Figure 4. Sample data sheet: Tim.

Problems of balance and limited range of motion may interfere with the acquisition of cane skills. The diagonal cane technique is sometimes more beneficial for the student with coordination problems. This technique provides a degree of protection and serves as a bumper. The cane is held diagonally across the body in a stationary position. This technique does not provide optimum protection; however, it is better than no technique and is often easier to learn.

When students have difficulty with coordination and with learning to rhythmically tap the cane, or have trouble interpreting tactile feedback, the use of the constant contact technique may be helpful. The cane stays in continuous contact with the ground while moving back and forth in an arc movement. This technique allows for more tactile information about varying surfaces, contours, and obstacles. A disadvantage of the constant contact technique is that the cane often gets stuck in cracks, holes, and so forth.

Modifying the cane itself is beneficial for many students. One modification is the "marshmallow tip" developed by Wurzburger (1980), a 1¼ inch diameter white nylon tip that provides the student with as much tactile input as possible. Its weight encourages the student to keep the cane on the ground, and the tip slides across the surface better than the traditional tip. Another cane adaptation was developed by Morse (1980) for a student who is deaf-blind. A diagonal cane extension was attached to the long cane at a point less than halfway from the ground, so that the secondary tip touched the opposite side from where the primary cane tip arc touched, thus providing body-width coverage without having to move the cane. This modification proved to be useful for the student who had trouble coordinating the back and forth movements of the touch technique. Another modification for a student with a physical disability might be to paint a support crutch white with a red tip, to signal the presence of a visual impairment. When properly used, the crutch will also identify obstacles.

For the student who is visually impaired and in a wheelchair, the teacher may attach curb detectors to the chair, to inform the student of obstacles and/or allow the student to trail a wall, curb, or building. Curb detectors are also useful in identifying intersecting corridors or doorways.

Adaptations to assist in route retention or in asking for help from the public are important. Cassette tape players with tapes of clear verbal instructions of a route can be carried by more advanced students, using a "Walkman." The tape may assist the student by identifying such things as landmarks, street crossings, and bus numbers. The student who is nonverbal may use a route card with the printed questions that ask for assistance at particular crossing, i.e., "Please help me cross Main Street," or "I need to take the 104 uptown and get off at Main Street." The cards have a tactile cue so the student knows which card to use. The cards should be as subtle as possible. For the student with low vision, using a thick black marker on a white card has been proven to be successful. Picture cards have also been utilized with the student who has low vision and is also a non-reader.

As a result of increased technology, individuals who are visually impaired are benefiting from electronic travel aids (ETAs) (see Warren, Horn, & Hill, Chapter 11, this volume). Some of these aids have potential use with the student with multiple handicaps. The Pathsounder, developed by Linsay Russell, is a small battery-operated sonar device that is chest mounted, and that warns the user of objects within the path of travel. The feedback is both auditory and tactile, through vibrations in a neckstrap. The Pathsounder has been used with students who are deaf-blind and students who are in a wheelchair.

Nurion Industries have recently developed a new ETA, the Polarion, a compact, hand-held or chest-mounted aid for persons with visual impairments. It detects objects at various ranges and emits a sound or vibrates. The chest mount or a headband sensor mount make it useful for persons using walkers, crutches, or wheelchairs, or for persons who are deaf-blind.

A more sophisticated technological advancement that enhances the mobility of students who are in wheelchairs is the Nurion Step-Forward device. This electronic aid utilizes ultrasonic and laser technology to provide the user with advance information about the environment. The sensor will detect obstacles and drop-offs in the path of the student.

The Mowat Sensor is another simple ETA that is hand-held and has a vibrating output. This is used as a secondary aid with the long cane to locate doorways, obstacles, other landmarks, and pedestrians.

For the student with a hearing loss in one ear, adaptations can be made such as having the student walk on the side of the street with his or her good ear to the traffic. Wearing thin-soled shoes assists in obtaining more tactile input while traveling. It is also important to understand how the use of a hearing aid seriously distorts sound localization abilities, especially in loud traffic and in inclement weather. An effort must be made to accommodate for the impact of the hearing loss.

Both programmatic and material adaptations should be specified and included in the instructional program. Generating functional adaptations and modifications of O&M teaching strategies and techniques for the student with multiple handicaps has only recently begun. With the increase in technology, future optimism for increased independence is justified.

SUMMARY

A model has been presented for the development of programs to teach O&M skills to students with severe multiple handicaps. Data documenting the use of this model can be found in Gee and Goetz (1985).

Five main factors are important in implementing the model. First, instruction is provided at times across the day when travel is necessary in order to participate in particular activities. Not all of the activities must be exceedingly motivating; however, the activities should not be unpleasant or aversive to the student. The presumed motivation for travel is the expectation of a change in activity. This method is in contrast to mobility instruction provided in isolation for a 45-minute period per day. A transdisciplinary approach is inherent to the model. Following a collaborative effort in program development, the O&M instructor provides continued inservice and feedback to the classroom teacher and staff regarding O&M techniques and performance criteria. The classroom teacher provides continued input on instructional strategies, data analysis, and performance criteria.

The second factor is the selection of a minimum of four different routes for instruction distributed across the student's day. Given class size and availability of staff for the assistance required during initial route travel, teachers are often unable to practice travel skills during every activity or every time the student needs to travel to another location. By choosing four routes for systematic instruction, however, students learn basic skills, can generalize those skills to new routes, and learn four travel routes as well.

Third, instruction is provided on a systematic basis with experimentally validated operant teaching procedures. All staff should be taught the same O&M procedures in order to provide consistent delivery of cues, prompts, and reinforcement. Instruction is delivered without the reliance on verbal instructions typically used by O&M instructors for students with only a visual disability.

The fourth important aspect of the instructional method is the selection of skills for instruction within long chains of travel. By starting with just one skill and assisting the student on all other aspects of the route, the teacher maintains a level of expectations established in the context instruction phase, while providing periodic opportunities along each route for the student to perform in order for travel to continue. As the first skill reaches criterion, the second skill is added, and so on through the program. This facilitates the acquisition of generalizable skills as well as functional, purposeful travel routes.

The fifth factor to remember is the context instruction phase. While the current data (Gee & Goetz, 1985) preclude a definitive analysis of the role of context instruction, a number of points merit speculation. Mobility skills can be divided into three very general categories. The first is the basic movement skills that involve performance of the behaviors required for travel (such as trailing, cane techniques, stairs, etc.). These skills are generalizable to all travel and mobility routes. Second, there are the skills related to memory, discrimination, and other sensory and conceptual abilities that, while generalizable on a schematic level, are also specific in performance to each route (e.g., markers designating where to turn to find a particular classroom). These skills could also be described as skills related to the *initiation* of mobility behavior. Most non-sighted travelers without other disabilities require some preview of a mobility route (e.g., tactile map, verbal directions and/or a certain number of practice runs) and an understood destination, prior to independent performance (Strelow, 1985). Because many students with severe handicaps may not understand tactile maps, verbal directions, or other concepts related to position and direction, context instruction provides them with the similar information—a destination and some initial reason for movement. After the initial objectives in the study by Gee and Goetz (1985) were met, context instruction was used as a method for introducing new routes in which the students easily generalized basic movement skills.

The third category of O&M skills—problem solving skills (i.e., responding to unanticipated changes in a route)—has not been discussed in this chapter. While these skills also relate to the ability to remember and use various strategies, they pose a particular challenge to many students with severe intellectual disabilities. One area of future research might focus on this aspect of O&M instruction. Indeed, more research into O&M instruction for this population is needed. With the introduction of the community-based model, most students will be expected to function within an increasing number of environments.

In conclusion, current curriculum models make the learning of O&M skills a necessary and important goal for all students. Continued research and program development in this field will advance knowledge of this field. The model presented above is somewhat complex. Data have demonstrated, however, the effectiveness of both natural contexts and the periodic placement of instructional trials within the travel route. Future research may also provide new adaptations which will make traveling even more efficient.

Further efforts directed at the development of transdisciplinary service delivery models will also provide O&M instructors and teachers with methods to serve most effectively students with severe multiple handicaps within variable school and community settings. The combination of the disciplines of O&M instructors and educators working with students with the most severe handicaps will, no doubt, produce new and innovative instructional and service delivery models.

REFERENCES

Bachman, J.C. (1961). Specificity vs. generality in learning and performing two large motor tasks. *Research Quarterly, 32,* 3–11.

Baumgart, D., Brown, L., Pumpian, I., Nisbet, J., Ford, A., Sweet, M., Messina, R., & Schroeder, J. (1982). Principle of partial participation and individualized adaptations in educational programs for severely handicapped students. *Journal of The Association for Persons with Severe Handicaps, 7,* 17–27.

Brown, L., Branston, M., Baumgart, D., Vincent, L., Falvey, M., & Schroeder, J. (1979). Using the characteristics of current and subsequent least restrictive environments in the development of curricular content for severely handicapped students. *AAESPH Review, 4,* 407–424.

Brown, L., Nisbet, J., Ford, A., Sweet, M., Shiraga, B., York, R., & Loomis, R. (1983). The critical need for nonschool instruction in educational programs for severely handicapped students. *Journal of The Association for Persons with Severe Handicaps, 8,* 71–77.

Bryant, N.W., & Jansen, W. (1980). Topic: The mentally retarded visually impaired person. In R. Welsh & B. Blasch (Eds.), *Foundations of orientation and mobility* (pp. 452–459). New York: American Foundation for the Blind.

Caton, H.R. (1977). The development of a tactile analog to the Boehm test of basic concepts. *Journal of Visual Impairment and Blindness, 71,* 382–386.

Cratty, B., & Sams, T. (1968). *Body-image of blind children.* New York: American Foundation for the Blind.

Eisenberg, R.A. (1979). *Orientation and mobility.* Unpublished manual. California State University, Los Angeles.

Folio, M.R., & Fewell, R.R. (1983). *Peabody Developmental Motor Scales and Activity Cards.* Allen, TX: DLM Teaching Resources.

Ford, A. (1983). *The performance of moderately and severely handicapped students in the community as a function of the cue available and the antecedent vs. consequential teaching procedures used.* Unpublished doctoral dissertation, University of Wisconsin, Dept. of Behavioral Disabilities, Madison, WI.

Ford, A., & Mirenda, P. (1984). Community instruction: A natural cues and corrections decision model. *Journal of The Association for Persons with Severe Handicaps, 9,* 79–88.

Foulke, E. (1971). The perceptual basis for mobility. *Research Bulletin of the American Foundation for the Blind, 23,* 1–8.
Gamble, S.M. (1980). Topic 6: The visually handicapped person with cerebral palsy. In R. Welsh & B. Blasch (Eds.), *Foundations of orientation and mobility* (pp. 445–452). New York: American Foundation for the Blind.
Gee, K., & Goetz, L. (1985). *Outcomes of instructing orientation and mobility across purposeful travel routes in natural environments.* Unpublished manuscript. San Francisco State University, Dept. of Special Education, San Francisco.
Gibson, J.J. (1979). *The ecological approach to visual perception.* Boston: Houghton Mifflin.
Goetz, L., Gee, K., & Sailor, W. (1985). Using a behavior chain interruption strategy to teach communication skills to students with severe disabilities. *Journal of The Association for Persons with Severe Handicaps, 10,* 21–30.
Goetz, L., Schuler, A., & Sailor, W. (1983). Motivational considerations in teaching language to severely handicapped students. In M. Hersen, V. Van Hasselt, & J. Matson (Eds.), *Behavior therapy for the developmentally and physically disabled* (pp. 57–77). New York: Academic Press.
Guess, D., & Helmstetter, E. (1986). Skill cluster instruction and the individualized curriculum sequencing model. In R. Horner, L. Meyer, & B. Fredericks (Eds), *Education of learners with severe handicaps: Exemplary service strategies* (pp. 221–250). Baltimore: Paul H. Brookes Publishing Co.
Hapeman, L. (1967). Developmental concepts of blind children between the ages of three and six as they relate to orientation and mobility. *International Journal for the Education of the Blind, 17,* 41–48.
Haring, N., Liberty, K., & White, O. (1980). Rules for data based strategy decisions in instructional programs: Current research and instructional implications. In W. Sailor, B. Wilcox, & L. Brown (Eds.), *Methods of instruction for severely handicapped students* (pp. 159–190). Baltimore: Paul H. Brookes Publishing Co.
Harley, R.K., Henderson, F.M., & Wood, T.A. (1975). The development of a scale in orientation and mobility for multiply impaired blind children. *Education of the Visually Handicapped, 7,* 1–5.
Harley, R., Wood, T., & Merbler, J. (1975). Programmed instruction in orientation and mobility for multiply impaired blind children. *The New Outlook for the Blind, 69,* 419–422.
Harley, R., Wood, T., & Merbler, J. (1980). An orientation and mobility program for multiply impaired blind children. *Exceptional Children, 46,* 326–331.
Harrell, R., & Rosenberg, R. (1986). *Best practices in orientation and mobility for individuals who are multihandicapped vision impaired.* Unpublished manuscript, California State University, Los Angeles, and Whittier Union High School District, California.
Haynes, U., Patterson, G., D'Wolf, N., Hutchison, D., Lowry, M., Schilling, M., & Siepp, J.M. (1976). *Staff development handbook: A resource for the transdisciplinary process.* New York: United Cerebral Palsy Association, Inc.
Hill, E.W. (1981). *The Hill performance test of selected positional concepts.* Chicago, IL: Stoelting Company.
Hill, E., & Blasch, B. (1980). Concept development. In R. Welsh & B. Blasch (Eds.), *Foundations of orientation and mobility.* New York, American Foundation for the Blind.
Hill, E., & Ponder, P. (1976). *Orientation and mobility techniques: A guide for the practitioner.* New York: American Foundation for the Blind.
Kay, L. (1974). A sonar aid to enhance spatial perception of the blind. *The Radio and Electronic Engineer, 44,* 605–627.
Langley, M.B. (1980). *Functional vision inventory.* Chicago, IL: Stoeling Company.

Lolli, D. (1980). Topic 5: Deaf-blind persons. In R. Welsh & B. Blasch (Eds.), *Foundation of orientation and mobility*. New York: American Foundation for the Blind.

Lyon, S., & Lyon, G. (1980). Team functioning and staff development: A role release approach to providing integrated educational services for severely handicapped students. *Journal of The Association for Persons with Severe Handicaps, 5,* 250–263.

Merbler, J., & Wood, T.A. (1984). Predicting orientation and mobility proficiency in mentally retarded visually impaired children. *Education and Training of the Mentally Retarded, 19,* 228–230.

Miller, H. (1982). Relationship between mobility level and development of positional concepts in visually impaired children. *Journal of Visual Impairment and Blindness, 78,* 149–152.

Minsky, M. (1975). A framework for representation knowledge. In P. H. Winch (Ed.), *The psychology of computer vision* (pp. 211–280). New York: McGraw-Hill.

Morse, K.A. (1980). Modifications of the long cane for use by a multiply impaired child. *Journal of Visual Impairment and Blindness, 74,* 15–18.

Rieser, A., Gruth, T.S., & Hill, B.W. (1982). Mental processes mediating independent travel: Implications for orientation and mobility. *Journal of Visual Impairment and Blindness, 76,* 212–218.

Sailor, W., & Guess, D. (1983). *Severely handicapped students: An instructional design*. Boston: Houghton Mifflin.

Sailor, W., Halvorsen, A., Anderson, J., Goetz, L., Gee, K., Doering, K., & Hunt, P. (1986). Community intensive instruction. In R. Horner, L. Meyer & H.D.B. Fredericks (Eds.), *Education of learners with severe handicaps: Exemplary service strategies* (pp. 251–288). Baltimore: Paul H. Brookes Publishing Co.

Shingledecker, C.A., & Foulke, E. (1978). A human factors approach to the assessment of the mobility of blind pedestrians. *Human Factors, 20,* 273–286.

Singer, R. (1966). Interlimb skill ability in motor skill performance. *Research Quarterly, 37,* 406–410.

Snell, M. (1983). *Systematic instruction of the severely and moderately handicapped*. Columbus OH: Charles E. Merrill.

Snell, M., & Browder, D. (1986). Community referenced instruction: Research and issues. *Journal of The Association for Persons with Severe Handicaps, 11,* 1–11.

Snell, M, & Gast, D. (1981). Applying time delay procedure to the instruction of the severely handicapped. *Journal of The Association for Persons with Severe Handicaps, 6,* 3–14.

Stokes, T., & Baer, D. (1977). An implicit technology of generalization. *Journal of Applied Behavior Analysis, 10,* 349–367.

Strelow, E.R. (1985). What is needed for a theory of mobility: Direct perception and cognitive maps—lessons from the blind. *Psychological Review, 92,* 226–248.

Swallow, R., Mangold, S., & Mangold, P. (1977). *Informal assessment of developmental skills for visually handicapped students* (AFB Practice Report). New York, NY: American Foundation for the Blind.

Touchette, P. (1971). Transfer of stimulus control: Measuring the moment of transfer. *Journal of the Experimental Analysis of Behavior, 15,* 347–354.

Webb, R.C. (1969). Sensory motor training of the profoundly retarded. *American Journal of Mental Deficiency, 74,* 283–295.

Welsh, R.D., & Blasch, B. (Eds.). (1980). *Foundation of orientation and mobility*. New York: American Foundation for the Blind.

Wurzburger, P. (1980). Wurzburger Mobility Aids. 3960 Cottonwood Drive, Concord, CA 94519.

CHAPTER 7

Integrated Programming for Students with Multiple Handicaps

Philippa H. Campbell

AN INCREASING NUMBER of students entering the educational system have multiple handicaps characterized by combinations of disorders of the motor and sensory systems. An increase of 7,000 students with multiple handicaps was reported to Congress by state departments of education between 1980 and 1985. The largest annual changes have occurred over the past three years, with an approximate 10% increase in numbers of children reported in each of those years (*Seventh Annual Report to Congress,* 1985).

Several trends account for this increase. The first is the increasing incidence of children with multiple handicaps, due to the greater number of low birth weight infants who survive the neonatal period (e.g., Grady, 1985). These survivors are likely to be either without significant handicaps or severely and multiply involved (Robertson & Finer, 1985). The second is that the types of multiply handicapping conditions are changing due to medical practices of neonatal care. For example, increases in the numbers of children with combined motor handicap and visual impairment have been documented (e.g., Fitzhardinge & Pape, 1982). This increase appears to be related to required treatments for respiratory difficulties that place an infant at risk for developing neonatal retinopathy (Hoyt, Nickel, & Billson, 1982; Pornat, 1984). A third trend is an increasing sophistication in the identification and diagnosis of sensory impairment with infants and difficult-to-test children. Disorders of both structural and functional vision and hearing are now more easily and reliably identified, resulting in more precise classification of children as having multiple handicaps (Griffiths, 1979).

Teachers and related service personnel, for the most part, have not been adequately trained to develop programming for children with combined disorders (Smith-Davis, Burke, & Noel, 1984). For example, a physical therapist may be skilled at providing intervention to enhance motoric functioning in a child with cerebral palsy, but may have limited skills in mobility training for children with visual impairment. Students with unique combinations of disorders in the motor and sensory systems require individualized methods of instruction. Expertise from a number

Partial support for the preparation of this chapter was provided through the Office of Education, Office of Special Education and Rehabilitation Services, Innovative Programs for Severely Handicapped (G008302839) and for Deaf Blind (G008430095) awarded to the Children's Hospital Medical Center of Akron.

of different disciplines must be shared and integrated to develop instructional methods that are appropriate for each student's unique learning needs. The purpose of this chapter is to present a model of integrated motor programming for students who have multiple handicaps. The model utilizes the expertise of parents and multidisciplinary professionals to design and implement programming that synthesizes a variety of strategies to teach students various functional skills.

DISCREPANCIES IN POSTURE AND MOVEMENT

Students with multiple handicaps may have disorders in sensory and/or motor functioning. The extent of damage to brain tissue during birth and the neonatal period, as well as the location(s) of that damage, establish the basis of the motor impairment. Visual and auditory impairments may occur as the result of damage to the brain, the optic or auditory nerves, or the visual and auditory structures themselves. Some sensory impairments occur at birth, while others are secondary to other events. The term *impairment* describes actual changes in the physical structures of the body. The extent to which these impairments become disabilities or handicaps, however, is dependent on the ways in which those impairments are managed—medically, educationally, and therapeutically. The management of posture and movement of a student may also significantly affect the level of disability. Most disorders of the motor system are the result of interactive relationships among several factors—the type of damage sustained by the child, the ways in which people respond, situations in the environment, and the interaction of all these factors with the sensory impairment will all influence the degree of functional disability demonstrated by a student (Campbell, 1986; S. Campbell, 1984).

Sensory Impairment

Children with auditory impairment alone acquire posture and movement skills within normal limits when compared with children without handicaps, demonstrating no disability in the area of motor functioning (Simeonsson, Huntington, Short, & Ware, 1982). Children with visual impairment demonstrate differences in posture and movement when their development is compared with that of children without handicaps (Adelson & Fraiberg, 1974; Fraiberg, 1977). Longitudinal studies indicate that children with visual impairment demonstrate significant delay in performing those skills that involve movement through space, but acquire postural control at ages comparable to children without handicaps (Adelson & Fraiberg, 1974; Fewell & Sandall, 1983; Zinkin, 1979). A child with visual impairment alone would be expected to learn to sit independently without delay, but would show significant delays in crawling and walking.

Differences in the development of posture and movement skills that can be predicted in children with visual impairment must be considered when developing programming for students with both movement and visual system disorders. Programming must take into account impairment in both areas of functioning. For example, a child without visual impairment may be allowed to reach and contact an object with a fisted hand. A child with visual impairment must learn to move the arm in space and to contact the object with an open hand. The child with intact vision can use the eyes to identify the object. The child without good vision is dependent on tactile information for object location and identification.

Muscle Tone

The primary disorder in deficient posture and movement involves muscle tone, the mechanism used to control tension in the muscle fibers (e.g., Bobath & Bobath, 1984; S. Campbell, 1984; Scrutton, 1984). Low birth weight infants are often born with low postural tone, or *hypotonia* (Prechtl & Nolte, 1984). Hypotonia is also characteristic of many chromosomal disorders, such as trisomy 21 or Down syndrome (Coleman, 1981). Children who demonstrate developmental delay in the early childhood years are also often mildly hypotonic (Molnar, 1982). However, full-term infants who have undergone severe neonatal asphyxia are more likely to demonstrate increased postural tone, or *hypertonus*, as are infants who have undergone other major structural damage to brain tissue (Gorski, 1984).

The presence of tone discrepancies impedes a child's ability to produce the muscle contractions necessary to withstand the effects of gravity. Two basic types of muscle contractions are involved. Active contractions result when a muscle shortens, thereby creating movement at a specific body joint. Cocontractions of muscles support a body joint, holding the joint in position against gravity. Shortening of the elbow flexors produces an active movement, bending the arm at the elbow joint, whereby cocontraction of the muscles around the elbow supports and stabilizes the elbow joint, for example, when leaning on the arm. Muscle tone provides the background for active contractions of muscles. These contractions are coordinated by a process of reciprocal inhibition, a neurophysiological mechanism that allows for balanced activity between muscle groups (e.g., Bobath, 1980; Bobath & Bobath, 1984). When the elbow flexors, for example, shorten to bend the elbow, the elbow extensors lengthen to allow the shortening to occur. This process of continual balancing between muscle groups results in coordinated posture and movement skills. Discrepancies in muscle tone, in the production of muscle contractions, or in the balance between those contractions (reciprocal inhibition) will result in: a) delayed performance of posture and movement skills; b) poorly coordinated patterns of movement; or c) combined problems in both skill and pattern.

Posture and Movement

Normally coordinated movement occurs as a result of the functional integrity of a number of different factors that underly the production of movement (e.g., S. Campbell, 1984; Campbell, 1987b). Those factors that are of the greatest importance with students with impaired posture and movement include: a) muscle tone; b) muscle strength; c) endurance; d) range of movement at body joints; and e) motor planning. Dysfunction in any of these factors will directly influence the pattern of movement that is produced. For example, a student with shortened hip flexor muscles may be able to stand independently, but may be able to do so only in a bent forward position.

The shortened hip muscles prevent full hip straightening (extension), therefore altering the pattern of movement used to stand erect.

Posture and movement can be viewed from two separate but related perspectives. The first is *skill performance*. What gross and fine motor activities can an individual perform and with what levels of independence? The second perspective focuses on the *qualitative dimensions* of performance. How well does the individual perform the skill? Some students are unable to perform posture and movement skills. Others perform skills but do so in unconventional (or abnormal) ways, using poorly coordinated patterns of muscular activity (Campbell, 1987a, 1987b; Campbell & Stewart, 1986). These unconventional patterns are due to atypical muscle tone in combination with the presence of one or more secondary factors (e.g., limited strength; motor planning) that affect the production of movement.

Students with a variety of problems may demonstrate delay in performance of posture and movement *skills*. Delayed acquisition is attributable to discrepancies in muscle tone (e.g., Bobath & Bobath, 1984; Wilson, 1984), to impaired vision (Adelson & Fraiberg, 1974; Zinkin, 1979), and to other factors that influence performance. Posture and movement are a significant part of an infant's early development. The coordination of muscular activity necessary to perform numerous skills is acquired during the first two years of life. Some of these developmental skills are essential for adult functioning. Others have immediate usefulness for an infant or young child, but have less utility for adults (Egan, 1979). Reaching, for example, is critical for performance throughout life, while crawling is used temporarily by a young child to move around the environment. *Developmental* and *functional* are two terms that are frequently used to further describe skills. *Functional* skills are those that are critical for performance throughout life. *Developmental* skills are those demonstrated by infants and young children during their early years.

PROGRAMMING FOR PERFORMANCE OF ESSENTIAL AND ELABORATED SKILLS

Effective programming for students with multiple handicaps occurs when professionals of various disciplines, in cooperation with parents, integrate information to select functional learning objectives. A number of different professional disciplines are likely to be involved in the educational programs of students with multiple handicaps, due to their complex and often varied learning needs. Student goals are best determined by the team of professionals and parents as a group, rather than by each discipline in isolation from other professionals. Goals state the functional skills that are necessary and desirable for a student to learn in order to function as independently as possible as an adult. A total program plan (e.g., an individualized education program, or IEP) integrates the expertise of each discipline into goal selection and establishes the basis for programming activities that will be implemented by parents and professionals over a given time period.

Many individuals with multiple handicaps may not be able to learn a wide array of functional movement skills, due to the degree of impairment in the motor and sensory systems. However, the performance of a few *essential* functional skills can enable independent functioning as an adult. *Essential skills* are simple forms of behavior that are important in and of themselves, but that also provide the basis for elaborated (and more complex) forms of behavior. These skills include: (a) looking; (b) vocalization; (c) functional reach; (d) simple manipulation; and (e) combined manipulation (Campbell, Becker, & Gent, 1985). Essential and elaborated skills are programmed for within content areas and across contexts. An overview of the relationships of posture and movement skills to performance within various content areas is illustrated in Figure 1.

Most students require programming in one or more of the following content domains: 1) communication; 2) environmental problem solving; 3) mobility; 4) social skills; 5) recreation leisure; 6) self management; and 7) occupational skills. Instruction in each of these domains may include activities that occur in a number of different *contexts*, including home, school, community, and work environments. The team involved in developing and implementing programming for a given student identifies both naturally-occurring and contrived activities that will be undertaken, and encourages use of the specified essential skill within those activities. Activities themselves are chronologically age appropriate, functional, and related to the domains being emphasized with a given student.

Upper Extremity Movement

Primary among critical movement skills is the use of the upper extremities for reaching activities. Upper extremity arm movements are components of numerous functional skills, as well as important movements used to overcome visual limitations. For example, a student who is unable to extend the arms will have difficulty locating objects around the body, or in using the arms for tracking when moving in a wheelchair. A nonverbal student who might communicate using object exchanges, or with an object or raised symbol communication board, will have difficulty if unable to extend the arms in reaching.

Many factors impede upper extremity movement in students with movement dysfunction. Muscle tone that is too low or too high may prevent a student from being able to reach at all. More often, however, a student may be able to move the arms, but will do so with compensatory or poorly coordinated patterns. A student may, for example, move the arms forward but not with fully extended elbows, or may be able to move the arm in one direction (e.g., frontwards) but not in other directions (e.g., backwards or sideways). Most reaching movements are performed against gravity. This means that students must have good strength and endurance in order to perform and sustain a reaching movement. Some students are able to reach out, but can only do so if the arm is supported so that the movement is not fully antigravity. For example, some students may be able to reach from a sidelying position, but are unable to reach from a sitting position in which movements are fully against gravity. Or, other students may be able to move their arms forward, but can only do so if the arms are supported by, for example, the wheelchair tray. Still other students may be able to

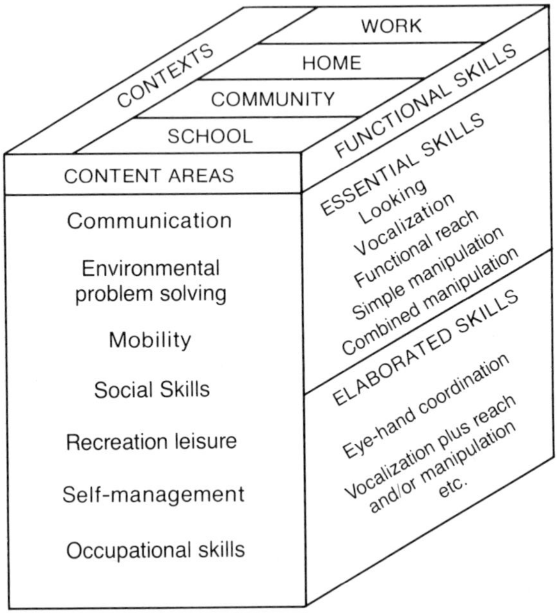

Figure 1. A guide for the selection of naturally occurring or continued activities.

perform the desired movement, but are unable to keep the arm in position for any length of time.

The shoulder girdle and upper extremities frequently become areas of compensation for students with low tone in the head and trunk muscles. Students may use the arms to support the trunk, either through shoulder girdle fixing to gain stabilization, or by leaning on the arms to gain extra support. In either of these situations, the arms are not available for reaching movements, and this is usually obvious when observing a student's posture and movement skills. However, the shoulder girdle and arms also may be used to support the head or the legs. One typical pattern that can be observed occurs when the shoulder girdle is elevated and perhaps tipped forward, bringing the arms behind the trunk. This pattern, while providing greater support for the head, also inhibits use of the arms for reaching since the arms are behind, rather than in front of, the trunk.

Manipulation

The purpose of most upper extremity movement is to *transport* the hands to a location for grasping and manipulation (Bower, 1979). Most assessment procedures used with students with various handicaps do not separate upper extremity, grasping, and manipulation skills, yet these divisions are important when planning programming for a student with combined sensory and motor impairments. Most functional activities can be performed by holding or grasping an object. Fewer skills require actual manipulation of an object with the hands. A student can eat independently using a grasping pattern to hold utensils; however buttoning, for example, requires manipulation of the button with the fingers. Some objects can be identified simply by holding them in the hand, but smaller or more detailed objects may require movement in the hand (manipulation) to provide the sensory information necessary for identification.

Access to the environment for a student with visual impairments comes from tactile and auditory stimuli. Auditory stimuli, without accompanying visual information, are elusive, particularly for an infant or young child. Sounds exist only for a moment in time and are typically made more interpretable through accompanying facial expression, gestures, or objects that are not available to the child who has a significant visual disability (e.g., Egan, 1979). Touch can compensate for unobservable visual information. An object that cannot be seen can be felt. The boundaries of an environment—the floors, walls, or doors—are identified through the use of movement leading to tactile exploration. For these reasons, a child who has both significant visual and motoric disabilities must be guided, using therapeutically correct procedures, to use upper extremity movement, grasping, and manipulation to the best advantage.

Grasping and manipulation skills may be inhibited if the student has either extremely high or extremely low postural tone. High tone often results in hands that are fisted and difficult to open. Students with low tone may have open hands, but may be unable to grasp objects or to hold onto them for any length of time, and manipulation abilities are either severely limited or absent. Fisted hands, in particular, are especially problematic if a student also has visual disabilities. The student may be able to reach with the arms and contact an object. However, little information about the properties of the object can be gained when contact is made with fisted hands; in essence, most objects have similar physical properties when contacted with closed hands.

Eye-Hand Coordination

The relationship between limited visual functioning and upper extremity movement is especially crucial. For example, a student may only be able to see an object if it is placed 4 inches from the face at midline. However, this same student may only be able to reach forward with the left arm in front of the left side of the body. Such a student can, in essence, reach where vision is not possible and see where reaching is not possible. Other students may be able to reach when the influences of gravity are eliminated, when, for example, the arms are supported by the tray, but also may only be able to see an object placed at face level. The interaction between visual and movement abilities is often more complicated that either problem in isolation. The limited compensatory function of the arms must be increased through programming, as must the limited visual functioning range, depending upon the nature of the visual disorder.

PROGRAMMING FOR UPPER EXTREMITY MOVEMENT

Upper extremity movement used for reaching in all directions away from the body (e.g., front, side, back) is critical for students with both visual and movement dysfunction. Frontwards reach, using a pattern of shoulder flexion with elbow extension and an open hand, is an especially important movement pattern. Performance of this pattern enables a student with visual dysfunction to search and locate objects that are in front of the body, as well as to perform most functional skills that require interaction with objects (e.g., self feeding, brushing hair or teeth, performing vocational tasks). A sideways reaching pattern is also important, but is most useful for tracking during mobility, whereas backwards reaching is less useful, especially for students who use wheelchairs. There are few effective alternate strategies for absent or limited upper extremity movements. In some instances, head or leg movements can be used. These are frequently difficult to perform, restricted in their usefulness, and poor substitutes for limited arm use. Therefore, every effort must be directed to enabling a student to use arm movement functionally.

Desired Movement Pattern

A sequence of assessment concerns and treatment goals that specifically relate to the motor components involved in enabling a student to perform upper extremity movements is illustrated in Figure 2. The steps include: 1) positioning to attain postural alignment; 2) therapeutic procedures to instate proper upper extremity movement; 3) therapeutic procedures to shape existing movement into more normally coordinated patterns; 4) modification of visual aspects of the task, including attention to object characteristics and placement, and involving the assistance of the vision specialist; and 5) incorporation of motivating outcomes to encourage reaching, calling upon the expertise of the parent and teacher. Each of these steps must be included in the intervention sequence for students with significant dysfunction in the motor system.

Appropriate intervention methods are designed by *integrating* programming strategies from physical and occupational therapy with those from education. Therapeutic strategies are more likely to enable a student to generate the desired pattern. The educational strategies integrate information specific to teaching students with visual impairment, as well as information that will encourage the development of a functional use of the movement patterns.

Functional Use of Movement

Performing the desired upper extremity movements is only one aspect of using functional reaching skills in the environment. The arm movement must result in contact with the object and, in some functional activities, in either grasping or holding. Figure 3 outlines a lattice for the functional use of forward reaching patterns (Campbell et al., 1985; Campbell & Wilcox, 1986). This lattice is designed to provide guidelines for adults who are identifying situations in which students can use forward reaching patterns in a variety of instructional contexts. Some examples of instructional activities are included in Table 1. Reaching can be required in many naturally occurring situations, or adults can contrive situations in which reaching can be practiced. For example, with a student who was working on the second step of the lattice, adults

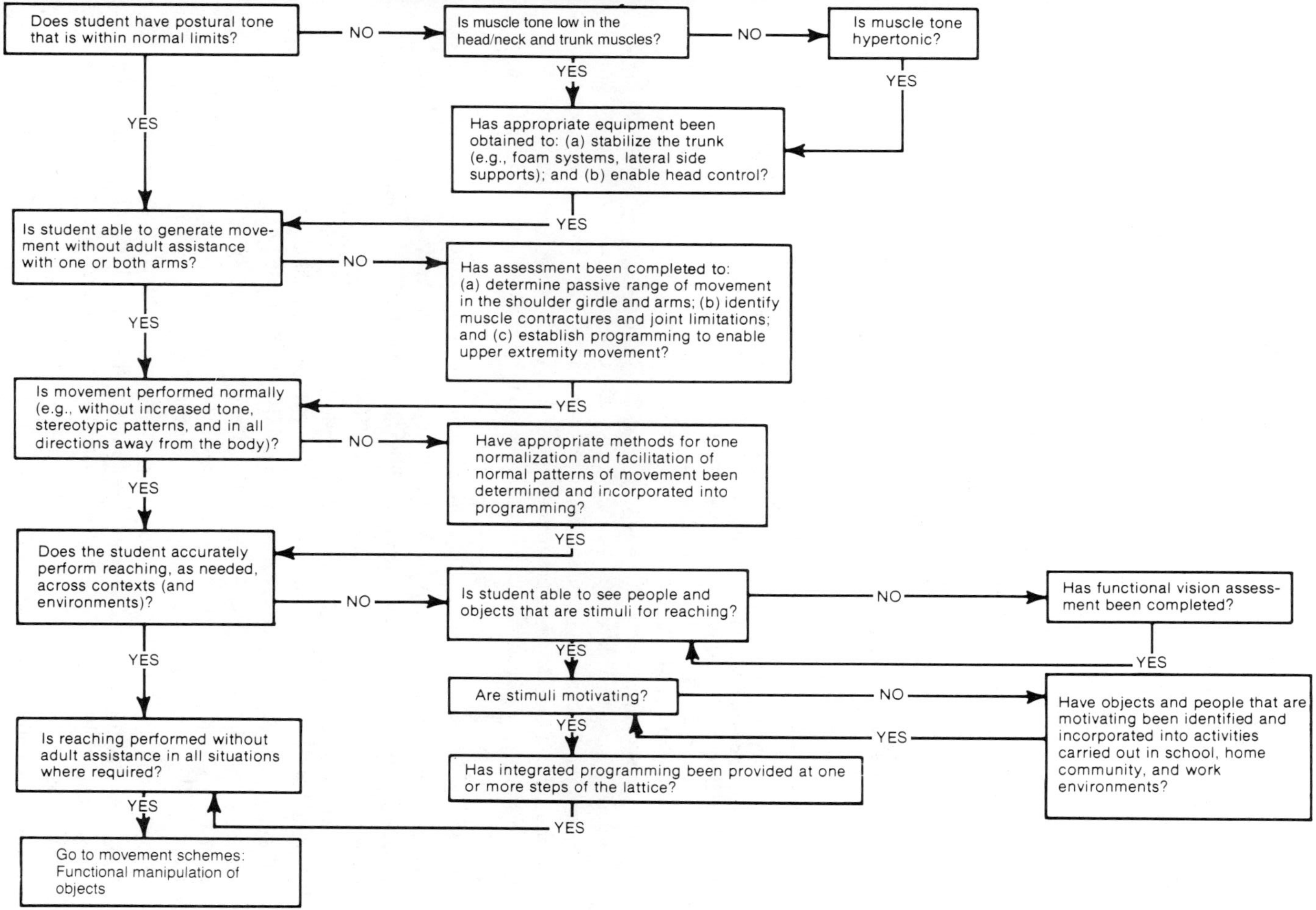

Figure 2. Appropriate intervention steps for teaching students to perform upper extremity movement.

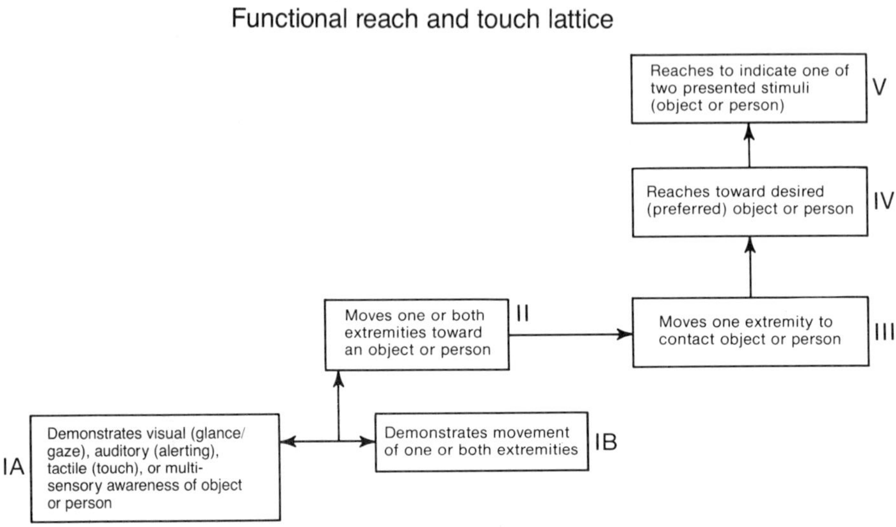

Figure 3. A diagram of the steps necessary to train forward reaching with the upper extremities, to provide guidance in selecting basic levels of required response to be incorporated into activities carried out at school, home, work, and in various community environments.

could require forward reach toward an instructional material needed in a particular activity, the spoon or cup when eating, or an adult (to signal to be lifted and/or for attention.) The actual activities in which forward reaching may be required are dependent on the contexts of instruction, the chronological age level of the student, and the content emphases in programming for a given student. (See Nietupski & Hamre-Nietupski, Chapter 9, this volume, for environmental inventory strategies to identify contexts for instruction.)

Eye-hand coordination is critical to functional reaching. The visual stimuli used in programming must be carefully selected on the basis of three dimensions: 1) functionality; 2) motivational properties; and 3) visual properties. Every dimension will not have to be systematically selected for each student. Activities provide the context for teaching functional use of reach. However, the activities themselves, or the materials used in those activities, may be functional but may not be motivating enough for some students. Programmers will need to establish the response first, using motivating materials, and then switch to materials that are functionally related to the programming activities being used. For example, some students are only motivated by food. Food is a functional motivator if the situation is mealtime, but is less functional as part of a mobility or work task. Two approaches can be taken in situations of this type. The reaching response (toward food) may be trained only during eating situations. This response, once established toward food, can then be required in less motivating circumstances. For example, a student might be required to reach forward and touch a switch to activate a motorized vehicle. The training might occur on the way to the cafeteria, thus allowing food to remain a functional motivator. A second approach, in a situation such as this, is to provide food as a motivator even if it is not immediately part of the training situation. For example, a student might be given food as a reward for activating a switch correctly. Ideally, most materials used to motivate a response can be made both functional and motivating. These materials would be used in programming before resorting to the use of materials with little functional relevance within the programming activity.

Objects and materials used with students having visual impairments must also be selected on the basis of visual properties. Functional vision inventories (such as that designed by Langley and DuBose, 1976) can provide important information about object properties. These include: a) placement; b) size and shape; c) color and pattern; d) room light and placement of the object in relation to lighting; and e) relevant cues (such as noise or movement). These dimensions, as well as others, will define the conditions under which a given student can see the object or materials toward which reach is being directed. These objects must also be functional and motivating. Objects that a student may be able to visually discriminate may not be motivating, or may be functionally inappropriate within the programming situation. However, the purpose of programming is to establish the critical skill of reaching. For this reason, a student should be initially trained to reach toward motivating materials that are appropriate in terms of their visual characteristics, even if these objects are not functionally related to an activity.

Discrepancies sometimes occur between the conditions under which a student can reach toward an object, and conditions under which that student can see objects or programming materials. For example, a student may be able only to reach toward the left side, but may best view objects when they are placed on the right side. Unique solutions to these discrepancies must be worked out by team members. The therapy program for a student who could only reach toward the left might emphasize teaching those movement components necessary to reach across the midline to the right side. Specifically, these might include: a) sideways weight shift across the hips (base of support) in sitting; and b) sideways movement (adduction) of the arm across the front of the body.

Another common difficulty is that students may be able to best view an object that is placed, for example, at midline, 8 inches away from the face, but may be unable to produce the antigravity arm movement required to reach at face level. Several solutions for this incompatibility are possible. For example, the surface on which an object is placed, such as a wheelchair tray or a table in front of a student, could be raised to shoulder level. The required movement of the upper extremities, with the tray at this height, minimizes the effects of gravity and makes the movement response easier to perform. Or a sidelying position might be used initially to develop the reaching pattern. In sidelying, the arm is not moving against the full influence of gravity, again making the movement response easier. An active therapeutic intervention program could be implemented to: a) develop extension in the upper back with stability

Table 1. Matrix of activities by domains for functional/reach lattice

Behavior		Communication	Environmental problem solving	Mobility	Recreation and leisure	Self-management	Social
IA.	Demonstrates visual, auditory, tactile or multisensory awareness of object or person.	Place a multisensory object (e.g. rattle, toy piano, vibrator, in child's hand. Facilitate exploration of item slowly. Initially use a familiar set of items (e.g. 5 items).	Use objects with a variety of textures, shapes and sounds (i.e. bristle blocks, velcro, flattened aluminum foil, bells, rattles, etc.) Place child's hand on object, and facilitate hand movement or explore objects.	Hang cradle gym above child's chair, within close proximity. Dangling items should be close enough for hand/arm contact through random movements.	Hang lullaby mobile over child's resting area & at a position to facilitate visual gaze. Use this activity at a time when the child is alert and rested.	When child is eating, present food items for child to smell, feel, and taste (where possible).	Play interactive games such as patty cake, peek-a-boo, and tickle-bee. Adult facilitates child's participation.
IB.	Demonstrates movement of one or both extremities.	Using multisensory toys, place item at child's midline. Respond to movement as if it were a request, and give child the toy.	Fasten a bright noisemaker (e.g. rattle) on child's hand. Vary hand of noisemaker. Movement will result in sound.	Hang a dangling object with noisemaker attached (i.e. scarf with bells sewn on it). Place item close enough to be kicked by foot or reached by hand movement. When child moves extremity, adult ensures noise and movement of hanging object.	Position child on a small trampoline. Any movement of extremities should be felt by slight bouncing of the trampoline.	Provide opportunity for finger feeding. When child moves extremity, provide refreshment.	Play peek-a-boo using a transparent scarf. With movement of extremity, adult lifts scarf and "peeks;" alternate turns with adult hiding face too.
II.	Moves one or both extremities toward an object/person.	Play "Up-Up-and-Away" When child reaches toward person—he or she is picked-up and	Hide a multisensory toy under a towel. When extremity is moved toward hidden object,	Before moving child from one location to another (e.g. to high chair for lunch), wait for	Use a switch set up to activate a toy. Guide child's hand to hit switch several times. After guides,	During dressing activities, child moves extremity towards clothing item (placed in front of	Position child near a docile pet (e.g., cat, dog, or if necessary a stuffed animal). Child

		swung through the air. Repeat sequence.	remove towel. Interact with child around the toy. Repeat hiding sequence.	movement of extremities.	adult activates switch when child initiates movement.	child), then item is put on.	should be close enough to contact animal even when extremity is moved.
III.	Moves one extremity to contact object/person.	See IB Contact required.	Stack blocks up. When child contacts objects, they will fall. Repeat at sequence (if done on table, falling blocks will make noise).	Adult reaches hands out to child. When child contacts adult's hand, child's movement to a new location is facilitated as necessary.	See above. Child must now contact switch for activation.	During washing (before meals), position child to contact faucet, soap, towels before using each item.	Child touches body part on another person; the interactor locates the same body part on the child (e.g. child touches adult's foot; adult finds child's foot).
IV.	Reaches toward desired (preferred) object/person.	Place bright object just out of child's reach. When child contacts object, he or she can interact with adult around them.	Place desired object on a scarf out of reach of child. Child retrieves object by pulling scarf.	During play, place toys out of child's reach. When child reaches toward a desired object, adult facilitates (if necessary) child's movement toward object.	Use a switch to activate a preferred toy/object (e.g. record player).	Facilitate self-feeding. Child reaches and contacts bowl, utensil or actual food items.	Have collection of toys, a box, and another child. Present desired object for child to reach and contact. Task is to put objects into box, alternating turns between the children.
V.	Reaches to indicate one of two presented objects/persons.	Same as IV, two objects presented (should include objects that are bright and noisey).	Have two large containers (i.e. plastic container, box). Place an object in/under each of the containers. Child reaches to retrieve object of choice and lifts or knocks over container to obtain item.		Give child choice of toys/people to play with during free time activities (example TV or stereo).	During lunch, present choice of what child wants to drink, eat first, etc.	Have collection of dress-up items and several children. Child indicates which of two items he or she wants to wear. Children alternate turns and dress-up.

of the shoulder; and b) develop forward movement of the arm against varying influences of gravity.

Students with multiple handicaps that include severe visual impairment will not be able to acquire eye-hand coordination with upper extremity movement. An object or material is located by guiding the hand to a temporal sound source, or through tactile means that use tracking and searching strategies. Examples of programming for coordination of reaching with manipulation skills are provided in the discussion of manipulation in this chapter.

Programming Strategies

The framework for intervention activities designed to teach a student to perform a desired upper extremity skill is formed by determining as great a number of activities as possible that are content-based (e.g., communication; recreation leisure) and are performed within a variety of programming contexts. These activities may be naturally occurring or may be contrived (designed) by team members to provide students with opportunities to practice upper extremity movement. Most students with multiple handicaps will require *integrated* teaching methods in order to use functional reaching to interact with and receive information from the environment. These intervention strategies must integrate information needed for a student's unique learning needs. These needs will be dependent on the number of impairments present (e.g., motor, visual, auditory) as well as the degree of impairment in each area. Professionals of different disciplines should combine their knowledge with that of parents to develop strategies appropriate for the unique learning needs of each student.

A few general principles can be applied when determining appropriate programming strategies to use with a given student. Strategies that have been uniquely designed to respond to the individual needs of a student are most effective. However, the following general principles provide guidelines for developing integrated strategies:

1. *Positioning:* Make sure that the student is maximally positioned, especially with regard to the head and trunk musculature. Upper extremity movement may have come to be used by the student only to support the trunk (either by supporting on the arms/hands or posturally fixing in the shoulder girdle and arms) if the trunk is not adequately supported through external means.
2. *Postural Tone:* Determine whether tone is low or high in the shoulder girdle and upper extremities, as well as what environmental factors may cause tone to fluctuate. Sometimes the initiation of the movement (reaching) itself may cause tone to increase. Particular problems in the shoulder girdle often include low tone (even when tone in the arms is high). Intervention should focus on providing adequate stabilization while inhibiting abnormal stabilization patterns (such as elevated shoulders, forward tipping of the shoulders, and/or "winging" of the shoulder blades, all of which result in a rounding of the upper back and shoulders). Trained therapists can assist in determining appropriate intervention methods.

3. *Prompting Sequences:* A least-to-most prompting sequence (e.g., Lent, 1979) is often used to teach a student without major motor impairment to perform a desired movement. In this approach, a student is asked to perform the movement, is verbally or physically cued, and then finally manually guided, if performance does not occur. For many students with multiple handicaps, this sequence may not be the most appropriate, in that often the problem lies in the physical initiation of the movement rather than in lack of motivation. Students receive little consistent opportunity to independently initiate and perform a required movement when a least-to-most prompting sequence is used. Some students with multiple handicaps seem to learn that if they wait long enough, the response will be performed for them through manual guidance. The following alternatives have proven helpful in this situation:
   a. *"Priming":* A student who lacks sensory-motor awareness of a movement can be guided in the desired movement pattern, using appropriate therapeutic facilitation methods, for two or more guided trials before being asked to respond independently. Immediately following the guided series of trials, the student is asked to perform the movement without adult assistance. This procedure can be combined with systematic methods of fading so that all adult assistance is not necessarily dropped between the guided trials and independent performance (Campbell, Place, & Gossett, 1986).
   b. *Movement Cuing:* Movement cuing is a therapeutic facilitation procedure that capitalizes on automatic placing reactions that occur without conscious direction in the arms when muscle tone is within normal limits (e.g., Bobath, 1980; Campbell, 1987b; Campbell & Forsyth, 1986; Smith, 1986). The programmer guides the desired reaching movement by physically cuing the arm into the direction of the reach, moving from the shoulder area down into the hand. A variety of different means can be used to provide the cue. One example is to sweep the programmer's hand under the arm that is being cued, while moving the arm into the direction of the reach.
4. *Object Placement:* The placement of an object is critical when teaching a student to reach. The object must be visible to the student and/or made visible through auditory cues. Placement itself can be a viable cue for students with object permanence skills. Objects should be placed in the same location(s), in relation to the student's body, each time they are presented. This helps a student with visual impairment to know where the object is likely to be, an important initial consideration in learning to search for objects. Holding the object location constant for initial training minimizes the cognitive requirements of the reaching task for a student with severe visual impairment. In this situation, the student is required to search for an object where it was last found, a simple form of object permanence. Adaptive aids can be used to ensure maximal object placement. Devices such as slanted trays (with lips) can be used to bring objects into closer visual range at face level, and boards marked with masking tape help locate objects in the same place for each presentation.

Measuring Results

Baseline and intervention data are collected for all activities carried out with students with severe and multiple handicaps (e.g., Gaylord-Ross & Holvoet, 1985; Haring, Liberty, & White, 1980). These data are necessary for two reasons: 1) determining whether a particular method is effective in teaching a desired movement response to a student; and 2) documenting student progress. Many students are very challenging! Methods that integrate information from a variety of disciplines may still be ineffective with particular students due to their unique learning needs. Team members need to know that programming is or is not effective in order to make constructive decisions to enhance student acquisition of skills.

Data that were collected in a program designed to teach a student to reach are illustrated in Figure 4. Reaching performance was the focus of therapeutic programming, and was also trained during communication and within classroom activities. The student was reinforced for reaching toward an object or person in condition A. The object had to be contacted for the student to be reinforced in condition B. Reinforcement was both functional and social and consisted of an adult interacting with the student around the object (or person) that had been reached toward. Two different programming strategies were used. The first procedure relied on a least-to-most prompting sequence. Each trial in the second procedure was preceeded by two guided trials, using therapeutic procedures to normalize muscle tone and facilitate a normally coordinated pattern of reaching. Data were recorded for both reaches toward

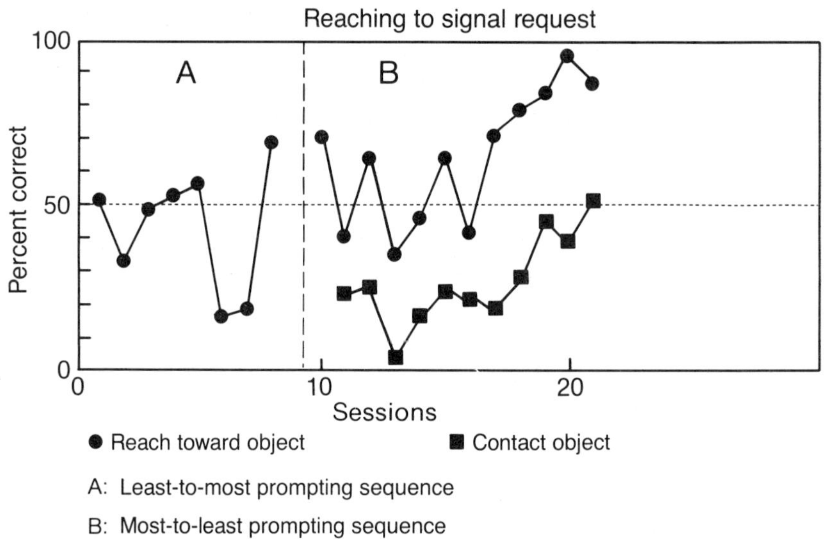

Figure 4. Effects of two different training procedures designed to teach a 3-year-old child (with visual, auditory, and severe movement impairment) to reach and contact an object as a nonverbal signal for request.

and contacts with the object during condition B. These data suggest that the second procedure was successful when used with this student.

PROGRAMMING FOR GRASP AND MANIPULATION SKILLS

Grasp and manipulation can be programmed for separately or in conjunction with upper extremity movement, after a student is able to reach toward an object or adult. Being able to both generate a movement toward an object and to contact the object are necessary before independent grasp and manipulation can be added (chained) to the sequence. Requiring both reach and grasp/manipulation can be too difficult for some students, as coordination of two different movement patterns is required. Lattices for simple and combined manipulation are illustrated in Figures 5 and 6. These lattices provide guidelines for teaching a student to perform specific movement responses with the hands and arms, and to use these movements for functional purposes.

The movements required for simple and combined manipulation have been described as *schemes* that are used for acting on objects in the environment (e.g., Piaget, 1952; Robinson & Robinson, 1983). Movement of the hand fulfills a variety of purposes, including: a) receipt of tactile and other sensory information; b) grasp (holding); c) simple manipulation of an object (e.g., opening a container or turning a doorknob); and d) environmental problem-solving through combinations of two or more different schemes (e.g., pushing a switch to turn on a communication device, then pushing a second switch to activate a voice synthesizer or a visual scanner). Performance of many functional skills requires only simple hand manipulation

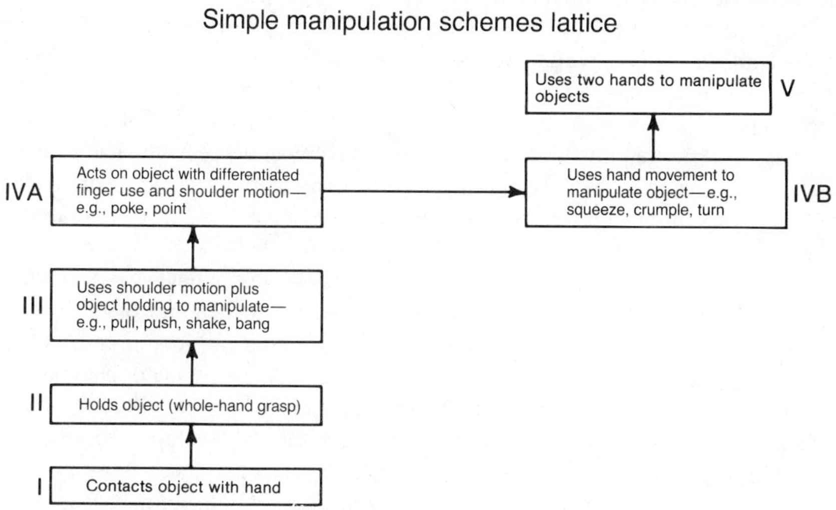

Figure 5. Several basic manipulation schemes required to interact with objects of different types are diagrammed on the basis of increasing levels of difficulty in motor coordination.

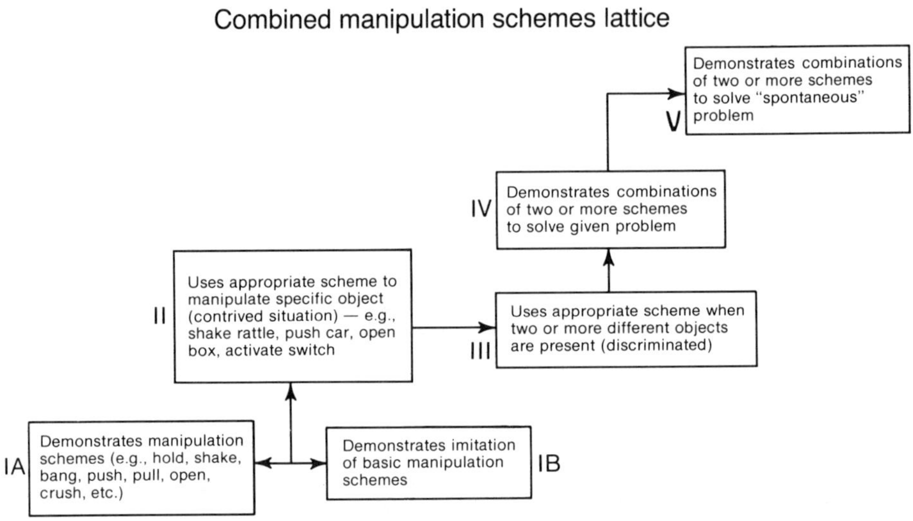

Figure 6. Combinations of movement schemes provide students with functional means to interact with objects in increasingly complex ways within various environments.

schemes, such as grasp, in combination with upper extremity movement. Complex fine motor abilities, requiring coordinated finger movements, are seldom possible for a student with severe impairment in posture and movement.

Desired Movement Pattern

The lattice for simple manipulation establishes steps for teaching a student to hold objects and to act on those objects using a variety of simple schemes. Programmers use this lattice as a guide with students who are unable to grasp and manipulate objects and/or who may have a repertoire of only one or two schemes for interacting with objects. The emphasis in simple manipulation is on the performance of a variety of movement patterns that involve some degree of movement of the hand. The extent to which these movements are used appropriately in relation to objects (e.g., functional manipulation) is not taken into account. Examples of activities that can be accomplished with simple manipulation schemes are provided in Table 2.

Students with severe movement dysfunction may be able to hold an object with a total hand (or palmar) grasp but may be unable to orient the hand for other forms of object contact (e.g., pincer grasp, between thumb and first finger, or pointing). Other students may use only one movement scheme, for example mouthing or banging, for every object with which they interact. All students need to be able to act on objects within a variety of environmental contexts, using a variety of simple manipulation schemes. Programmers are guided by the lattice to select and teach those types of simple manipulation schemes that a student can perform in both contrived and naturally occurring situations.

Many students with severe movement dysfunction may be unable to perform the finely coordinated movements of the hands and fingers necessary to acquire a wide variety of motorically coordinated and complex manipulation schemes. Holding (or grasping) an object, however, is possible for almost all students (or can be bypassed through use of adaptive aids, such as special spoons in feeding, or a flexion mitt with velcro to hold objects in the glove). Ideally, a student should be able to hold an object without an increase in muscle tone throughout the arm. Many students with hypertonus in the extremities, for example, grasp (or hold) an object using muscles in the whole arm. Grasping is accompanied by forward tipping of the shoulder, elbow (and sometimes wrist) flexion, and movement of the arm behind the trunk (or against a back support, if one is present that restricts arm movement). This pattern, while successful in holding an object, *inhibits* use of the arm for the movement required by the activity. For example, a student who grasps a spoon with this type of pattern is then not able to bring the spoon to the mouth, using a hand-to-mouth pattern, since the arm is behind, rather than in front of, the body. Grasping movements must be performed in isolation from total arm movement. For this reason, grasping seems to be best taught as the end component of a reaching chain. A student who can reach without assistance can be guided through the required manipulation. Or, a student can be guided through the reaching and required to perform the manipulation without assistance.

Some students, especially those with low muscle tone and poor stability in the upper back muscles, may have difficulty lifting objects once they are grasped. These students lack the strength and coordination to move the arm and the weight of the object against the influences of gravity. Activities can be modified, where possible, to use only lightweight objects for grasping. Therapy programs to strengthen the upper spine and back muscles and gain shoulder stability will be necessary to assist students such as these to hold objects of all weights.

Students with severe visual impairment will also need to use their hands to search for and locate objects in their immediate environments. Locating and searching are carried out with open hands, where possible, to provide a means for receiving information about the environment. Students can be taught to reach toward and locate an object that is placed in the same position each time. An ideal starting point for object placement is in front of and to the left of a student. This position forms the initial starting point for systematic searching, which typically occurs using a left-to-right searching pattern. Eventually, a student will use one arm and hand, crossing the body midline to search systematically from left to right to locate objects that are placed in unknown positions. Once located, an object would then be grasped or manipulated. Ideal searching patterns may not be possible for all students, depending on the degree of dysfunction in movement that may also be present in the shoulders and arms. Teachers and therapists who work with students with visual impairment will need to analyze the movement patterns present, as well as those required in searching, to develop patterns that can be functionally used by individual students.

Table 2. Matrix of activities by domains for simple manipulation

	Behavior	Communication	Environmental problem solving	Mobility	Recreation and leisure	Self-management	Social
I.	Contacts object with hand.	Hold mirror in front of child. As child touches mirror, comment on body part, "pointing" to it.	See Social II: Peek-a-boo with scarf.	Hold child on lap; when child makes contact with your arms, bounce child. Repeat.	Present child with a bright noisy roly-poly toy so that when child contacts the toy, a noise is produced.	During grooming activities, place items in front of child. When he or she contacts object, facilitate child's use of item (i.e., mirror, comb, brush).	Face exploration—facilitate child's exploration of own face and others' faces. Locate eyes, nose, mouth, hair, etc.
II.	Holds object (whole hand grasp).	Provide attention when child grasps object.	Adults holds out small object for child to grasp. Hands child a second object (transfer of hands/object).	Adult sits child on swing, aids to grasp the ropes. Push child a little.	Adult sits child on swing, aids to grasp the ropes. Push child a little.	Before and after meal times, child can use grasp for washing (e.g. grasp faucet, soap, washcloth, toothbrush, etc.).	Play peek-a-boo with scarf. Facilitate removal of scarf from child's face and adult's face when child grasps edge.
III.	Uses shoulder motion plus object holding to manipulate (e.g. pull, push, shake, bang).	Place push toy in front of child. When child reaches to object, adult aids child to push toy (e.g. large truck), other toys, busy box, pop-ups, toy piano.	Adult hides a cracker and a raisin in a container away from the child. Place container on a towel within child's reach. Child must pull towel to self to get to container.	Child sits or lies on floor with a truck. Child scoots to push truck with upper or entire body. May also use a ball.	Child holds two blocks and bangs in imitation of adult.	Child will participate in simple dressing and undressing tasks (e.g. pull off shoes & socks, put slippers & hats on).	Play turn-taking games with a series of objects (e.g. putting blocks in and out of box; pushing car to and fro).

IVA.	Acts on object with differentiated finger use and shoulder motion (e.g. poke).	Use simple puzzle with handles on each piece. Child reaches for puzzle piece, puts in/out with assistance as necessary.	After III, child uses hands to hold and open container. Child uses pincer grasp to get cracker and raison and transfer to mouth.	Adult supplies child with small ball or block, bean bag, and a medium ball for child to throw or push into a colorful bag. Adult may aid child in releasing object.	Child sits at table with paper and crayon. Adult may need to start child's scribbling motion. Child holds crayon and moves arm and hand in all directions.	Self-feeding with finger foods—include scooping as well as pincer grasp.	Play with a doll or stuffed animal with the child. Let child pull object to self for a hug, explore toy's face with hands, etc.
IVB.	Uses hand movement to manipulate object (e.g. squeeze, crumple, turn).	Child manipulates noise-maker to obtain adult attention (ring bell; play piano; squeeze horn).	Adult presents child with two cups and places a bead or small food into one of the cups. Child must grasp cup, find and remove small item. Then child must return the item to the cup.	Sit child in toy car. Give child a noisy toy to hold. When child bangs, squeezes, or shakes toy and makes a noise, push the car.	Present child with bright toy that can be squeezed, poked, and shaken. Let child explore toy.	During grooming activities child can squeeze toothpaste, crumple paper towel, turn faucet on/off, etc.	Place a bucket of blocks within reach. Allow child to dump, throw, mouth, stack and drop blocks back into bucket.
V.	Uses two hands to manipulate objects.	Child "talks" on phone and receives adult attention.	Adult presents child with peg and rings. Child uses hands to remove and replace rings on the peg.	Grasp adult/peers hands to get up, and/or for walking.	Roll giant ball in game with other children/adult.	Facilitate two-hand drinking (from cup or bottle).	(See Recreation and Leisure)

Functional Use of Movement

The lattice for combined manipulation schemes (Levels I and II) overlaps with the simple manipulation lattice (Level IV). Students need only to perform two or more different schemes before programming can emphasize the appropriate use of those to attain desired ends (e.g., Robinson & Robinson, 1983). Independent performance of most functional skills requires combinations of movement schemes. A student must grasp, scoop, and bring a utensil (spoon) to the mouth to be independent in self-feeding. Simple food preparation activities, such as fixing a bowl of cold cereal, require opening (box, milk), pouring (cereal, milk) and then combining these manipulation schemes with those necessary to eat the food. Additional examples of activities across a variety of content domains can be found in Table 3.

Programming for all students with multiple handicaps must emphasize the performance of the required movement and the functional use of as many movement schemes as possible. The exact schemes to be taught are those necessary to enable a student to perform age-appropriate curricular activities. All students should be taught, where possible, to grasp and release objects. Other schemes to be taught can be generated from analyses of activities being carried out with a student (e.g., Baumgart et al., 1982) and/or can be selected from lists such as those included in Table 2. Independent and appropriate use of manipulation schemes is an important component of many functional skills, but is critical for those students who also have visual impairment. These students are learning about object properties and purposes through interaction with objects to a greater extent than are students who are not visually impaired. Limited object manipulation abilities also result in decreased information about the physical environment.

Programming Strategies

Ideally, students should be trained to perform object holding and manipulation skills as independently as possible. Full independent performance, however, may be impossible for some students with severe movement dysfunction or with combined vision and movement impairment. Adaptive aids (and cues) can be used to assist students to perform without adult assistance. Aids can be used to totally "replace" a required response and/or in combination with training procedures designed to allow as much independence as possible. Basic aspects of programming, however, must still be completed before special devices will be effective. Postural control must first be ensured through appropriate positioning. Strategies to influence postural tone with movement must also be implemented.

Replacement Aids. Occupational therapists can assist with the design of aids that will help overcome physical limitations that prevent a student from grasping or manipulating. Special spoons attach to the hands. A universal holder or a flexion mitt can be used with other students to hold objects of all types. Since many manipulation schemes actually involve movement of an upper extremity (or extremities), assisting a student to grasp through use of adaptive aids often makes it possible for the student to perform manipulation schemes. Feeding is a good example. Many students are able to bring their hands to their mouths and can learn to eat independently when special spoons are used to "bypass" grasping.

Devices that totally bypass both grasp and object manipulation by substituting head movement are often necessary for some students. These devices include head pointers and/or electronic switches operated through head or eye movement. This type of substitution has several drawbacks, even though a student may be able to interact with the environment in specific situations (e.g., communication) using these devices. Use of these devices enables a student to act on the environment, but not to receive information about objects in the environment. Head pointers usually perform only the function of pointing to objects or using pressure against an object (e.g., activating a typewriter or computer keyboard with a headstick). Eye-hand coordination tasks are often quite difficult when using a headstick. Microswitches, while helpful with some students, are removed from the object that is being acted on (e.g., toy, computer, communication aid, mobility aid) and require knowledge of cause and effect with detached objects for accurate operation. Younger students, or those with severe handicaps that involve cognition, may not yet have acquired the cognitive skills necessary to operate the device, and will require substantial training for device use to be functional. Finally, cues or additional aids may be necessary for a student who also has severe visual impairment. Head sticks can be used to locate and search for objects, but microswitches are not as functional in this type of situation.

Aids That Simplify a Task. Other types of devices may simplify tasks and make them possible for a student with vision or movement dysfunction. "Handles" made from large loops can enable a student without grasp to hook an arm through the loop to bring an object close to the body, or to perform aspects of dressing independently. Tactile cues (or raised symbols) can be placed on objects for students who are learning to locate and search for specific items. Selection of objects to be used can also simplify a task without the use of "special aids." For example, a student may be able to operate a microwave oven with a touch panel, but not one with a dial. Blenders and other appliances may be operated using a microswitch, and without further modification, by plugging the appliance through an aid such as the Training Aid 2 (Prentke-Romich, 1985). Use of an electric can opener or a variety of aids that are manufactured to be used by individuals with only one functional arm or hand can also help students with multiple handicaps to perform tasks independently. Aids that are manufactured for individuals with visual limitations can also be incorporated into training programs. Occupational therapists and vision specialists can be used as resources to help develop aids and/or provide catalogues and other information from manufacturers.

Training Strategies. A number of strategies may be used to train object holding and manipulation. Selection of objects for grasp/manipulation tasks is of critical importance for success. Objects should be visible to a student, motivating, and part of a functional task. Appropriate aids and cues should be used to enhance visibility and/or

Table 3. Matrix of activities by domain for combined manipulation schemes

Behavior	Communication	Environmental problem solving	Mobility	Recreation and leisure	Self-management	Social
IA. Demonstrates manipulation schemes (e.g. hold, shake, bang, pushes, pull, open).	Child bangs hands together to indicate "more" toy, food, game.	Adult hides own face with hands. Child pulls hands away from adult's face.	Child holds adult's hand before being moved from one activity to another.	Child bangs workbench with hammer, hits piano keys, beats drum.	Child assists adult in holding cup, bottle, or spoon while feeding.	Child pushes ball, car, truck back and forth with peer and/or adult.
IB. Demonstrates imitation of basic manipulation schemes.	Same as IA above or Social IB.	Same as IA above.	Same as IA above.	Same as IA above.	Same as IA above.	Child waves to a variety of people with prompts by adult.
II. Uses appropriate scheme to manipulate specific object (e.g. shake, rattle, push car).	Child pushes ball to adult to signal playing ball.	Child picks up bucket to dump out blocks.	Child seated on a scooter board and uses feet to push self along with adult assistance.	Child pushes truck, shakes tambourine, hugs stuffed animal.	Present child with bowl and spoon at snack time. Child uses spoon to scoop food and eat.	Child participates in routines/fingerplay with others (e.g. How big are you? Where is Thumbkin? Peek-a-boo!).

III.	Uses appropriate scheme when two or more different objects are present (discriminates).	Child pushes car and bangs tambourine to gain adult's attention/ assistance.	Hide toys (e.g. in box, under towel, in drawer). Child searches for item, then manipulates object appropriately.	With child lying on the floor, place a truck and a pull toy by child. Adult may need to assist child in pushing truck away and pulling toy toward.	When presented with two objects (e.g. doll and ball) child hugs doll and pushes ball.	Present child with different pairs of items (e.g. comb, cup, spoon, toothbrush, towel). Have child show adult what is done with each item.	Child sits with adult and/or peer. Child is presented with a truck and a tambourine. Child manipulates object, then gives to partner, who manipulates. Continue, presenting different objects and alternating turns.
IV.	Demonstrates combination of 2 or more schemes to solve given problem.	Same as mobility IV.	Place small toy in box with lid. Place box out of child's reach on a towel that is within the child's reach. Child pulls towel to get box, opens to get toy.	Child holds arms up to indicate wants on sliding board and then touches/ hits the sides of the sliding board to indicate desire to slide down.	Present child with a bucket of blocks. Child must dump or take blocks out of bucket then stack them or build with them.	Assist child in pouring juice into cup and then drinking.	Present child and peer or adult with a set of pop beads. Child must push beads together and pull beads apart with interactant to make necklaces or ropes.
V.	Demonstrates combination of two or more schemes to solve "spontaneous" problem.	When an adult or peer ceases interaction with the child, he or she will vocalize and tap the table to regain the interactant's attention.	Child drops cup and spills juice on table. Child must pick up cup, gain adult's attention to get a towel, then wipe up juice.	Child is in chair but needs to use the restroom. Child must position walker, get from chair to walker, turn self around in walker and go to restroom.	Child is participating in an arts/craft activity and sponge-paints. Child grasps sponge, dips it into paint, then dabs it onto paper.	Child is eating a snack. Juice is out of reach. But he or she wants a drink. Child vocalizes, reaches toward cup/bottle.	Child is interacting with peers and wants to play with another toy that is out of reach. Child pushes own toy away, vocalizes and reaches toward desired toy.

make easier the movements that are required to interact with the object. Training should follow careful planning.

1. *Physical guidance:* Required movement patterns may be physically guided at any step of the sequence where a student demonstrates difficulty. For example, a programmer would allow a student to reach toward and contact an object independently, might then physically guide the holding of the object, and allow the student to complete the functional manipulation (e.g., move object to mouth, pull object toward body) independently.
2. *Facilitation:* Many therapeutic procedures are used to facilitate the performance of a desired movement pattern through very precise physical guidance (e.g., Bobath & Bobath, 1984; Campbell, 1987a; S. Campbell, 1984; Scrutton, 1984; Smith, 1986). Knowledge of the development of posture and movement abilities and of neuromuscular function will aid therapists in selecting appropriate facilitation procedures. Facilitation methods are specific to the individual patterns of posture and movement demonstrated by a student. Physical and occupational therapists can help design appropriate methods, and can teach others proper implementation with particular students.
3. *Movement cues or physical prompts:* Cuing a student to perform a desired movement can assist some students. Tapping or brushing across the upper part of the hand can, for example, cue a student to open the hand. Verbal descriptions of a movement, provided from the perspective of the student, may function as movement cues for students with sufficient comprehension of language (Hari and Tillemans, 1984). For example, a programmer might pair brushing across the upper hand with the verbal description "I open my hand" to cue a student to perform the desired movement response.
4. *Imitation or modeling:* Some students can be helped to learn a particular component of a functional object manipulation task and/or the whole task through imitation of a model. Other students in the room may be the models, or a programmer can specifically model for a student. This type of strategy is complex for many students with multiple handicaps. Obviously, a student has to be able to view the model (in order to imitate). Students must also be able to produce the physical movement(s) to be imitated. In other words, the movement to be imitated must be within the repertoire of a student. Thirdly, students must be able to follow a model, which represents a fairly complex cognitive ability (e.g., Bricker, Levin, & Macke, 1984; Robinson & Robinson, 1983). Posture and movement abilities in general are not typically learned through imitation, although selected skills have been trained in this manner. More often, movement patterns are learned through practice. Modeling can effectively teach some students selected and isolated manipulation schemes, but more often is less effective than other strategies used with individuals with severe or multiple handicaps.

Measuring Results

Measuring the effects of training for the performance of simple as well as elaborate manipulation schemes enables programmers to determine the effectiveness of procedures being used. Sequential performance data from four months of classroom programming provided for a student with multiple handicaps are illustrated in Figure 7. This student was diagnosed with cerebral palsy, severe visual impairment (partially corrected) with functional vision limitations, and seizure disorder. Programming was initially focused on reaching and contact with the object. Subsequent levels of programming trained: a) the use of simple manipulation schemes in interaction with objects and materials used in classroom activities; and b) the use of combinations of two schemes, present in student's repertoire, to attain appropriate consequences.

EFFECTIVE AND INTEGRATED PROGRAMMING

Providing functional and relevant programming for students with severe and multiple impairments requires a synthesis of expertise from a variety of professional disciplines as well as from parents. Programming goals and objectives teach skills that will be functional for students throughout their lives. Reach, grasp, eye-hand coordination, and object manipulation are essential acquisition skills, especially for students with combined visual and movement impairment. Early acquisition of these skills can enhance cognitive experience by providing students with the means for direct interaction with objects in their environment.

All skills must be incorporated into functional curricular domains, rather than trained in isolation from meaningful content or separate from the environmental context in which those skills will be used. Skills are critical components of functional activities. Curricular domains, such as personal care, environmental control, mobility, communication, recreation-leisure, and work provide the basis for the selection of programming content. Incorporation of essential skills into functional content areas, embedded in activities that are carried out in a variety of environments, provides the context for teaching functional movement skills. Analyses of movement responses that are required within activities assist programmers to target skills to be trained and adapt materials and devices.

Ascertaining the postural abilities of a student with movement dysfunction is the starting point in training any desired movement response. Postural alignment can be attained independently (through the use of muscles) or artificially (through the use of adaptive positioning equipment). Most students with severe movement dysfunction will require proper positioning, with assistance of positioning equipment, before coordinated movement responses will be feasible. Positioning a student in proper body alignment will increase the probability of the performance of coordinated movement, as well as prevent the development of secondary motor impairments (e.g., orthopaedic deformities, changes in muscles and joints).

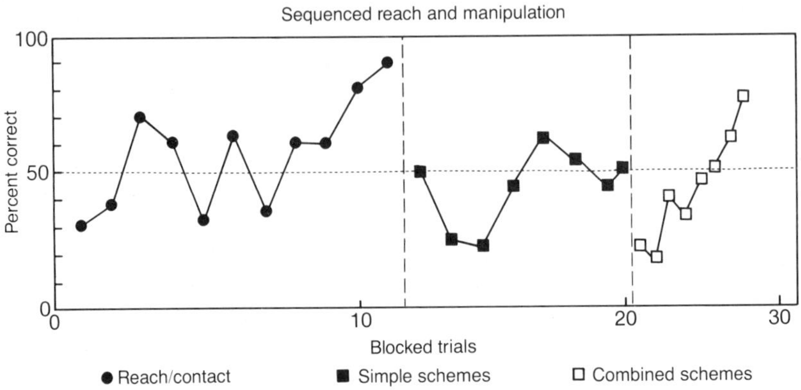

Figure 7. Sequenced programming strategies that chain performance of simple and combined manipulation schemes with reach and contact movement.

Each professional discipline brings a distinct knowledge base to the challenge of designing unique and appropriate programming strategies. The most effective programming strategy for a given student (and a particular task) is individually designed to represent a synthesis of techniques drawn from relevant professional disciplines. A vision specialist contributes techniques appropriate to a student's functional vision abilities. A physical or occupational therapist brings techniques to influence postural tone, facilitate desired movement patterns, and make use of adaptive equipment and aids. Parents contribute knowledge of past training history and of possible reinforcers, while educators can assist in designing learning programs that structure cognitive demands and incorporate applied behavior analysis. Information from each of these sources is synthesized into one integrated instructional approach to teach a student to perform a desired response. The effectiveness of the approach is then evaluated with appropriate measurement strategies.

The often complex learning needs of students with multiple handicaps provide a challenge for parents as well as for professionals from a variety of disciplines. Learning and independence result when parents and professionals form true partnerships to respond to these complex needs by sharing information and implementing uniquely designed and *integrated* instructional programs.

REFERENCES

Adelson, E., & Fraiberg, S. (1974). Gross motor development in infants blind from birth. *Child Development, 45,* 114–126.

Baumgart, D., Brown, L., Pumpian, I., Nisbet, J., Ford, A., Sweet, M., Messina, R., & Schroeder, J. (1982). Principle of partial participation and individualized adaptations in educational programs for severely handicapped students. *The Journal of The Association for the Severely Handicapped,* 7(2), 17–27.

Bobath, K. (1980). *A neurophysiological basis for the treatment of cerebral palsy.* London: William Heinemann Medical Books Ltd.

Bobath, K., & Bobath, B. (1984). The neuro-developmental treatment. In. D. Scrutton (Ed.), *Management of the motor disorders of children with cerebral palsy* (pp. 6–18). Philadelphia: J. B. Lippincott.

Bower, T.G.R. (1979). Visual development in the blind child. In V. Smith and J. Keen (Eds.), *Visual handicap in children* (pp. 145–155). Philadelphia: J. B. Lippincott.

Bricker, W.A., Levin, J.A., & Macke, P.R. (1984). Early language development. In M.J. Hanson (Ed.), *Atypical infant development* (pp. 281–311). Baltimore: University Park Press.

Campbell, P.H. (1987a). Physical management and handling procedures with students with movement dysfunction. In M. Snell (Ed.). *Systematic instruction of persons with severe handicaps* (3rd ed.) (pp. 174–187). Columbus, OH: Charles E. Merrill.

Campbell, P.H. (1987b). Programming for students with dysfunction in posture and movement. In M. Snell (Ed.), *Systematic instruction of persons with severe handicaps* (3rd ed.) (pp. 188–211). Columbus, OH: Charles E. Merrill.

Campbell, P.H., Becker, M., & Gent, P. (1985). *The integrated curriculum*. Akron, OH: Children's Hospital Medical Center of Akron.

Campbell, P.H., & Forsyth, S. (1986). Active mat treatment programs. Akron, OH: Children's Hospital Medical Center of Akron.

Campbell, P.H., Place, P., & Gossett, K. (1986). *Comparisons of two methods to teach reaching behavior.* Manuscript submitted for publication.

Campbell, P.H., & Stewart, B. (1986). Measuring changes in movement skills with infants and young children with handicaps. *Journal of The Association for Persons with Severe Handicaps, 11*(3), 153–161.

Campbell, P.H., & Wilcox, M.J. (1986). *An integrated functional curriculum for young children with multisensory impairments*. Unpublished manuscript.

Campbell, S. (1984). *Pediatric neurologic physical therapy* (Vol. 5). New York: Churchill Livingstone.

Coleman, M. (Ed.). (1981). *Neonatal neurology.* Baltimore: University Park Press.

Egan, D.F. (1979). The early development of visually handicapped children. In V. Smith & J. Keen (Eds.), *Visual handicaps in children* (pp. 139–144). Philadelphia: J. B. Lippincott.

Fewell, R.R., & Sandall, S.R. (1983). Curricula adaptations for young children: Visually impaired, hearing impaired, and physically impaired. *Topics in Early Childhood Special Education, 2,* 51–66.

Fitzhardinge, P.M. & Pape, K.E. (1982). Follow-up studies in the high-risk newborn. In G.B. Avery (Ed.), *Neonatology* (2nd ed.). Philadelphia: J. B. Lippincott.

Fraiberg, S. (1977). *Insights from the blind: Comparative studies of the blind and sighted infants*. New York: Basic Books.

Gaylord-Ross, R.J., & Holvoet, J.F. (1985). *Strategies for educating students with severe handicaps*. Canada: Little, Brown & Company.

Gorski, P.A. (1984). Infants at risk. In M.J. Hanson (Ed.), *Atypical infant development* (pp. 57–80). Baltimore: University Park Press.

Grady, D. (1985, August). Preemies: A 2-billion dollar dilemma. *Discover,* 53–65.

Griffiths, M.I. (1979). Associated disorders in children with severe visual handicaps. In V. Smith & J. Keen (Eds.), *Visual handicaps in children* (pp. 139–144). Philadelphia: J. B. Lippincott.

Hari, M., & Tillemans, T. (1984). Conductive education. In D. Scrutton, (Ed.), *Management of the motor disorders of children with cerebral palsy* (pp. 19–35). London: Spastics International Medical Publications.

Haring, N.G., Liberty, K.A., & White, O.R. (1980). Rules for data-based strategy decisions in instructional programs: Current research and instructional implications. In W. Sailor, B. Wilcox, & L. Brown (Eds.), *Methods of instruction for severely handicapped students* (pp. 159–192). Baltimore: Paul H. Brookes Publishing Co.

Hoyt, C.S., Nickel, B.L., & Billson, F.A. (1982). Ophthalmological examination of the infant: Developmental aspects. *Survey of Ophthalmology, 26*, 177–189.

Langley, B., & DuBose, R.F. (1976). Functional vision screening for severely handicapped children. *New Outlook for the Blind, 8*, 346–350.

Lent, J. (Ed.). (1979). *Project MORE*. Bellevue, Washington: Edmark Associates.

Molnar, G. (1982). Intervention for physically handicapped children. In M. Lewis & L. Taft (Eds.), *Developmental disabilities: Theory, assessment, and intervention*. Jamaica, N.Y.: Spectrum Publications.

Piaget, J. (1952). *The origins of intelligence in children*. New York: Norton Books.

Pornat, R. (1984). Care of the infant with retinopathy of prematurity. *Clinics in Perinatology* (Vol. II, No. 1).

Prechtl, H.F.R., & Nolte, R. (1984). Motor behaviour of preterm infants. In H.F.R. Prechtl (Ed.), *Continuity of neural functions from prenatal to postnatal life* (pp. 79–92). Philadelphia: J. B. Lippincott.

Prentke-Romich. (1985). *The TA–2*. Prentke Romich Company, 8769 Township Road 513, Shreve, OH 44676.

Robertson, C., & Finer, N. (1985). Term infants with hypoxic-ischemic encephalopathy: Outcome at 3.5 years. *Developmental Medicine and Child Neurology, 27*, 473–484.

Robinson, C., & Robinson, J. (1983). Sensorimotor functions and cognitive development. In M. Snell (Ed.), *Systematic instruction of the moderately and severely handicapped* (2nd ed.). Columbus, OH: Charles E. Merrill.

Scrutton, D. (Ed.). (1984). *Management of the motor disorders of children with cerebral palsy*. Philadelphia: J. B. Lippincott.

Seventh Annual Report to Congress on the implementation of Public Law 94–142: The education for all handicapped children act (1985). Washington D.C.: U.S. Department of Education.

Simeonsson, R.J., Huntington, G.S., Short, R.J., & Ware, W.B. (1982). The Carolina record of individual behavior: characteristics of handicapped infants and children. *Topics in Early Childhood Special Education, 2*, 43–55.

Smith, M.M. (1986). Sensory-motor facilitation based on the postural reflex mechanism. In *Selected proceedings from Babro Salek Memorial Symposium* (pp. 81–112). Newark, NJ.

Smith-Davis, J., Burke, P.J., & Noel, M. (1984). *Personnel to educate the handicapped in America: Supply and demand from a programmatic viewpoint*. College Park: University of Maryland.

Wilson, J.A. (1984). Cerebral palsy. In S. Campbell (Ed.), *Pediatric neurologic physical therapy* (pp. 353–413). New York: Churchill Livingstone.

Zinkin, P.M. (1979). The effects of visual handicap on early development. In V. Smith & J. Keen (Eds.), *Visual handicap in children* (pp. 132–138). Philadelphia: J. B. Lippincott.

SECTION III

INSTRUCTIONAL METHODS

CHAPTER 8

A Movement-Based Approach to The Education of Students Who Are Sensory Impaired/Multihandicapped

Jan Writer

THE MOVEMENT-BASED approach to instruction considers motor experiences to be the foundation upon which all other learning is built (van Dijk, 1967). Education is viewed as a process of enhancing both the quality and the quantity of interactions that students have with persons, objects, and events in their environment. The primary role of the teacher in this process is two-fold: a) to provide reference points that enable students to organize their world, and b) to encourage and motivate students to communicate and relate to the world around them (Turiansky & Bove, 1975; van Dijk, 1966).

The student and his or her unique wants, needs, and interests are at the core of this approach. Education is not imposed on children, in that activities are done *with* them rather than *to* them (van Dijk, 1968). The development of a reciprocal relationship between a child and an adult, whereby they move and act together, enables the child to discover his or her own body as an instrument with which to explore the world. To attain such a relationship with students, educators should approach all children in their "total existence" and provide them with functional means to have an impact upon their environment across the activities of the natural daily routine (van Dijk, 1965c).

This chapter presents ways in which the movement-based approach may be applied in the design and implementation of educational programs for students who are sensory impaired/multihandicapped. The movement-based approach to education was first postulated in the literature by Dr. Jan van Dijk as a vehicle for enhancing the functional communication and social abilities of children who are deaf-blind. Turiansky and Bove (1975) emphasize that this approach is "not a method or a technique but a philosophy, a total way of looking at each child in combination with a flexible theoretical framework" (p. 60). This philosophy has been successfully applied over the past two decades with children and youth who manifest varied disabilities, including persons with mental handicaps, orthopaedic impairments, communication handicaps, behavioral disorders, vision impairments, hearing impairments, and multisensory impairments. The majority of students with whom this approach has been utilized are those who experience multiple disabilities that include sensory impairments and/or severe communication deficits.

THE INTERACTION BETWEEN THE CHILD AND THE ENVIRONMENT

Systematic interactions between the child and the environment are the foundation of the movement-based approach. The process of reciprocal interactions is viewed as essential for normal learning to take place (Bijou & Baer, 1961; Bricker & Dennison, 1978; Cooper, 1979; V. Guldager, 1969). The more varied a child's interactions with the environment are, the greater the learning will be (Hart & Risley, 1976).

The child must be actively involved in the educational process for learning to take place (Gill & Dihoff, 1982; McGrane, Pierson, Read, Tarleton & Vierra, 1984). Van Dijk (1965c) believes that by moving and interacting with adults in their environment, children discover that their bodies are the vehicles with which to explore the world. This system of learning through doing enables children to acquire concepts, form social relationships, and influence the environment.

The Role of Movement in Education

Movement is involved in everything children do. It is the means by which they discover their world and express their individuality. Movement has an impact upon all critical areas of educational need. Geary (1980b) states that during the first two years of life, cognition, communication, and motor learning are harmonious in their relationship, and that a problem in one area will disrupt the other two areas. Ward (1981) views movement as the foundation for language and thinking. She feels that movement and perception are interrelated in that motor development is stimulated by, and in turn stimulates, the development of vision and hearing.

Piaget (1964) stresses the importance of motoric interaction and object manipulation in the development of symbolic representations and related cognitive skills requisite to the development of language. Van Dijk (1967, 1968) states that the process of evoking a motor-reaction from an object provides information about its qualities and characteristics. He views movement as the basis for the development of object meaning, as he feels things become meaningful to children only when they can do something with them.

Movement also affects the child's interpersonal relationships. Folio (1976) observes that interaction and communication with the world can be developed only in a "moving-acting" relationship with others. Van Dijk (1968) underscores the importance of movement in personality development when he states that "what we want of children is that they show interest, that they are really willing to have contact with the people in their environment. We want them to communicate, we want them to have the intention to go places, to show that they are a person" (p. 1).

The Impact of Sensory and Orthopedic Impairments on Movement and Learning Children who are multihandicapped frequently have difficulty moving effectively and efficiently. Some experience orthopaedic disabilities such as cerebral palsy. Many have dyspraxia, which causes them to be clumsy in organizing their movements (de Leuw, 1970). Even children who have no known motor impairments often experience movement dysfunction, due to the impact of sensory impairments on their ability to interact appropriately with the environment.

Maron (1982) observes that sensorially impaired students learn best by direct, first-hand experiences in real-life situations. He notes that learning by doing serves to compensate for reduced visual and auditory input. Since many children who are multihandicapped are not motivated by a spontaneous need for movement, the educator must awaken this need (V. Guldager, 1969; van Dijk, 1968).

The Development of Body Image Children who have limited contact with the environment will encounter difficulty developing a concept of themselves as physical and mental beings (V. Guldager, 1969). They will lack the experiences necessary for the growth of a healthy self-concept and body image. Van Dijk (1965a) observes that children who are multihandicapped often have problems differentiating between themselves and other persons and things in their environment. Their inward directedness sometimes causes them to view things as extensions of their own bodies. Werner and Kaplan (1963) believe that the understanding of the separation of self from the environment is requisite to the development of representational and symbolic abilities underlying language.

Van Dijk (1965a) states that the differentiation between self and things requires that the child move both toward things and with things in changing situations. He suggests that an adult move with the child: a) to offer experiences with the environment; b) to develop a dialogue between the child and the world in which he or she is a part; and c) to develop a nonverbal dialogue between the child and another person. Folio (1976) further recommends that the physical guidance of body parts be used in the initial stages of teaching new skills so that the child can gain a feeling for correct movement sequences. Stillman and Battle (1984) note that the shift from personal need satisfaction to the acquisition of knowledge about things in the environment also requires a focus on building the child's intrinsic motivational systems, rather than developing a reliance on extrinsic reinforcement.

Impact of Sensory Impairments Kennedy (1973) states that the negative aspects of sensory deprivation in students who are multihandicapped are multiplicative, as "the deficit from one handicap cannot be subtracted from the functioning of experience of an individual because other aspects are involved" (p. 99). Folio (1976) observes that children who have more than one sensory impairment generally have more motor problems and delays in overall development.

Children who have severe visual impairments are more likely to have movement dysfunction than children who are hearing impaired. Ward (1981) stresses the importance of the link between vision and grasping. She feels that vision controls manual activity, as the coordination of vision with grasping allows the child to act deliberately on the environment. Bower (1977) notes only two areas in which he feels that a lack of vision affects motor skills: (a) behaviors connected with reaching, and (b) behaviors connected with independent locomotion.

G. Stone (1979) notes that all motor output is in response to sensory input; therefore, a distortion of sensory input can result in neuromotor dysfunction. Barraga (1976) sees a strong interrelationship between movement and learning, and suggests that " . . . movement alone, if carefully designed, could facilitate the same quality of psychomotor development that is achieved by children who have both vision and movement" (p. 26). She feels that the effectiveness with which children who are visually handicapped organize perceptions and learn through other senses is contingent upon the willingness of others around them to teach movement and to provide the desire and reason for exploration.

Sensory impairments may precipitate additional learning problems in children. Woznak and Lasky (1980) state that visual perception is directly related to the child's ability to attend to, interpret, and respond to stimuli. Sopers (1971) feels that children whose sensory limitations impair their ability to form an accurate world image often remain at a physical stage in which things have meaning only if they appeal to the child's own body (i.e., if the child can hold them or feel them on his or her body). Scholl (1973) perceives the resultant self-stimulatory activity as an attempt by children to satisfy the need for movement and environmental exploration. He recommends that movement be encouraged through play, interaction with peers, and sensory stimulation.

Sensory impairments may also affect the child's ability to acquire functional communication skills. Guess (1980) notes that the child's ability to receive stimuli through vision, hearing, touch, taste, and smell plays an important role in language development. He states that damage to a sensory mechanism "may not only impair the ability of the child to learn a language but may also influence the choice of appropriate modes to teach the child, irrespective of the particular language competencies to be acquired" (p. 197). Damage to the child's hearing creates an obvious impairment in the ability to acquire speech- and language-related skills. Damage to the child's vision may also result in restricted social communication skills.

Impact of Orthopaedic Impairments Children who have orthopaedic impairments are restricted in their ability to move and interact with the environment; thus many traditional avenues of learning are closed to them. Motor dysfunctions not only impair children's ability to respond to the environment; these impairments create a disturbance in the way children perceive the world (C. Stone, 1977; 1979).

Van Dijk (1965c) describes motor activity as one of the early ways of knowing about the world and the things in it, and stresses that fine and gross motor movements must be developed before the child can begin a more formal education. Folio (1976) notes that the child's systematic interactions with the environment produce the internal development of perceptual abilities that aid in the foundation of intellectual performance. Children who have severe orthopaedic impairments must, therefore, be encouraged to initiate and employ independent movement across all activities of the ongoing daily routine in order to reduce the potential impact of physical limitations on their overall growth and development.

The problems experienced by children with orthopaedic handicaps become more complex when a concomitant sensory impairment also exists. Very often children become the unwilling recipients of environmental stimulation, in that things are done *to* them rather than *with* them. This inhibits their ability to attach meaning to stimuli and to act upon such stimuli in systematic ways. Children who are not afforded the opportunity to exert any control over what is happening to them will sometimes attempt to obtain control in inappropriate ways, such as by screaming, hitting, pushing, scratching, or biting. At other times they may remain passive, allowing things to happen to them but not benefiting from the experience.

A lack of functional communication skills is a major problem for children who have severe physical limitations. Such children may experience difficulty both in understanding the expectancies for their behavior and in expressing their individual wants, needs, and interests. Their attempts at interacting may be discouraged by persons who find it difficult to reach out and involve them in communication, and by those who are unable or unwilling to respond to their nonverbal messages (O'Brien & Andresen, 1983).

VAN DIJK METHODOLOGY OF MOVEMENT-BASED COMMUNICATION AND EDUCATION

The movement-based approach to education currently utilized in the United States has its roots in the teachings of Jan van Dijk and his associates at the Institute for the Deaf in Sint Michielgestel, Holland. They developed their techniques with children who were deaf, and later refined them for application with children who were deaf-blind. Although the target population of van Dijk and his colleagues did not include children who had orthopaedic impairments, their practices and procedures have been expanded upon by educators in this country to apply to these students. It should be noted that the majority of articles from which the movement-based approach emanates were written in the mid- to late 1960s and the early 1970s. The methodologies espoused by the authors have, therefore, been modified and augmented over time.

Stillman and Battle (1984) state that the movement-based approach provides a methodology for establishing the structure of the child's day, as opposed to merely offering a sequence of activities to be conducted separate from daily routines. Van Dijk (1965a, 1965b, 1965c, 1965d, 1966, 1967, 1968, and 1969) stresses the need for initiating activities in natural contexts during the times when they would normally take place. He also feels that the objects and events presented to the child should be functional ones that the child has both reason and motivation to engage in. Unfortunately, the movement-based approach is frequently misconstrued as being a hierarchy of isolated activities (e.g., rocking, crawling, clapping hands) that are conducted in isolated places (e.g., on mats and benches), rather than the practical vehicle that it is for increasing the child's level of response across home, school, and community environments. Van Dijk (1967) cautions against teaching communication skills in isolation from other critical areas of development, and reminds educators that language is imbedded in the totality of everything the child does.

Basic Components of the Movement-Based Approach

The movement-based approach is designed as a vehicle to elicit conversation between the child and the outside world. Van Dijk (1965c) views communication with the world as interpersonal communication that evolves from the child's interactions with the environment and the people in it. He feels that open communication can occur only in a "moving-acting-relationship-toward-each-other" (p. 46).

Van Dijk (1967) describes human development as "the task of growing to an increasing distance" (p. 82). By this he refers to the child's need to differentiate that he or she is separate from things in the environment. A child may require close physical contact with an adult, moving together at the same time, in the initial stages of training. As he or she develops, the child will be able to perform at greater distances: a) in proximity (distance between the child and other persons); and b) in time (time between the environmental model and the child's response to it).

Van Dijk (1967) describes the acquisition of distance in communication as a process of moving from concrete attitudes to abstract ones. He states that concrete attitudes occur when children are able to communicate about things that they can see, feel, or hear. Abstract attitudes evolve when the children are able to converse about things beyond their immediate environment. Symbolic language becomes possible when children are able to separate themselves from the "here and now" and communicate about objects, people, and events not present.

The Nonverbal Child's Outgrowth Toward the World of Symbols Van Dijk (1967) use the term "nonverbal" to describe the communication of children unable to use words, rather than the more common term "pre-linguistic," as he observes that some children never do become aware of the symbolic values of language. Fieber (1976) notes that, although not every child develops language, every child communicates, but not always with symbolic behaviors. The communication of children who are multihandicapped may assume the form of spoken words, manual signs, natural gestures, the tensing of a muscle, the movement of a hand, a shift of gaze, or even a smile. Each communication effort should be considered both valid and valuable.

The movement-based approach delineates several roughly sequential levels of communication that the child progresses through in the development of symbol consciousness. Stillman and Battle (1984) emphasize that there are no formal boundaries between the levels, in that programs for an individual child frequently include activities from more than one level. Van Dijk's program is composed of six major levels: nurturance, resonance, coactive movement, non-representational reference, deferred imitation, and natural gestures. These levels will be redefined and expanded upon in a later section dealing with the application of the movement-based approach across the activities of the ongoing daily routine.

Nurturance Nurturance is the development of a warm social bond between the child and another person. Van Dijk (1967) describes nurturance as a sense of security, a feeling of "being at home with yourself and another" (p. 88). The love, affection, and pleasurable stimulation received from another person forms the basis of a trusting relationship.

Resonance Resonance is a term from physics that denotes "an effect produced in response to vibrations from another body" (Darnell, 1982, p. 33). Sopers (1971) describes resonance as rhythmic movements that reverberate from the child's movements when a pleasurable stimulus is suddenly stopped. There is little or no distance between the child and the adult at this level. Resonance is typically evoked by total body movements, but may also be prompted by other forms of sensory stimulation. Stillman and Battle (1984, p. 163) cite three major reasons for engaging a child in resonance activities: a) to elicit attention to and participation in interactions with others; b) to develop the child's understanding of how his or her actions can affect the environment; and c) to encourage the formulation of positive relationships with others.

Turiansky and Bove (1975) describe the need for the educator to enter the child's world at the resonance level and to develop a nonverbal dialogue. Stillman and Battle (1984) state that the educator should respond to the child's existing behavior as though it were communicative, rather than attempting to teach specific communication behaviors per se. The educator should seek to elicit natural responses from the child and not impose or shape artificial ones.

Coactive Movement Coactive movements are ones that the child executes parallel to (side by side with) a peer or adult model. These movements are done simultaneously but require physical separation between the child and the model. Some children may require that the movements be initiated with full physical prompts, tactual cues, and/or manual signals, prior to the demonstration of true coactive movement. Van Dijk (1965b) observes that many students found working in groups to be stimulating, and would perform coactive movements in groups that they would not do in one-to-one situations.

Full body movements (walking, jumping) are typically used in the initial phase of training at this level. These movements may be expanded upon by introducing obstacles for the child to maneuver around. The most functional application of coactive movements involves instruction in the use of objects during routine events (e.g., wiping the table after lunch; returning materials to their proper storage areas; putting clothes on after swimming). Coactive movement is also referred to as *concurrent imitation*.

Non-representational Reference Non-representational reference involves the child's indicating and positioning his or her body parts (arms, legs, head, etc.) in response to a three-dimensional model (person, doll, clay figure). Fieber (1976) identifies three major behaviors that these activities seek to evoke: (1) recognition and indication of body parts in more detail; (2) the use of pointing behaviors; and (3) increased distance in time and space between the child and the communication referent. Turiansky and Bove (1975) cite the primary function of non-representational reference as building body image by referring to specific parts of the child's body. They feel that the use of stick figures and line drawings in the later stages of training also facilitates children's development of a symbolic representation of themselves.

Deferred Imitation Deferred imitation requires that the child replicate a model after it has been produced and is no longer present. Stillman and Battle (1984) list four major areas of focus in the development of imitative behavior: (1) the child's understanding of the correspondence between his or her actions and the observed actions of others; (2) the child's ability to depict dynamic qualities of observed actions; (3) the educator's ability to use imitation as a tool to demonstrate how the child should do things; and (4) the child's ability to expand his or her mental imagery for things seen, heard, and/or felt.

Imitative movements are usually taught beginning with full body movements (standing up, sitting down, walking) and then progressing to limb movements and hand movements. Symmetrical body movements (e.g., pushing an object with two hands) are easier for the student to replicate than are asymmetrical body movements (e.g., kicking a ball). Movements made on the body (e.g., putting a hat on) are also considered more basic than movements made without body contact (e.g., signing "want"). Van Dijk (1966) recommends that imitation activities be conducted with familiar objects in which the motor components are obvious (e.g., a favorite toy, a comb, a glass). He stresses that the child be engaged in these activities during ongoing events of the natural daily routine.

Natural Gestures A natural gesture is a motor representation of how the child typically uses an object or participates in an event. Many of the signs employed in American sign language for the deaf (AMESLAN) evolve from the natural gestures of adults. For example, the AMESLAN sign for "car" employs the bilateral holding and moving of an "invisible" steering wheel. Although this represents how the adult uses (drives) a car, it would not be a natural gesture for a child who does not drive a car.

Van Dijk (1965a) states that natural gestures evolve from children's experiences with the motor qualities of things. The educator must observe how children spontaneously interact with things in their environment to determine what will be natural gestures for them. Van Dijk (1968) notes that natural gestures, in which the manual movement is almost the same as the object action, are a part of normal development.

Stillman and Battle (1984) feel that the focus of training with the child should be on the spontaneous production of gestures, rather than on teaching gestures in structured situations. Van Dijk (1968) suggests that the educator initiate the gesture immediately prior to the time when the child expects something (e.g., anticipates getting a drink at snack time). The gesture is first made with the object present, so that the child may make a visual or tactual association before getting it. After the child has paired the gesture with the object, the gesture is made without the object present to promote asking behavior.

Van Dijk (1968) notes that after the child is able to spontaneously utilize a variety of natural gestures during the context of the ongoing daily routine, the gestures can be shaped into manual signs through the processes of denaturalization and decontextualization. *Denaturalization* involves the gradual shaping of the natural gesture into the standardized sign through systematic tactual cuing and modeling. *Decontextualization* involves the development of anticipation and mental imagery on the part of the student. This process enables the student to ask for desired items and actions that are outside of the natural context (e.g., asking for food whenever hungry, not just when food is visible).

APPLICATION OF THE MOVEMENT-BASED APPROACH

The act of communication is interwoven with everything that is done with children. The words that are spoken, the vocal intonation and facial expressions used, the way a student is held or touched, the manual gestures and signals employed, the objects and activities that are utilized, *all* communicate messages. The ability of the student to accurately interpret and respond to environmental messages is contingent upon the effectiveness with which these messages are conveyed. McInnis and Treffry (1982) recommend that educators constantly keep in mind that every experience students engage in should be part of a "planned framework designed to promote the development of communication skills" (p. 8). These skills should, in turn, enable students to become more independent across the environments in which they live, work, and play.

Effective communication requires that educators learn to communicate with the "all" of themselves—with the words they speak, their vocal intonation, their facial expression, the gestures they use, the visual/tactual signals they provide, their body posture, the way they position and handle children, and the materials and stimuli they present to students (Writer, 1984). Children who are multihandicapped require a multiplicity of communication cues to maximally understand the expectancies for their behavior. The spoken word or the manual gesture will often not suffice to convey the intended message to these students.

Students who are nonverbal will use modes other than spoken, signed, or written words to express their wants, needs, and feelings. These alternative modes may include clapping to indicate happiness, gesturing to indicate a preferred object's function, or pointing to a desired object or event. Some students may initially employ only basic signaling behavior to indicate pleasure (smiling) or displeasure (crying).

There are students who may outwardly appear to have no communicative responses: they neither laugh nor cry; they do not use speech, gestures, or signals. It is these students at whom the educator must learn to look more closely, as they may be responding with their bodies in ways that are not readily discernible. When the total person is observed, subtle responses may be noted. A student may be moving his or her body, if ever so slightly, toward pleasurable stimuli and/or away from displeasurable stimuli. If the student is held in the educator's arms, a change in muscle tone may be noted (e.g., relaxing for pleasurable stimuli and/or tensing for displeasurable stimuli).

McInnis and Treffry (1982) state that communication is dependent upon the students' ability to perceive accurately the results of early attempts at interacting. Students who are multihandicapped will require adult guidance in these interactions, as they frequently receive distorted feedback from the environment. In order to enhance students' communication efforts, educators must determine which communication cues or cue combinations they rely upon to take in information from the world around them, and then use these cues to provide input. It is also important to ascertain what modes the students employ to express their wants, needs, feelings, and interests. This necessitates that educators learn to "listen" to students in non-traditional ways—with their eyes, with their ears, with their hands and bodies (e.g., by sensing changes in movement and muscle tone), and with their knowledge of the student as a unique individual.

Although each student has distinctive communicative needs and capabilities, some basic goals may be postulated (Shane, 1979; Writer, 1984):

1. Receptive Communication Goals
   a. To understand and respond to the expectancies for one's behavior; and
   b. to obtain information from the world around oneself.
2. Expressive Communication Goals
   a. To express wants, needs, and feelings; and
   b. to describe the "here and now."

The Development of Nonverbal Communication Skills

Stillman and Battle (1986) describe the development of representational behavior as a process of distancing and differentiating between oneself and the external world. They cite three behaviors which illustrate the student's shift in focus from self to the outside world: 1) a decreased reliance on immediate/familiar contexts to anticipate external events; 2) an increased ability to imitate the observed actions of people and objects; and 3) an increased ability to understand the correspondence between one's own actions and observed actions. Stillman and Battle (1986) note the major components of this process as being: a) anticipation of events, b) imitation of behavior, c) differentiation between symbolic "vehicles" employed in varied contexts and at varied points in time, and d) reciprocity of communication, as observed in actions to initiate, sustain, terminate, and/or protest the termination of a communication exchange.

The point of reference for the development of communication abilities should be the student's body and his or her existing repertoire of movements. Communication may be enhanced by increasing the efficiency with which the student can employ functional communication modes and media in conversations with others.

Receptive and Expressive Communication Modes Sailor et al. (1980) define a communication mode as "the form in which the content of a message is expressed" (p. 72). Varied modes may be used by students to understand the expectancies for their behavior (receptive communication) and to express individual wants and ideas (expressive communication). Receptive communication modes may be divided into four broad categories: 1) tactual/kinesthetic cues; 2) vocal/visual signals; 3) coactive cues or models; and 4) natural gestures.

Tactual/Kinesthetic Cues Tactual/kinesthetic cues provide the basis for initial receptive communication. These cues utilize the student's own body as the focal point of reference. When a mother cradles and rocks her baby in her arms, a feeling of pleasure and security is communicated to the child. When the educator holds and moves the student in a way that is pleasurable to the child, a similar feeling of joy and reassurance is conveyed. This harmonious, cooperative movement forms the basis for both receptive communication and the development of a primary social bond between the student and another person.

The student's generalized response to total body movement may later be refined to the development of specific motor responses following consistent tactual cues. If, prior to picking a student up from a supine position, the educator consistently places one hand under the student's upper back and the other hand under the student's knees, exerts upward pressure, then releases pressure; the student will eventually learn to anticipate being picked up, following the tactual (pressure) cues. At a later stage, the student may learn to execute a motor act, subsequent to a light, tactual cue (e.g., raise his or her head, following a touch to the forehead; sit down, following a touch to the buttocks).

Vocal/Visual Signals Vocal signals provide the student with cues related to the identification of individual persons (e.g., recognition of the mother's voice). These cues also provide information on the emotional status of the immediate situation through variation in vocal intonation (e.g., "angry" voice versus "happy" voice). Visual signals provide the student with information from a variety of sources that include: (a) changes in physical situation (e.g., movement from house to school bus = go to school); (b) situational cues (e.g., movement from task area in classroom to leisure area = time to play); (c) object cues (e.g., placement of adapted bowl on wheelchair tray = time to eat); and (d) manual signals (e.g., pointing to a glass of milk = drink milk; tapping seat of chair = sit in chair).

Coactive Cues or Models Coactive or paired movements between the educator and the student provide simultaneous cues for the student's expected behavior (e.g., the parent and the student carry their dinner dishes to the sink at the same time). This form of side-by-side movement encourages the student to follow the adult, and enhances the student's awareness of what the adult's body is doing. Coactive movements also further the development of social relationships and assist in the student's development of body image.

Natural Gestures Natural gestures pantomine how the student spontaneously interacts with the environment. These movements are the beginning of true representational behavior. Natural gestures are individual to each student. They should never be artificially created by the educator and imposed on a student, as a student at this level of prelinguistic communication skill development is not able to functionally integrate abstract (i.e., artificial) symbols.

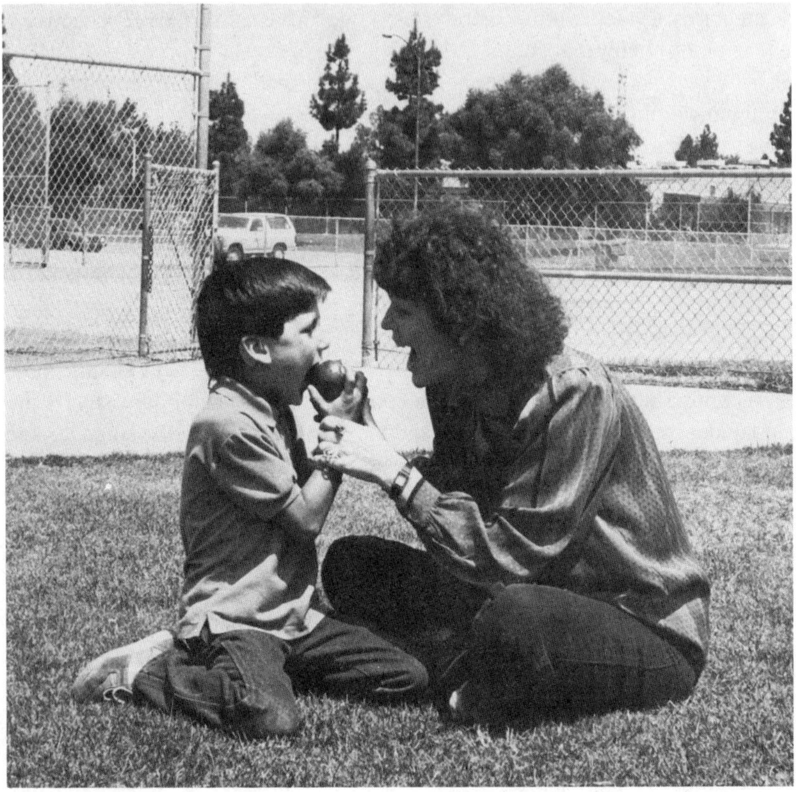

Figure 1. A teacher uses coactive movements and tactual cues to prompt a child to bite into an apple.

Expressive communication modes may be divided into two broad categories: 1) vocal signals; and 2) physical signals. Stillman, Aylmer, and Vandivort (1983) define expressive signals as "purposeful, goal-directed actions which the child anticipates will result in a certain effect, but which require the participation or cooperation of another person in order to be achieved" (p. 2).

Vocal Signals Consistent vocalization patterns may be used as an expression of feeling, state, or attitude (e.g., student laughs to indicate pleasure and makes throaty, guttural sounds to indicate displeasure). Vocal signals, in the form of projected voice, may also be employed to obtain the attention of another person.

Physical Signals Physical signals involve the way the students move their bodies during expressive communication attempts. These movements may include:

1. Total body movements (e.g., student consistently moves body toward preferred objects/events and away from undesired objects/events; student consistently relaxes body in presence of pleasurable stimuli and tenses body in presence of irritating stimuli).

2. Manual signals—student does the following:
   a. Tugs, pulls, pushes (e.g., leads) people to a desired object or event;
   b. touches a desired object or hands it to a person to elicit an event (e.g., hands adult a glass to indicate a desire for a drink); and/or
   c. points (with index finger or whole hand) to: (1) obtain a desired object/event; and (2) direct attention to something shared.
3. Facial expressions (e.g., student opens eyes wide and smiles to express the desire to initiate/continue a conversation).
4. Eye movements (e.g., student looks at a desired object in an attempt to have the adult retrieve it).
5. Natural gestures (e.g., student holds both arms up over his or her head as an indication that he or she wants a hot sweater taken off).

Communication Media Communication media are objects, materials, and symbols that are employed in the conveyance of a message. A hierarchy of media from the most concrete (representational) to the most abstract (symbolic) follows:

1. Real-life objects
2. Representational objects
3. Photographs of real-life objects
4. Line drawings of real-life objects
5. Colored pictures
6. Black and white pictures
7. Pictographs
8. Printed or brailled words

Shane (1979) and Sims-Tucker and Jensema (1984) state that pictures are more concrete than line drawings for some students. Writer (1984) assumes a different viewpoint and observes that students who are multihandicapped typically demonstrate concept knowledge of line drawings prior to the acquisition of concepts with pictures from magazines or kits. She postulates that line drawings are more representational than pictures, due to their similarity to the real-life objects that the student employs, particularly when: (a) drawn in the student's presence, and (b) drawn in the same color(s) as the real-life object. Writer felt that pictures, on the other hand, are more abstract for students, as they frequently differ in color, shape, and general characteristics from the objects that the student encounters in the environment.

Graphic media (photographs, line drawings, and pictures) may be effectively utilized by students to communicate with persons who are nonhandicapped. To facilitate conversation, printed word strips should be placed under media to clarify intent (e.g., "I want to swing" under a drawing of a swing).

Real-Life Objects Communication skills development should be initiated with familiar, real-life objects that the student employs in natural environments (e.g., the student's own shirt, rather than a doll's shirt; the actual school bus, rather than a picture of a school bus). The focus of initial training should be on the development of concepts, as opposed to labels. Many students are capable of acquiring labels (e.g., signing "glass" when presented with a picture of a glass, pointing to a plastic shoe when verbally told "to point to the shoe") without acquiring the corresponding concepts that the label implies (e.g., a glass is something you drink liquid from; a shoe is something you wear on your foot).

Photographs of Real-Life Objects Once the student has acquired concepts of real-life object functions, photographs of those objects may be used as an alternative medium. The photographs should be of the actual objects that the student employs, rather than photographs purchased in a kit. To provide maximal clarity, objects should be photographed against a solid, contrasting background (e.g., photograph a white bowl against a black or dark blue background).

Photographs should be presented along with the corresponding real-life object, prior to the presentation of the photograph alone. If the student is visually impaired or has difficulty discriminating the single-object photographs, blow-ups of the photographs might be used.

Representational Objects A representational object may be either: a) a real object that represents an event; or b) a miniature of a real object. Students typically learn to associate real-life objects with events early in the development of both receptive and expressive communication skills (e.g., glass = "I'm thirsty"; clothes bag handed student at end of day = time to walk to the bus, then go home).

A more abstract form of representational objects is a miniature that closely resembles the real-life stimuli (e.g., a miniature jogging shoe that resembles the jogging shoes that the student wears). To be truly representational, the miniature must look and feel like the real-life object that the student uses (i.e., a miniature jogging shoe would not be representational to a student who only wears brown, orthopaedic shoes). Van Dijk (1984) feels that these objects can serve as a viable alternative medium for the student whose visual impairment precludes the use of graphic media. As with photographs, representational miniatures should be presented with the corresponding real-life object, before the presentation of the miniature alone.

Line Drawings of Real-Life Objects Line drawings are black-on-white outlines of the real objects routinely employed by the student. Color cues may be added, as deemed appropriate for the individual student. A hierarchy of techniques for generating line drawing follows, with the most concrete method cited first:

1. Line drawing that the student makes.
2. Line drawing made in the presence of the student with: a) student participating; b) student watching.
3. Line drawing made outside of the student's presence.
4. Commercially made line drawing.

Students who are blind might employ two-dimensional imprints of real-life objects embossed on special plastic sheets by means of a Thermoform machine as a substitute for line drawings. Outlines of objects made with yarn or a textured material which corresponds to that found on the real-life object could also be used.

Representational Pictures Representational pictures include pictures and photographs found in magazines and commercial kits. The student who has demonstrated

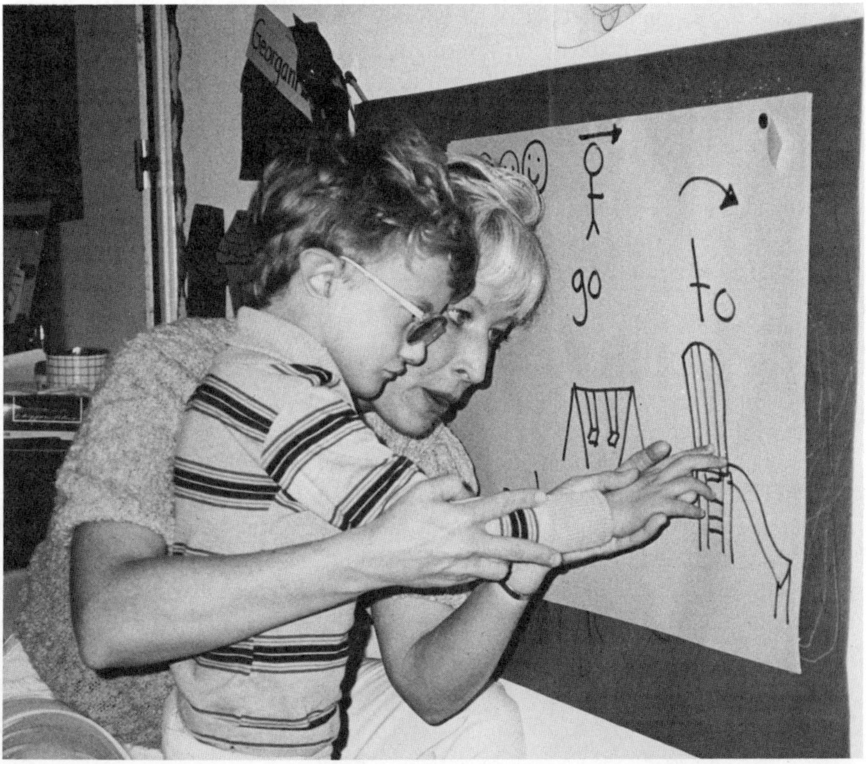

Figure 2. A teacher uses line drawings and limb movements to inform a child that they are going to the park.

concept knowledge of photographs and line drawings might successfully use representational pictures. These pictures may serve to expand the student's knowledge of the properties of familiar objects and events, and can offer a broad array of conversational choices.

Pictographs A pictograph is a graphic symbol that represents an object, person, activity, or event. Rebus symbols, Bliss symbols, and other pictographics have been successfully employed with some students during the transition stage between pictures and the printed word. Although they have proven useful in the development of more advanced language concepts, pictographs may be too abstract for many students who are multihandicapped.

APPLICATION OF THE MOVEMENT-BASED APPROACH DURING ROUTINE ACTIVITIES

Recognition of each student as unique requires flexibility in the design and implementation of functional communication systems for individual children and youth. The educator must continuously bear in mind that all levels of instruction are both ongoing and overlapping. Students who are multihandicapped will typically demonstrate communicative behavior on several different levels at the same point in time, contingent upon such variables as the physical situation, the student's motivation to communicate, and the student's personal preference for the person he or she is communicating with.

The six major levels of van Dijk's program described earlier will be subsumed and expanded upon under the following headings: 1) nurturance, 2) anticipation, 3) coactive movements, 4) deferred imitation, and 5) natural gestures. Representative instructional activities will be described at each level.

Nurturance

The establishment of a primary social relationship between the student and another person is essential to both the growth of functional communication skills and the growth of the student as a total person. Condon (1979) considers this social attachment to be the most important prerequisite of communication and language.

Van Dijk (1984) offers three suggestions for helping students at this level achieve an affective, social relationship: 1) limit the number of people working with the child; 2) build a routine of daily activities around the child, and 3) distribute external stimuli to avoid either overstimulation or understimulation. Robinson and Allen (1975) caution that the educator can attempt to hold students, but should not restrain their arms and legs—students should be held with "open arms," allowing them the option to remain or leave.

Anticipation

The development of anticipation responses involves the building of habits. The student gradually learns that specific behaviors are followed by recurrent, hence predictable, events. If a preferred toy (e.g., an electric train) is activated every time the student pushes a switch, he or she will soon learn to associate the pushing of the switch with the activation of the train; thus, a habit is formed.

One of the most critical elements in the development of initial anticipation responses is the start-stop format used for the presentation of stimuli. The student is briefly engaged in a pleasurable activity, then the activity is stopped. During the interval between the cessation and reactivation of the desired stimuli, the educator looks for a consistent, spontaneous movement response from the student that signals anticipation of the resumption of the activity. Through consistent structuring of routine events, students may demonstrate anticipation in response to sensory stimulation, total body movements, limb movements, situational cues, manual signals, or communication media.

Anticipation in Response to Sensory Stimulation Anticipation responses to sensory stimulation may result from the consistent presentation of light, tactual cues (e.g., a spoonful of food is touched to the student's lower lip and the student opens his or her mouth to receive the food), or the presentation of pleasurable stimuli (e.g., the student smiles while warm lotion is stroked on his or her arm; the adult ceases stroking;

the student then raises the arm in anticipation of a resumption of the stroking). The student should begin to demonstrate voluntary motor responses to consistently applied sensory stimuli during this stage of communication skill development.

Passive acceptance of pleasurable stimuli should progress to more active participation on the part of the student. Through systematic sensory stimulation, the student receives information from the environment (via sight, hearing, touch, smell, taste, or movement), and learns to act upon that information through voluntary motor responses. For example, the educator may observe that a student consistently smiles when talcum powder is rubbed on his or her arm. The educator might subsequently rub talcum powder on the student's arm, wait for the student to smile, suddenly cease the rubbing, and look for a motor response that indicates the student would like the "talc rub" to continue.

It is important that students who are multihandicapped be allowed adequate time to voluntarily respond to systematic sensory stimulation. If a student fails to respond after five or more trials, a light tactual cue might be utilized. Should the student continue to show no response to the cessation of stimuli, it could mean that: a) a more intense stimulation is needed (e.g., a deeper pressure rub or a longer period of stroking); b) a longer reaction time is needed; and/or c) the stimuli are no longer pleasurable to the student.

Van Dijk (1968) emphasizes the importance of affording the students opportunities to integrate different sensory pathways by enabling them to attach meaning to the sensory data provided. Fieber (1976) proposes that sensory integration could be facilitated by allowing the student to participate in the selection and application of stimuli. She recommends a program of gradual sensory enrichment in which the student remains relaxed and is not bombarded with sensory input.

Educators need to recognize that voluntary movement on the part of a student functioning at this "sensory stimulation" level will only be attained if the student truly wants a stimulus to continue. Movements should not be imposed or conditioned. The student must learn that the movement of the body in a consistent manner can initiate predictable forms of stimulation. Such a program will enable the student to progress through a hierarchy of reactiveness toward environmental stimuli that includes: a) sensation or awareness, b) activation of stimuli, and c) integration of stimuli.

Anticipation in Response to Total Body Movement Anticipation responses to total body movement include the resonance movements described previously. These responses are evoked through harmonious interaction between the student and another person. Movements used should be ones that are within the student's repertoire and/or range of capability, and that the student enjoys. Rocking, swinging, bouncing, and swaying are frequently used with younger students. Varied equipment (e.g., rocking chairs, swings, hammocks, trampolines) may be employed to prompt similar pleasurable responses in older students.

The adult should select a total body movement that the student enjoyed during the nurturance interactions. The procedure that is subsequently applied is the same as the one previously described with sensory stimuli—the adult actively engages the student in a pleasurable movement, then suddenly stops the movement and looks for a motor response from the student (e.g., the student laughs while swinging; the swinging is stopped; the student then leans his or her trunk forward in anticipation of swinging). The use of the start-stop format helps to shift the student from self-directed input to environmental input.

Anticipation in Response to Limb Movements Anticipation responses to limb movements also involve the initiation and cessation of stimuli. For example, if the student has been engaged in repetitive range-of-motion exercises involving the legs, the adult might periodically cease the exercise and tactually cue the student to move his or her legs in the same direction of the movement that follows. Independent anticipation of movement in such exercises involves active participation on the part of the student, which results in more optimal muscle tone as well as increased range of motion. Other examples of routine activities that could lead to anticipatory limb movements include raising an arm, prior to placing it in the sleeve of a coat, and reaching out to bat a preferred toy or activate an electronic switch.

Anticipation in Response to Situational Cues Anticipation responses to situational cues result from the establishment and maintenance of consistent daily routines, and consistently employed activity areas (e.g., leisure area, sensory stimulation area, work area) within the student's environment. The student learns that the same types of activities are conducted in the same place with the same persons each day. This consistency helps fulfill the student's need for structure, and aids in the acquisition of concepts of time, order, and place. As the student learns the routines, anticipation of daily events and social interactions will develop (e.g., first comes work, then snack, then music).

Anticipation in Response to Manual Signals Anticipation responses to manual signals develop through the paired association of signals (e.g., pointing) with predictable behavioral intentions (e.g., being expected to pick up the object pointed to). Auditory signals may be paired with manual signals to clarify performance expectancies (e.g., tapping the side of the sink to indicate that the student should put his or her dirty lunch dish in it; tapping the seat of the chair to indicate that the student should sit in it).

Anticipation in Response to Communication Media Anticipation responses to media may be evoked through either sequential or singular presentation of objects, photographs, and/or drawings. Sopers (1971, pp. 33–34) describes the use of media as a vehicle for characterizing persons, things, and events in the student's environment. He discusses three major areas in which communication media could be used to elicit anticipation, and potential techniques for each:

1. Characterizing people: a) bring something typical and unique about the person to the attention of the student (e.g., ring, beard), and b) engage the student in a movement with the personal feature (e.g., twist the ring, stroke the beard).
2. Characterizing animals and things: draw the student's attention to a unique feature using movement, as described above.

3. Characterizing events: a) start with "going out" activities and have the student take an object that is routinely used at the destination (e.g., shopping bag = grocery store, baseball bat = park, lunchbox = school); and b) provide the student with an object that represents other routine events, immediately prior to the event (e.g., bowl = eat meal, bus pass = ride bus, sponge = clean table, headset = listen to music).

The consistent pairing of a communication medium (object, photograph, or drawing) with an activity will allow the student to anticipate the activity upon seeing the corresponding stimulus. The student first associates the presentation of the medium with a change in activity. Next the student may actually anticipate the activity that follows (e.g., a student who is prompted to touch a photograph of a toilet, prior to walking to the bathroom, may begin to independently walk to the bathroom upon presentation of the photograph). At a later stage, the student may employ the stimuli to signal for the activity (e.g., hand an adult the photograph of the toilet as an indication of the desire to use the bathroom).

Students can learn to anticipate the sequence of routine activities by using "anticipation shelves" and "calendars" (Geary, 1980a; Sopers, 1971; Sternberg, Battle & Hill, 1980; Stillman & Battle, 1984; Writer, 1984). Anticipation shelves contain a representative object for each major activity of the day, arranged in chronological order. White plastic frozen dinner plates laid side by side are often used to replace the more stationary object self (see Figure 3). The objects selected for use should be ones that the student associates with major daily activities. An item of apparel that is related to an activity could be substituted for an object on the shelf (e.g., a sweatband worn on the wrist to gym; a baseball cap worn home on the school bus; an apron worn to the kitchen).

All representational items should be sequenced in the frozen dinner plates (or on the shelf) in the order in which they are used by the student during the daily routine. Prior to the first major activity of the day, the student is prompted to take the first object from the trays/shelf and transport it to the place where it will be used. When the student completes the activity, he or she transports the representational object to its proper storage area. This procedure is then repeated for each object in the sequence.

Photographs of real-life objects or events may replace objects on the shelf. These may be especially effective in depicting events that are difficult to represent with an object cue (e.g., swinging in an outdoor swing, participating in a regular education classroom, using a bathroom located outside of the classroom). In the aforementioned examples a photograph of the swing, a photograph of the regular education teacher, and a photograph of the toilet might be used.

Anticipation calendars employ photographs and/or line drawings of events that routinely occur during the day or the week. Daily calendars are sequenced in the same manner as the anticipation shelves (see Figure 4). Weekly calendars depict daily routines in vertical rows under the days of the week.

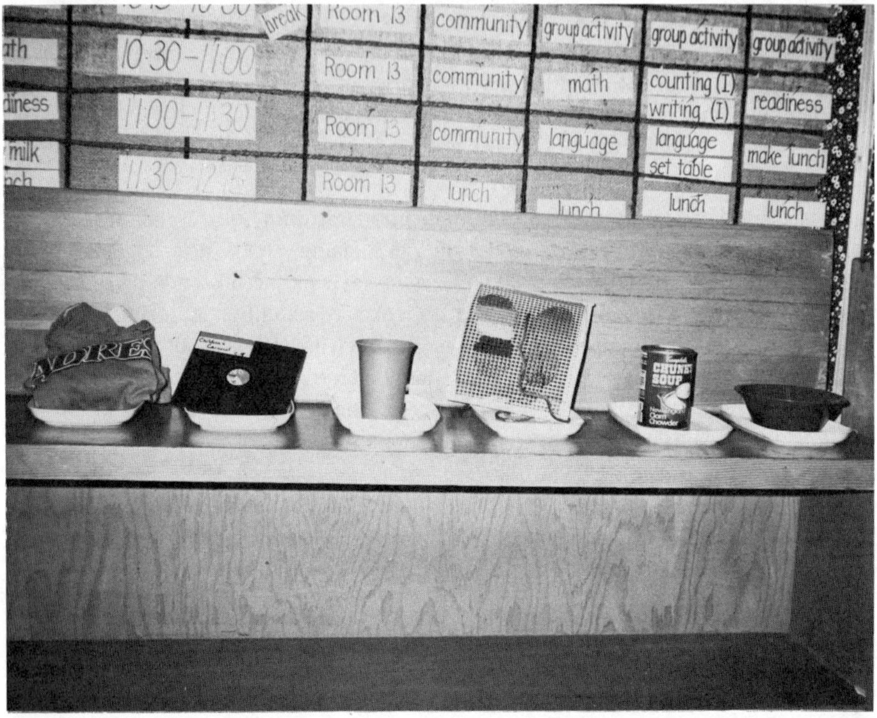

Figure 3. An anticipation shelf with objects representing major activities of the morning routine (physical education, computer time, snack, leisure, food preparation, and lunch).

Photographs and drawings can also be used to enable students to anticipate the sequence of events that occurs in functional activities (e.g., setting the table, brushing teeth, doing the laundry). Individual photographs/drawings of each step in the sequence should be given to the students to put in correct order, prior to participating in the event. The media sequence could then be used to prompt performance during the activity.

Coactive Movement

Coactive movements allow students who are functioning at a prelinguistic communication level to see the behavior that is expected of them at the same time that they are called upon to execute it. These movements subsequently afford students who have problems with visual memory and/or skill sequencing the opportunity to perform successfully without direct, physical assistance. Coactive movements may involve total body movements, body movements utilizing objects, limb movements, or hand movements.

Total Body Movements These movements provide the most complete model for the student to replicate. Examples of coactive body movements include the student walking next to an adult or peer from the classroom to tne lunchroom, and the student swinging on a swing next to a peer.

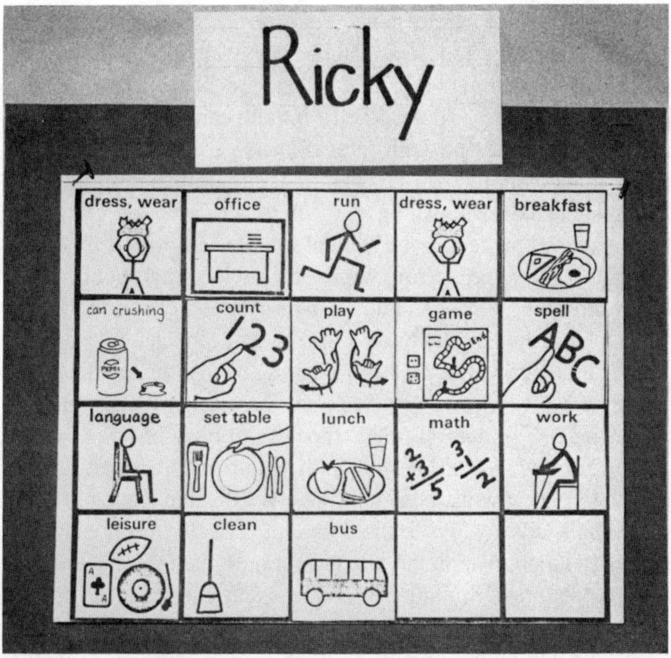

Figure 4. A daily calendar with line drawings depicting major activities of a student's school routine. (Communication calendar designed by Kim Jubala, Lafayette Elementary School, San Diego.)

Body Movements Utilizing Objects These movements can be used to help promote functional independence in routine activities. They are also more meaningful for some children than total body movements. Examples of coactive movements with objects might include the student and a peer simultaneously picking up their lunch trays and transporting them to the kitchen, or the student picking up a toy he or she has played with and putting it in a toy box, at the same time as an adult model.

Limb Movements These movements require the student to perform asymmetrical actions with his or her body. They frequently constitute manual signals, such as the student and an adult waving "goodbye" at the same time, or the student and a peer simultaneously pointing to the same object.

Hand Movements These movements can facilitate the transition to a spontaneous use of natural gestures and manual signs. Examples of coactive hand movements might be the student and an adult washing their hands at the same time, or the student and an adult simultaneously making a natural gesture for a preferred object.

Deferred Imitation

Deferred imitation requires the passage of time between the modeling of a behavior and the student's replication of it. Van Dijk (1969) notes the importance of teaching imitation through the use of natural movements (i.e., movements that occur during events of the daily routine) versus artificial ones (e.g., hand clapping, hand raising).

The development of imitation precedes the acquisition of more symbolic forms of communication. Students who are able to imitate can independently expand their gestural or oral vocabularies through interactions with persons and events in their environment. A student should first be encouraged to imitate movements requiring a single motoric response (e.g., pushing a switch to activate a toy). Complexity of response can be increased by having the student imitate activities involving an increasing number of movements (e.g., from wiping the table with a sponge to picking up a soiled article of clothing with one hand, transferring it to the other hand, and then depositing it in a hamper); and by having the student replicate the activity over progressively longer time periods (e.g., from washing hands immediately after the adult model to making a sandwich five minutes after the teacher makes one).

Visual cues play an important role in the development of imitative skills. Imitation of actions that provide visual cues typically occurs before imitation of actions that lack visual cues. Imitation with visual cues involves the duplication of a behavior that can be seen (e.g., the adult walks to the door and waits for the student to follow; the adult places a dirty lunch dish on the kitchen counter, then the student places a dirty lunch dish on the counter). Imitation without visual cues requires that the student remember what was seen, heard, or felt (e.g., the adult walks down the hall, opens the lunchroom door and enters, then the student walks down the hall and enters the lunchroom; the adult places a dirty lunch dish in the sink, then the student places a dirty lunch dish in the sink).

Natural Gestures

Natural gestures may provide the student with a viable alternative form of prelinguistic communication. As no assistive media are required, the student can spontaneously communicate with all persons in the environment. The inherent "naturalness" of the gesture (i.e., its direct correspondence to the student's own actions during an activity) makes it easy for both the student and the adult to use and understand.

Functional natural gestures are most readily developed through the integration of coactive movements and imitation in the instructional process. The adult should first produce the gesture coactively with the student, gradually fading the amount of prompting required. The adult next encourages the student to imitate the natural gesture, immediately prior to playing with the object or participating in the event. The student should eventually be required to spontaneously use the natural gesture when referring to the object or event.

FACTORS THAT FACILITATE COMMUNICATION SKILL DEVELOPMENT

Communication is a social process that is prompted in children in warm and playful situations. The student who is relaxed and happy is a more receptive learner than one who is tense and anxious. It is important that the educator and the student share pleasurable experiences that serve to strengthen the interpersonal relationship between the student and others, and that provide a secure foundation from which the student may explore and interact with the outside world.

Spoken words should be paired with all nonverbal cues provided throughout the day. Some students understand and respond to speech. Vocal intonation can also provide students with valuable information as to the expectancies for their behavior. The educator should be cautioned not to use superfluous verbiage with students. Provide only those cues (verbal, gestural, and/or tactual) that convey the essence of the message being expressed.

There are many factors that can facilitate and enhance communication skill development in students who are multihandicapped. These include contextual instruction, development of a functional vocabulary, provision of opportunities to make choices, and teamwork.

Contextual Instruction

Communication cues should be provided to students during the course of the normal daily routine, when students are involved in natural events (Bowling, 1970; Fieber, 1976; Goetz, Schuler & Sailor, 1981; Gold & Rittenhouse, 1978; Halle, 1982; Kaczmarek, 1985; Oliver & Halle, 1982; van Dijk, 1967; Wacker & Hoffman, 1984). The importance of contextual instruction is central to the development of functional movement-based responses. Instruction in natural situations with natural stimuli not only provides students with meaningful skills that they can use in natural environments, it also facilitates the development of concepts.

Development of a Functional Vocabulary

Students need to be offered continuous opportunities to express their wants, needs, feelings, and ideas. The initial response "vocabulary" (e.g., movements, gestures, signs) chosen for a given student must be individualized to represent those things that he or she has reason, desire, opportunity, and ability to communicate. Observation of the student's spontaneous behavior (e.g., the activities the student engages in, the objects the student repeatedly returns to) can provide a basis for vocabulary selection. A student who demonstrates limited voluntary movement may need to be systematically presented with a variety of stimuli to determine the most appropriate communication cues and/or media to employ.

Goetz et al. (1981) recommend that initial communicative responses be ones that evoke direct physical changes in events (e.g., "want ball" versus "red" or "on"). Hopper and Helmick (1977) note that responses that allow students to control aspects of their environment are the most meaningful and motivating, and hence are the first to be spontaneously produced. Additional considerations for developing a functional core vocabulary for students are:

1. The vocabulary should be immediately useful to the student.
2. There should be many opportunities for the student to employ the vocabulary in school, home, and community environments.

3. Words, concepts, and signals chosen should be ones the student is already trying to express.
4. Use of the vocabulary should result in natural consequences that are reinforcing for the student.
5. The vocabulary should be easily integrated into existing programs for functional skills development.
6. The communication modes and media employed should be appropriate, given the severity of the student's sensory and/or orthopaedic impairments.

[Gaylord-Ross & Holvoet, 1985; Goetz et al., 1981; Guess, Sailor, and Keogh, 1978; Harlan & Carlson, 1979; Hopper and Helmick, 1977; Kennedy, 1973; May, 1980; Salisbury, Wambold & Walter, 1978]

Provisions of Opportunities to Make Choices

To encourage vocabulary usage, students should be afforded the opportunity to make choices throughout their day. Shevin and Klein (1984) view choice making as playing an essential role in the development of independence in society, as it serves to build both self-reliance and self-initiation. Guess and Siegel-Causey (1984) identify five major opportunities for students to make choices within routine activities: 1) choosing among activities, 2) deciding whether or not to engage in activities, 3) deciding when to terminate an activity, 4) selecting alternative means of accomplishing an objective, and 5) choosing partners for activities.

Instruction in choice making might begin by having the student indicate his or her desire to participate in an event when provided with only one stimulus (e.g., touching a favorite toy, prior to playing with it; looking at a cracker, prior to receiving it for a snack). Once the student has learned that signals (pointing, touching, looking) can be used to obtain preferred objects, the choice may be expanded to two items (e.g., a choice between white milk and chocolate milk at lunch; a choice between two leisure activities before free time). The number of choices offered can gradually be expanded as the student demonstrates concept acquisition.

It is not advisable to employ aversive stimuli (e.g., chopped onions, hot sauce) as "undesirable" choices in an effort to accelerate skill acquisition. The use of negative stimuli could either reduce or extinguish the student's willingness to initiate interaction.

The Importance of Teamwork

Effective educational programming for students who are multihandicapped requires a cooperative effort on the part of all persons to work with them—parents, teachers, aides, support staff, and administrators. A good communication network must be developed in which information is exchanged and ideas shared. It is particularly important that the teacher, aides, and parents of a student be mutually consistent in their approach, as they are the primary persons who interact with the child. If a special procedure is being used at school (e.g., coactive movement, use of graphic media), the parents must be trained in its application so they can use it at home with their child. Conversely, if a special procedure is being used in the home (e.g., anticipation to sensory stimulation during bathing and dressing), the educators must be aware of it so that they may utilize it at school.

The major factor that facilitates communication skill development in students who are multihandicapped is teamwork, with everyone working together for the good of the student. These persons, as a team, must learn to communicate and listen with the "all" of themselves. They must become more aware of what the student is already communicating, and together help to make that communication effort more effective and efficient.

FUTURE PROGRAM AND RESEARCH DIRECTIONS

Little empirical research exists on the efficacy of the movement-based approach as presented by van Dijk and his colleagues. A few studies on varied aspects of the approach have been conducted, but their findings must be held suspect as the procedures utilized violated the basic tenet that all activities be performed in real-life situations during the natural daily routine. The value of this approach, however, has been observed and verified by classroom teachers through objective documentation of changes in students' performance over time.

A major problem that exists in designing research to investigate the movement-based approach is the difficulty encountered when trying to isolate its impact on student performance from the impact of other efficacious practices and procedures. Major components of the program that are shared with other approaches for fostering functional skills development include: a) use of real-life materials and situations; b) contextual instruction; c) relevancy and functionality in program planning and implementation; and d) encouragement of independent performance across all activities in which the student is engaged. It would be extremely difficult to eliminate the influence of other approaches when probing specific aspects of the movement-based approach.

The true value of the movement-based approach is as a tool to be used in combination with other functional practices and procedures in the promotion of meaningful interactions with the environment and enhanced communication with other persons. Investigation of the approach should be directed at assessing changes in the behavior of students with whom more traditional approaches to communication and social skills development have been applied. Since the movement-based approach seeks to impact the "total child," baseline and intervention data should include information on the student's performance across critical areas of concern (fine/gross motor skills, perceptual motor abilities, communication, cognition, interpersonal skills) and areas of educational need (domestic skills, vocational skills, community functioning, recreation and leisure skills). Tools and procedures that could be used to generate data are: a) videotaped, protocol-based assessments; b) measures of independent functioning in routine activities, including ecological inventories and discrepancy analyses; c) multi-modal assessment tools (e.g., Callier-Azusa Scale, Comprehensive Test of Adaptive Behavior, Hawaii Early Learning Profile); d) categorical assessment tools (e.g., 1985 Callier-Azusa Scales for the Assessment of Communicative Abilities); and 3) systematic documentation of student performance over time. Communication skills should never be observed in isolation, as they affect, and are affected by, other aspects of the student's total being and environment.

It is anticipated that a better understanding of the principles and practices involved in the movement-based approach will provide educators with viable alternatives for creating successful interactions between their students and the world around them. This is an approach that requires understanding, rather than time, from educators, in that techniques are integrated into existing functional educational activities. The facilitation of personal independence within these activities will subsequently reduce the discrepancies between students who are multihandicapped and their nonhandicapped peers.

REFERENCES

Barraga, N.C. (1976). *Visual handicaps and learning: A developmental approach.* Belmont, CA: Wadsworth.

Bigge, J. (1982). Accompanying disabilities. In J. Bigge (Ed.), *Teaching individuals with physical and multiple disabilities* (pp. 45–74). Columbus, OH: Charles E. Merrill.

Bijou, S., & Baer, D.M. (1961). *Child development I: A systematic and empirical theory.* New York: Appleton-Century-Crofts.

Bottorf, L., & DePape, D. (1982). Initiating communication systems for severely speech impaired persons. *Topics in language disorder,* 2(2), 55–71.

Bower, T.G.R. (1977). *A primer of infant development.* San Francisco: W.H. Freeman.

Bowling, W.L. (1970). The introduction of signs and fingerspelling to a deaf-blind child. *Education of the Visually Handicapped,* 2(3), 89–90.

Brannan, C. (1982). A survey of programs and services to hearing-impaired/mentally retarded children. In D. Tweedie and H. Shroyer (Eds.). *The multihandicapped hearing impaired: Identification and instruction* (pp. 29–36). Washington, DC: Gallaudet College Press.

Bricker, D., & Dennison, L. (1978). Training prerequisites to verbal behavior. In M.E. Snell (Ed.), *Systematic instruction of the moderately and severely handicapped.* Columbus, OH: Charles E. Merrill.

Brown, L., Nietupski, J., & Hamre-Nietupski, S. (1976). Criterion of ultimate functioning. In M.A. Thomas (Ed.), *Hey, don't forget about me* (pp. 2–15). Reston, VA: Council for Exceptional Children.

Burton, J.Y. (1979). Beginning communication: Presymbolic skills with multihandicapped children. In Texas Regional Center for Services to Deaf-Blind Children (Eds.), *Educational methods for deaf-blind and severely handicapped students* (Vol. 2, pp. 98–100). Austin, TX: Texas Education Agency.

Campbell, C.R., & Stremel-Campbell, K. (1982). Programming "loose training" as a strategy to facilitate language generalization. *Journal of Applied Behavioral Analysis, 15,* 295–301.

Cavallaro, C.C. (1983). Language interventions in natural settings. *Teaching exceptional children, 16*(1), 65–70.

Chapman, R.S., & Miller, J.F. (1980). Analyzing language and communication in the child. In R.L. Schiefelbusch (Ed.), *Nonspeech language and communication: Analysis and intervention* (pp. 161–196). Baltimore: University Park Press.

Condon, R. (1979). Prelanguage development: Communication training for the deaf-blind. In Texas Regional Center for Services to Deaf-Blind Children (Eds.), *Educational methods for deaf-blind and severely handicapped students* (Vol. 1, pp. 125–134). Austin, TX: Texas Education Agency.

Cooper, J.A. (1979). Communication training for the deaf-blind. In Texas Regional Center for Services to Deaf-Blind Children (Eds.), *Educational method for deaf-blind and severely handicapped children* (Vol. 2, pp. 111–119). Austin, TX: Texas Education Agency.

Culatte, B., & Blackstone, S. (1980). A program to teach non-oral communication symbols to multiply handicapped children. *Journal of Childhood Communication Disorders, 4*(1), 29–55.

Curtis, W.S., Donlon, E., & Tweedie, D. (1975). Learning behavior of deaf-blind children. *Education of the Visually Handicapped* 7(2), 40–48.

Curtis, W.S., & Donlon, W.T. (1984). A ten-year follow-up study of deaf-blind children. *Exceptional Children, 50*(5), 449–455.

Darnell, C.P. (1982) Bringing the best and brightest to UT. *Alcalde, 71*(2), 32–34.

Day, P.S. (1983). Assessment of deaf-blind children. In S. Ray, M.J. O'Neill, & N.T. Morris (Eds.) *Low incidence children: A guide to psychoeducational assessment* (pp. 141–198). Natchitoches, LA: Steven Ray Publishing.

deLeuw, L. (1970). *Exceptional disorders in the language acquisition of deaf-blind and multiply handicapped deaf children.* Paper presented at the European Regional Conference for Educators of the Deaf-Blind, Paris, France.

Dennis, R., Reichle, J., Williams, W., & Vogelsberg, R.T. (1982). Motoric factors influencing the selection of vocabulary for sign production programs. *Journal of The Association for the Severely Handicapped, 7*(1), 21–32.

Farrell, D., & Sherman, B. (Eds.) (1978). *A prelanguage curriculum guide for the multihandicapped.* Denver: Mountain Plains Regional Center for Services to Handicapped Children.

Fieber, N. (1976). *Movement in communication and language in deaf-blind children.* Unpublished manuscript, Meyer Children's Rehabilitation Institute, University of Nebraska Medical Center, Omaha.

Fieber, N. (1979). Sensorimotor cognitive assessment and curriculum for the multihandicapped child. In Texas Regional Center for Services to Deaf-Blind Children (Eds.), *Educational methods for deaf-blind and severely handicapped students* (Vol. 1, pp. 84–123). Austin, TX: Texas Education Agency.

Flathouse, V. (1979). Multiply handicapped deaf children and Public Law 94–142. *Exceptional Children, 45*(7), 560–565.

Folio, R. (1976). Significance of motor development in the deaf-blind child. In J. Gray & J. Schefler (Eds.), *Proceedings: The Institute of Deaf-Blind Studies.* Austin: Texas Education Agency.

Franklin, B. (1979). Auditory Assessment. In *Educational methods for deaf-blind and severely handicapped students* (Vol. II, pp. 38–51). Austin: The Texas Education Agency.

Fraser, B.A., & Hensinger, R.N. (1983). *Managing physical handicaps: A practical guide for parents, care providers, and educators.* Baltimore: Paul H. Brookes Publishing Co.

Gaylord-Ross, R.J. & Holvoet, J.F. (1985). *Strategies for educating students with severe handicaps.* Boston: Little, Brown.

Geary, S. (1980a). *An overview of the Van Dijk approach to language development.* Unpublished manuscript, Mountain Plains Regional Center, Denver.

Geary, S. (1980b). *Interface of cognitive, motor, and language development: Piaget, Kephart, and Van Dijk.* Unpublished manuscript, Mountain Plains Regional Center, Denver.

Geary, S. (1980c). *Suggestions for implementation of a Van Dijk pre-language program.* Unpublished manuscript, Mountain Plains Regional Center, Denver.

Gill, G., & Dihoff, R. (1982). Nonverbal assessment of cognitive behavior. In B. Campbell &

V. Baldwin (Eds.), *Severely handicapped/hearing impaired children: Strengthening service delivery* (pp. 77–113). Baltimore: Paul H. Brookes Publishing Co.

Goetz, L., Schuler, A.L., & Sailor, W. (1981). Functional competence as a factor in communication instruction. *Exceptional Education Quarterly, 2*(1), 51–60.

Gold, M., & Rittenhouse, R. (1978). Task analysis for teaching eight practical signs to deaf-blind individuals. *Teaching Exceptional Children, 10*, 34–38.

Griffith, P.L. (1980). Sign systems for non-oral children: What teachers need to know. *Journal of Childhood Communication Disorders, 4*(2), 98–110.

Griffith, P.L., Robinson, J.H., & Panagos, J.H. (1983). Tactile iconicity: Signs rated for use with deaf-blind children. *Journal of The Association for Severely Handicapped, 8*(2), 26–38.

Gruenwald, N., Schroeder, J., & Yoder, D. (1982). Considerations for curriculum development and implementation. In B. Campbell & V. Baldwin (Eds.), *Severely handicapped/hearing impaired students: Strengthening service delivery* (pp. 163–179). Baltimore: Paul H. Brookes Publishing Co.

Guess, D. (1980). Methods in communication instruction for severely handicapped persons. In W. Sailor, B. Wilcox, & L. Brown (Eds.), *Methods of instruction for severely handicapped students* (pp. 195–225). Baltimore: Paul H. Brookes Publishing Co.

Guess, D., Benson, H.A., & Siegel-Causey, E. (1985). Concepts and issues related to choice-making and autonomy among persons with severe disabilities. *Journal of The Association for Persons with Severe Handicaps, 10*(2), 79–86.

Guess, D., Sailor, W., & Baer, D.M. (1978). Children with limited language. In R.L. Schiefelbusch (Ed.), *Language intervention strategies*. Baltimore: University Park Press.

Guess, D., Sailor, W., & Keogh, W. (1978). Generalization of speech and language behavior: Measurement and training tactics. In R. Schiefelbusch (Ed.), *Basics of language intervention*. Baltimore: University Park Press.

Guess, D., & Siegel-Causey, E. (1984). Behavioral control and education of severely handicapped students: Who's doing what to whom? and why? In D. Bricker & J. Filler (Eds.) *Serving the severely retarded from research to practice*. Reston, VA: Council for Exceptional Children.

Guldager, L. (1969). The deaf-blind: Their education and their needs. *Exceptional Children, 36*(3), 203–206.

Guldager, V. (1969). *Body image and the severely handicapped rubella child*. Watertown, MA: Perkins School for the Blind.

Halle, J.W. (1982). Teaching functional language to the handicapped: An integrative model of natural environment teaching techniques. *The Journal of The Association for the Severely Handicapped, 7*(4), 29–37.

Hammer, E.A. (1977). Appraisal: A process for identifying problems and potentials of the severely handicapped. In N.G. Haring (Ed.), *Developing effective individualized instructional programs for severely handicapped children and youth* (pp. 51–57). Washington, DC: Department of Health, Education, and Welfare, Office of Education, Bureau of Education for the Handicapped.

Hammer, E.A. (1982). The development of language in the deaf-blind multihandicapped child: Progression of instructional methods. In D. Tweedie & E.H. Shroyer (Eds.), *The multihandicapped hearing impaired: Identification and instruction* (pp. 193–200). Washington, DC: Gallaudet College Press.

Hamre-Nietupski, S., Stoll, A., Holtz, K., Fullerton, P., Ryan-Flottom, M., & Brown, L. (1977). Curricular strategies for teaching selected nonverbal communication skills to nonverbal and verbal severely handicapped children. In L. Brown, J. Nietupski, S. Lyon, S. Hamre-Nietupski, T. Crowner, & L. Gruenwald (Eds.), *Curricular strategies for teaching functional object use, nonverbal communication, problem solving, and mealtime skills to severely handicapped students* (Vol. 2, pp. 94–250). Madison, WI: Department of Specialized Educational Services, Madison Metropolitan School District.

Harlan, N.T., & Carlson, F. (1979). Approaches to nonoral communication. In Texas Regional Center for Services to Deaf-Blind Children (Eds.), *Educational methods for deaf-blind and severely handicapped students* (Vol. 1, pp. 282–295). Austin: Texas Education Agency.

Harris, D., & Vanderheiden, G.C. (1980). Enhancing the development of communicative interaction. In R.L. Schiefelbusch (Ed.), *Nonspeech language and communication* (pp. 229–257). Baltimore: University Park Press.

Hart, B., & Risley, T.R. (1976). Community-based language training. In T.D. Tjossem (Ed.), *Intervention strategies for high risk infants and young children* (pp. 187–198). Baltimore: University Park Press.

Hart, V. (1977). Training of personnel. In E.L. Lowell & C.C. Rovin (Eds.). *State of the art: Perspectives on serving deaf-blind children* (pp. 238–245). Sacramento: California State Department of Education.

Healy, H., & Stainback, S.B. (1980). *The severely motorically impaired student*. Springfield, IL: Charles C Thomas.

Heward, W.L., & Orlansky, M.D. (1984). *Exceptional children: An introductory survey of special education*. Columbus, OH: Charles E. Merrill.

Hopper, C., & Helmick, R. (1977). Nonverbal communication and the severely handicapped: Some considerations. *AAESPH Review, 2*(2), 47–52.

Horrocks, B.L., & Hollis, J.H. (1979). Nonspeech language training. In R.L. York & E. Edgar (Eds.), *Teaching the severely handicapped* (Vol. 4, pp. 219–237). Columbus, OH: Special Press.

Jensema, C.K. (1974). Post-rubella children in special education programs for the hearing impaired. *The Volta Review, 76*(8), 466–473.

Jensema, C.K. (1981a). Report of communication method usage by teachers of deaf-blind children. *American Annals of the Deaf, 126*(1), 8–10.

Jensema, C.K. (1981b). Report of communication method usage by teachers of deaf-blind children—Part II. *American Annals of the Deaf, 126*(1), 392–394.

Jensema, C.K. (1981c). Report of communication method usage by teachers of deaf-blind children—Part III. *American Annals of the Deaf, 126*(5), 488–491.

Jensema, C.K. (1981d). Report of communication method usage by teachers of deaf-blind children—Part IV. *American Annals of the Deaf, 126*(7), 798–801.

Jurgens, M. (1977). *Confrontation between the young deaf-blind child and the outer world*. Sint-Michelsgestel, Netherlands: Instituut voor Doven.

Kaczmarek, L.A. (1985). Integrating language/communication objectives into the total preschool curriculum. *Teaching Exceptional Children, 17*(3), 183–189.

Kamaii, C. (1971). Evaluating learning in preschool education: Socioemotional, perceptual motor, cognitive development. In B. Bloom, J. Hastings, and G. Madans (Eds.), *Handbook on formative and summative evaluation of student learning* (pp. 281–344). New York: McGraw-Hill.

Karlan, G.R., & Lloyd, L.L. (1983). Considerations in the planning of communication intervention: Selecting a lexicon. *Journal of The Association for the Severely Handicapped, 8*(2), 13–25.

Kennedy, A. (1973). Language awareness and the deaf-blind child. *Teaching Exceptional Children, 6*(2), 99–102.

Kennedy, M.C. (1975). Communication and the deaf-blind child. In C. Fiociello (Ed.), *Language development of multi-handicapped children* (pp. 36–49). Dallas, TX: South Central Regional Center for Services to Deaf-Blind Children.

Kohl, F.L., Wilcox, B.L., & Karlan, G.R. (1978). Effects of training conditions on the generalization of manual signs with moderately handicapped students. *Education and Training of the Mentally Retarded, 13*(3), 327–335.

Kollinzas, G. (1983). The communication record: Sharing information to promote sign language generalization. *The Journal of The Association for the Severely Handicapped, 8*(3), 49–55.

Kriegsmann, E., Gallaher, J.C., & Myers, A. (1982). Sign programs with nonverbal hearing children. *Exceptional Children, 48*(5), 436–445.

Luftig, R.L., Page, J.L., & Lloyd, L.L. (1983). Ratings of translucency in manual signs as a predictor of sign learnability. *Journal of Childhood Communication Disorders, 6*(2), 117–134.

Maron, S. (1982). Adaptations for the sensorially handicapped. In J.G. Greer, R.M. Anderson, & S.J. Odel (Eds.), *Strategies for helping severely and multiply handicapped citizens*, (pp. 331–372). Baltimore: University Park Press.

May, J. (1980). *Teaching strategies for non-vocal communication.* Unpublished manuscript, University of Washington, Center for Inservice Training and Program Development, Seattle, WA.

McDonald, E. (1977). Design and application of communication boards. In G.C. Vanderheiden, & K. Grilley (Eds.), *Non-vocal communication techniques for the severely physically handicapped* (pp. 105–119). Baltimore: University Park Press.

McGrane, S., Pierson, M., Read, P., Tarleton, L., & Vierra, D., (1984). *Alternate ways: A guide for working with the nonoral student.* San Diego: San Diego City Schools, Programs for the Handicapped.

McInnis, J.M., & Treffry, J.A. (1982). *Deaf-blind infants and children: A developmental guide.* Toronto: University of Toronto Press.

Mira, M., & Hoffman, S. (1974). Educational programming for multi-handicapped deaf-blind children. *Exceptional Children*, 40(7), 513–514.

Morrison, D., Pothier, P., & Horr, K. (1978). *Sensory-motor dysfunction and therapy in infancy and early childhood.* Springfield, IL: Charles C Thomas.

Mount, M., & Shea, V. (1982). *How to recognize and assess pre-language skills in the severely handicapped.* Lawrence, KS: H & H Enterprises.

Musselwhite, C.R., & St. Louis, K.W. (1982). *Communication programming for the severely handicapped: Vocal and non-vocal strategies.* San Diego, CA: College-Hill Press.

Myers, S.D. (1981). A general overview of disabilities and handicaps. In S.R. Walsh and R. Holtzberg (Eds.), *Understanding and educating the deaf-blind/severely profoundly handicapped* (pp. 43–50). Springfield, IL: Charles C Thomas.

O'Brien, L., & Andresen, J. (1983). A family matter: Stimulating communication in the young cerebral palsied child. *Teaching Exceptional Children, 16*(1), 47–50.

Oliver, C.B., & Halle, J.W. (1982). Language training in the everyday environment: Teaching functional sign use to a retarded child. *The Journal of the Association for the Severely Handicapped, 7*(3), 50–62.

Piaget, J. (1964). *The origins of intelligence in children.* New York: W.W. Norton & Co.

Reichle, J.E., Williams, W., & Ryan, S. (1981). Selecting signs for the formulation of an augmentative communication modality. *Journal of The Association for the Severely Handicapped, 6*(1), 48–56.

Reichle, J.E., & Yoder, D.E. (1979). Assessment and early stimulation of communication in the severely and profoundly mentally retarded. In R.L. York & E. Edgar (Eds.), *Teaching the severely handicapped* (Vol 4, pp. 180–218). Columbus, OH: Special Press.

Reichle, J.E., Yoder, D.E., & Kreul-Starr, M. (1977, November). *Communication behaviors in severely and profoundly developmentally delayed children: Assessment and intervention.* Paper presented at the National Convention of the American Speech and Hearing Association, Chicago, IL.

Richards, J.B. (1887). The education of the feeble-minded. In *Proceedings of the Association of Medical Officers of Institutions for Idiotic and Feeble-Minded Persons*. Philadelphia, PA: J.B. Lippincott.

Robbins, N. (1977). Educational assessment of deaf-blind and auditorily-visually impaired children: A survey. In E.L. Lowell & C.C. Rovin (Eds.), *State of the art: Perspectives on serving deaf-blind children* (pp. 108–142). Sacramento: California State Department of Education.

Robinson, P., & Allen, P. (1975). *An educational approach utilizing developmental sequencing and coactive movement theory*. Unpublished manuscript, Indiana Department of Public Instruction, Northern Regional Service Center, South Bend, IN.

Russel, M. (1984). Assessment and intervention issues with the nonspeaking child. *Exceptional Children, 51*(1), 64–71.

Sailor, W., & Guess, D. (1983). *Severely handicapped students: An instructional design*. Boston: Houghton Mifflin.

Sailor, W., Guess, D., Goetz, L., Schuler, A., Utley, B., & Baldwin, M. (1980). Language and severely handicapped persons: Deciding what to teach to whom. In W. Sailor, B. Wilcox, & L. Brown (Eds.), *Methods of instruction for severely handicapped students* (pp. 71–105). Baltimore: Paul H. Brookes Publishing Co.

Salisbury, C., Wambold, C., & Walter, G. (1978). Manual communication for the severely handicapped: An assessment and instructional strategy. *Education and Training of the Mentally Retarded, 13*(4), 393–399.

Scholl, G.T. (1973). Understanding and meeting developmental needs. In B. Lowenfeld (Ed.), *The visually handicapped child in school* (pp. 61–92). New York: John Day.

Scott, E.P., Jan, J.E., & Freeman, R.D. (1977). *Can't your child see?* Baltimore: University Park Press.

Shane, H.C. (1979). Approaches to communication with the severely handicapped. In R.L. York & E. Edgar (Eds.), *Teaching the severely handicapped* (Vol. 4, pp. 155–179). Columbus, OH: Special Press.

Shea, V., & Mount, M. (1982). *How to arrange the environment to stimulate and teach prelanguage skills in the severely handicapped*. Lawrence, KS: H & H Enterprises.

Shevin, M., & Klein, N.K. (1984). The importance of choice-making skills for students with severe disabilities. *Journal of The Association for Persons with Severe Handicaps, 9*(3), 159–166.

Sims-Tucker, B.M., & Jensema, C.K. (1984). Severely and profoundly auditorially/visually impaired students: The deaf-blind population. In P. J. Valletutti & B.M. Sims-Tucker (Eds.), *Severely and profoundly handicapped students: Their nature and needs* (pp. 269–317). Baltimore: Paul H. Brookes Publishing Co.

Smithdas, R.J. Reflections of a deaf-blind adult (1980). *American Annals of the Deaf, 125*(8), 1015–1017.

Sopers, M.R. (1971). *The deaf-blind child*. Sint-Michielsgestel, Netherlands: Instituut vor Doven.

Stein, L.K., Palmer, P., & Weinberg, B. (1982). Characteristics of a young deaf-blind population. *American Annals for the Deaf, 127*(7), 828–837.

Sternberg, L., Battle, C., & Hill, J. (1980). Prelanguage communications programming for the severely and profoundly handicapped. *Journal of The Association for the Severely Handicapped, 5*(3), 224–233.

Sternberg, L., McNerney, C.D., & Pegnatore, L. (1985). Developing co-active imitative behaviors with profoundly mentally handicapped students. *Education and Training of the Mentally Retarded, 20*(4), 260–267.

Sternberg, L., Pegnatore, L., & Hill, C. (1983). Establishing interactive communication behaviors with profoundly mentally handicapped students. *Journal of The Association for the Severely Handicapped, 8*(2), 39–46.

Stillman, R., Aylmer, J., & Vandivort, J. (1983, June). *The functions of signalling behaviors in profoundly-impaired, deaf-blind children and adolescents*. Paper presented at the Annual Meeting of the American Association on Mental Deficiency, Dallas, Texas.

Stillman, R.D., & Battle, C.W. (1984). Developing prelanguage communication in the severely handicapped. An interpretation of the Van Dijk method. *Seminars in Speech and Language, 4*(3), 159–170.

Stillman, R.D., & Battle, C.W. (1986). Developmental assessment of communicative abilities in the deaf-blind. In D. Ellis (Ed.), *Sensory impairments in mentally handicapped people.* San Diego, CA: College-Hill Press.

Stone, C. (1977). Motor skills. In N.G. Haring (Ed.), *Developing individualized educational programs for severely handicapped children and youth* (pp. 58–90). Washington, DC: Department of Health, Education, and Welfare; Office of Education; Bureau of Education for the Handicapped.

Stone, C. (1979). An overview of normal and abnormal motor functioning: Implications for educational programming. In Texas Regional Services to Deaf-Blind Children (Eds.), *Educational methods for deaf-blind and severely handicapped children* (Vol. 2, pp. 3–22). Austin: Texas Education Agency.

Stone, G. (1979). Sensory stimulation, sensory integration theory. In Texas Regional Center for Services to Deaf-Blind Children (Eds.), *Educational methods for deaf-blind and severely handicapped students* (Vol. 1, pp. 72–277). Austin: Texas Education Agency.

Stremel-Campbell, K., Cantrell, D., & Halle, J. (1977). Manual signing as a language system and as a speech imitator for the nonverbal severely handicapped student. In E. Sontag, J. Smith, & N. Certo (Eds.), *Educatinal programming for the severely and profoundly handicapped* (pp. 335–347). Reston, VA: Division on Mental Retardation, Council for Exceptional Children.

Turiansky, K., & Bove, M. (1975). Methods of language development—Van Dijk. In C. Ficociello (Ed.), *Language development of multi-handicapped children* (pp. 60–72). Dallas, TX: South Central Regional Center for Services to Deaf-Blind Children.

Tweedie, D. (1982). Structuring the communication program for the needs of multihandicapped hearing impaired children. In D. Tweedie and E.H. Shroyer (Eds.), *The multihandicapped hearing impaired: Identification and instruction,* (pp. 185–192). Washington, DC: Gallaudet College Press.

Tweedie, D., & Baud, H. (1981). Future directions in the education of deaf-blind multihandicapped children and youth. *American Annals of the Deaf, 126*(7), 829–834.

Tweedie, D., & Shroyer, E.H. (Eds.), (1982). *The multihandicapped hearing impaired: Identification and instruction.* Washington, DC: Gallaudet College Press.

Vanderheiden, G.C., & Grilley, K. (Eds), (1977). *Non-vocal communication techniques and aids for the severely physically handicapped.* Baltimore: University Park Press.

Van Dijk, J. (1965a). The first steps of the deaf-blind child towards language. *Proceedings of the Conference on the Deaf-Blind,* Refsnes, Denmark (pp. 47–50). Boston: Perkins School for the Blind.

Van Dijk, J. (1965b). Introduction to the film. *Proceedings of the Conference on the Deaf-Blind, Refsnes, Denmark* (pp. 50–53). Boston: Perkins School for the Blind.

Van Dijk, J. (1965c). Motor development in the education of deaf-blind children. *Proceedings of the Conference on the Deaf-Blind, Refsnes, Denmark* (pp. 41–47). Boston: Perkins School for the Blind.

Van Dijk, J. (1965d). *Report of a seminar on the teaching of deaf-blind children held at Kalundborg, Denmark.* Boston: Perkins School for the Blind.

Van Dijk, J. (1966). The first steps of the deaf-blind child towards language. *The International Journal for the Education of the Blind, 15*(4), 112–114.

Van Dijk, J. (1967). The non-verbal deaf-blind child and his world: His outgrowth toward the world of symbols. *Proceedings of the Jaarverslag Instituut voor Doven, 1964–1967* (pp. 73–110), Sint-Michielsgestel, Netherlands.

Van Dijk, J. (1968) *Movement and communication with rubella children.* Paper presented at the

National Association for Deaf-Blind and Rubella Children, Annual General Meeting, Sint-Michielsgestel, Netherlands.

Van Dijk, J. (1969). *Educational approaches to abnormal development: Some aspects of the psychology of the senses in relation to the sensory-deprived child.* Dallas, TX: South Central Regional Center for Services to Deaf-Blind Children, 2930 Turtle Creek Plaza.

Van Dijk, J. (1984). *Research on rubella children.* Paper presented at the Eighth Conference on Deaf-Blind Education, New York Institute for the Blind, Rochester, NY.

Van Son, Y. (1983). *Pre-linguistic communication techniques and procedures for severely multihandicapped children.* Unpublished manuscript, University of San Diego, San Diego.

Vernon, M. (1982). Multihandicapped deaf children: Types and causes. In D. Tweedie and E.H. Shroyer (Eds.), *The multihandicapped hearing impaired: Identification and instruction* (pp. 11–28). Washington, DC: Gallaudet College Press.

Von Bruns-Connolly, S., & Shane, H. (1978). Communication boards: Help for the child unable to walk. *Exceptional Parent, 8,* 19–22.

Wacker, D.P., & Hoffman, R.C. (1984). Severely and profoundly mentally retarded students. In P.J. Valletutti & B.M. Sims-Tucker, *Severely and profoundly handicapped students: Their nature and their needs* (pp. 11–83). Baltimore: Paul H. Brookes Publishing Co.

Walsh, S.R. (1982). The educational implications of deaf/blindness. In S.R. Walsh & R. Holzberg (Eds.), *Understanding and educating the deaf-blind/severely and profoundly handicapped: An international perspective* (pp. 25–37). Springfield, IL: Charles C Thomas.

Walsh, S.R. & Holzberg, R. (1981). *Understanding and educating the deaf-blind/severely and profoundly handicapped: An international perspective.* Springfield, IL: Charles C Thomas.

Ward, M. (1981). An overview of motor development: Implications for educational programming. In S.R. Walsh & R. Holzberg (Eds.), *Understanding and educating deaf-blind/severely and profoundly handicapped: An international perspective* (pp. 100–113). Springfield, IL: Charles C Thomas.

Werner, H., & Kaplan, B. (1963). *Symbol formation.* New York: John Wiley & Sons.

Wilson, K.D. (1980). Selection of a core lexicon for use with graphic communication systems. *Journal of Childhood Communication Disorders, 4*(2), 111–123.

Woznak, D., & Lasky, E.Z. (1980). Levels of visual abstraction and the assessment of language comprehension in trainable mentally retarded children. *Journal of Childhood Communication Disorders, 4*(1), 12–18.

Writer, J. (1984, November). *Non-oral, prelinguistic communication skills development in children and youth who are severely multihandicapped.* Paper presented at the Eleventh Annual TASH Conference, Chicago, IL.

Writer, J. (1985). Research on educational practices and procedures employed with children and youth who are deaf-blind: Past, present, and future perspectives. In J.E. Stahlecker, L.E. Glass, & S. Machalow (Eds), *State-of-the-art: Research priorities in deaf-blindness* (pp. 79–122). San Francisco: University of California, Center on Mental Health and Deafness.

Wulz, S.V., Myers, S.P., Klein, M.D., Hall, M.K., & Walde, L.J. (1982). Unobtrusive training: A home-centered model for communication training. *Journal of The Association of the Severely Handicapped, 7*(2), 36–47.

CHAPTER 9

An Ecological Approach to Curriculum Development

John A. Nietupski and Susan M. Hamre-Nietupski

CASE STUDY #1: A SENSORY-DEVELOPMENTAL APPROACH

Laura is a 10-year-old child who is severely handicapped and has dual sensory impairments. She has residual hearing, which is enhanced through the use of bilateral hearing aids and an auditory trainer. Her residual sight is enhanced by corrective lenses through which she is able to perceive light and dark, and to discriminate objects on the basis of their outline.

Laura attends a program in which a sensory-developmental approach is emphasized. Accordingly, her individualized education program (IEP) goals, drawn from the developmental checklist used by the school program, are to: 1) tolerate different textures; 2) develop pre-speech babbling skills; 3) develop equilibrium responses and protective extension; 4) discriminate shapes and sizes; and 5) improve fine motor skills such as reach and grasp. Specific daily activities include touching sandpaper shapes; feeling hot and cold water at the sink and water table; tumbling in vats of Styrofoam peanuts and plastic balls in the "sensory learning environment" and experiencing different food textures/tastes at snack and lunch times. During communication time, the therapist encourages babbling through tickling and grab-bag exploration of different textured toys and other materials. The communication therapist occasionally works on the pre-speech oral skills of tongue and lip movements through exercises such as licking peanut butter off the upper lip or the roof of the mouth, blowing bubbles, and smacking lips. Snack periods are used to expose Laura to different food tastes, smells and textures. Occupational and physical therapy time is devoted to twirling in a suspended swing, rocking on a large ball, and rolling over a bolster in the prone position. Virtually all of Laura's instruction occurs in the classroom, the sensory learning environment, or the therapy room.

CASE STUDY #2: AN ECOLOGICAL APPROACH

James also is a 10-year-old child with severe handicaps and dual sensory impairments. He, too, has residual sight and hearing that are enhanced through the use of auditory and vision aids.

James attends a school program that emphasizes an ecological approach. His IEP goals, developed jointly with parents and therapists, address four major life-skill domains/curricular areas: domestic living, recreation/leisure, community functioning, and vocational. Specific IEP goals include: *Domestic:* 1) to put on shoes and socks, and 2) to spear bite-sized food with fork. *Community-Functioning:* 1) to walk from one area of a store to another by trailing the wall, and 2) to select items from a store shelf. *Recreation/leisure:* 1) to operate a musical Simon toy, and 2) to operate pop and snack vending machines. *Vocational:* 1) to staple and assist in delivering handouts needed by the school office personnel and regular education teachers in the building. A communication goal integrated throughout the above activities is to sign "help" when needing assistance.

James' daily instructional activities occur in both school and nonschool settings. Domestic living skills instruction occurs in the classroom, lunchroom, locker room, and, twice per week, in an actual community home. James and his classmates are taught to use the school vending machine during "break times" and community vending machines on their weekly community training experiences. They practice finding items on shelves in the simulated classroom store, and once per week in an actual community store. James practices his trailing/mobility skills in the school and during all community/domestic training sessions. James is taught the vocational stapling skill in his classroom, the school office, and the lead teacher's office. The therapists integrate instruction on motor and communication skills into the ongoing activities in the school and community.

The two case studies presented above, while perhaps exaggerated in order to accentuate the differences, reflect two major instructional approaches advocated for use with pupils who are severely handicapped, including students with dual sensory impairments (Brown, Branston et al., 1979; Brown, Branston-McLean et al., 1979). One approach, loosely termed sensory-developmental and embodied in Case Study #1, suggests that curriculum content should be based on developmental sequences in fine and gross motor, receptive and expressive communication, social, sensorimotor, cognitive, and self-help curricular areas. The educator's task under such an approach is to determine a student's developmental level and select those skills for instruction that would represent the next logical developmental milestone if that student were a nonhandicapped individual. Thus, educators take students from the bottom-up, from simple to more complex skills within each curricular area, following established developmental guidelines. Specialists from the communication, mobility, occupational, or physical therapy areas likewise assess developmental level and independently teach within a developmental framework.

The second major approach, termed *ecological* and embodied in Case Study #2, represents a radical departure from the sequential, bottom-up sensory-developmental approach. In essence, proponents of an ecological approach seriously question whether following normal developmental progression represents the most effective instructional approach for students with severe handicaps (Guess, Sailor, & Baer,

1977; Holvoet, Guess, Mulligan, & Brown, 1980). It is argued that, rather than narrowing the discrepancy between the behavior of individuals who are nonhandicapped and those who have severe handicaps, a developmental approach serves to widen this discrepancy (Brown, Branston-McLean, et al., 1979). Further, the limited amount of instructional time available, coupled with the often lengthy time needed to acquire skills, results in students who never become "ready" for instruction on skills that are appropriate to their chronological age and that lead toward more independent functioning in the community during post-school years.

As a result of these concerns, an ecological approach, discussed in detail below, has been proposed. This ecological or "top-down" approach provides a strategy for educators to determine the skills needed by *nonhandicapped* individuals to function independently in a variety of vocational, domestic, recreation/leisure, and community environments currently available or likely to be encountered in the future by students with severe handicaps. This information then forms the basis for individualized curriculum content for students with severe handicaps, including dual sensory impairments. Under this model, specialists such as communication, occupational, and physical therapists first determine the skills relative to their disciplines that are needed in vocational, domestic, community and recreation/leisure environments, and then teach students in the context of normalized experiences.

Proponents of an ecological approach argue that by referencing curriculum content to the skills needed by the nonhandicapped population, students are more likely to receive instruction on *functional* skills—skills that will be useful immediately or in the near future, across a range of natural environments. Thus, upon graduation from school programs, students are more likely to have acquired skills that will contribute to more independent functioning in the real world. Since the schools' responsibility, according to Public Law 94–142, is to teach skills needed to optimize independence (Hawkins & Hawkins, 1981), an ecological approach, much more so than a sensory-developmental approach, provides a means by which schools can meet that responsibility.

Those who favor an ecological approach also do so because of the *individualized* nature of the resulting curriculum. As stated by Snell (1983), "Because of cultural and geographic differences from one family and setting to another, all skills that are relevant for one student cannot be assumed to be relevant for another" (p. 78). Individualized and localized, rather than standardized, curricular sequences are needed. An ecological approach allows for such individualized curricula, due to its reliance upon careful observation of the skills demanded in particular nonschool environments.

The purpose of this chapter is to provide instructional personnel with a step-by-step process for developing ecologically valid curriculum content for students who are severely handicapped and have dual sensory impairments. In the following section, this process will be articulated and illustrated through several examples. Thereafter, the empirical support for an ecological approach will be discussed, along with future research needs with regard to this area.

APPLICATION TO EDUCATIONAL SETTINGS

Figure 1 delineates a step-by-step process for generating curricular content using an ecological approach. Each step in the process will be discussed below.

Step 1: Delineate Curriculum Domains

The first step in the ecological curriculum development process involves the specification of those domains to be addressed in a student's IEP. It is recommended that four domains be addressed: vocational, domestic, community, and recreation/leisure. These four domains represent major persisting life needs of all persons, including those with severe and dual sensory impairments. That is, all individuals are expected to participate to the extent possible in work, domestic living and community environments and in recreational/leisure pursuits. A domain approach facilitates the integrated use of communication, motor, social, and other skills within the context of natural, functional activities. Thus, when being taught to shop in a department store (community domain activity), a student also might be receiving instruction on: 1) the gross motor skills of walking across various types of terrain (streets, stairs, sidewalks, escalators, and elevators); 2) the fine motor skills of obtaining money from a wallet or purse and putting change in one's pocket; 3) the communication skill of indicating the desire to make a purchase to the clerk or cashier; and 4) the social skill of signaling good-bye when leaving the cashier. Traditional skill areas are not ignored under a domain approach, but integrated into meaningful activities so that students are able to discern the reason for performing these skills.

Step 2: Delineate Environments

Once the domains are delineated, instructional personnel should identify the environments in which students currently function and the subsequent environments likely to be experienced in the future. For example, the current environment in the domestic domain for James, the student in Case Study #2, might be his home. However, at

---

Step 1:	Delineate curriculum domains (Vocational; Domestic; Community; Recreation/Leisure)
Step 2:	Delineate the variety of current and subsequent natural environments in each domain in which students function/might function
Step 3:	Inventory and delineate the sub-environments within each environment
Step 4:	Inventory and delineate the activities performed by nonhandicapped persons in those sub-environments
Step 5:	Prioritize activities in order to delineate IEP goals
Step 6:	Delineate the skills needed in order to perform the activities
Step 7:	Conduct a discrepancy analysis in order to determine required skills not currently in the student's repertoire
Step 8:	Determine necessary adaptations
Step 9:	Develop an instructional program

Figure 1. The nine steps of the ecological curriculum development process.

some point in the future, a group home or supervised apartment might be appropriate for his domestic living arrangement.

Practitioners might focus more of their attention on the present environment in situations where such an environment is to be experienced for an extended period of time. For example, since James is 10 years old, he will probably remain at home until age 21. Thus, activities targeted for instruction primarily will be drawn from the current domestic environment. As he becomes older, however, an increasing amount of instructor attention should be devoted to inventorying and teaching activities needed in a subsequent living arrangement, such as a group home or sheltered apartment.

Step 3: Inventory and Delineate Sub-environments

Within most environments, several distinct areas, or sub-environments, can be delineated. For example, sub-environments in the home might include the bathroom, bedroom, kitchen, living room, porch, basement, and yard areas. Likewise, the community domain environment of a restaurant can be divided into the cashier, seating, and salad bar areas, the cloakroom, and the restroom.

Step 4: Inventory and Delineate Activities

Within each sub-environment, nonhandicapped individuals perform a myriad of activities. The ecological inventory process requires careful observation of nonhandicapped individuals in each sub-environment. By specifying the activities performed by nonhandicapped individuals, a practitioner can develop a rich source of information regarding possible curricular content. Figures 2, 3, 4, and 5 present sample ecological inventories in the vocational, domestic, community and recreation/leisure domains.

Step 5: Determine Priorities Among Activities and Select IEP Goals

As indicated in Figures 2–5, ecological inventories present instructional personnel with an enormous number of potential teaching targets. Obviously, a teacher cannot possibly address all needed activities within any one given period of time. Thus, a system for setting activity priorities and selecting IEP goals is critically needed.

No empirically derived rules currently exist for setting such activity priorities and selecting IEP goals. However, several authors have suggested strategies for creating activity priorities (Ford et al., 1984; Wuerch & Voeltz, 1982). Six of the more pertinent suggestions for selecting priorities include:

1. Parental preference
2. Student preference/reinforcement value
3. Instructional personnel preference
4. Frequency of occurrence (within or across environments or sub-environments)
5. Safety concerns
6. Social significance

Each of these considerations is discussed briefly below.

DOMAIN: *Vocational*
- Environment: *School cafeteria* (current)
  - Sub-environment: *Dish area*
    - Activity: Remove paper/plastic from trays and plates and discard
    - Activity: Stack plates, cups, saucers
    - Activity: Sort dirty silverware into silverware baskets
    - Activity: Rinse plates, cups, saucers, silverware, and trays
    - Activity: Scrub out pans with sponge/scrubber
    - Activity: Fill dishwasher trays with plates, etc.
    - Activity: Operate dishwasher to wash items on tray
    - Activity: Stack dishes, cups, saucers, etc., on carts in designated area for each item
    - Activity: Operate garbage disposal
    - Activity: Roll napkin around a set of spoon, fork, knife
  - Sub-environment: *Serving line area*
    - Activity: Remove empty pans from serving line, place on cart
    - Activity: Replace empty pans with full pans of same item
    - Activity: Replace dishes, saucers, cups, and silverware rolls as the supply runs low
    - Activity: Scoop and place portions of vegetables, potatoes, or casserole on plates
    - Activity: Hand plate of food to student
    - Activity: Take money/ticket and operate cash register
  - Sub-environment: *Seating area*
    - Activity: Wipe off tables (top and seat)
    - Activity: Sweep floor
    - Activity: Unfold and set up tables
    - Activity: Fold up tables and return to wall
    - Activity: Throw remaining trash items in trash can
    - Activity: Fill wash bucket with soapy water
    - Activity: Wash floor with bucket and mop
    - Activity: Replace plastic trash/pop can liners
    - Activity: Remove and tie filled trash/pop can liners
    - Activity: Replace pop in pop machine
    - Activity: Replace candy/snacks in candy/snack machine
    - Activity: Toss returnable pop cans into pop can receptacle
  - Sub-environment: *Loading dock/supply area*
    - Activity: Toss filled trash liners in dumpster
    - Activity: Place liner with returnable pop cans in appropriate area
    - Activity: Open/close key-type lock on pop/snack supply bin
    - Activity: Stack cases of pop/snacks/candy on two-wheel dolly
    - Activity: Push dolly to/from vending machine area

Figure 2. The ecological inventory process: Vocational domain.

Parental Preference This refers to assigning priorities on the basis of parental input about desired educational goals. Parental input too frequently is ignored in the selection of IEP goals (Alberto & Troutman, 1982). Frequently, educators select IEP goals and then ask parents to sign the IEP document. Thereafter, the lack of carryover at home is lamented. Perhaps the problem is not, as it has often been unfairly characterized, lack of concern/commitment on the part of parents. Rather, the fault may be

DOMAIN: *Domestic*
Environment: *Natural home* (Current)
Sub-environment: *Bedroom*
Activity: Make bed after awakening
Activity: Obtain outfit (pants/shirt/socks, underwear/shoes)
Activity: Put on clothing items
Activity: Remove clothing items
Activity: Put away clothing items in correct drawer
Activity: Pick up toys and return to toy chest
Activity: Hang up hanging clothes
Activity: Place shoes on shoe rack
Sub-environment: *Kitchen*
Activity: Dry dishes and silverware
Activity: Put silverware in tray in drawer
Activity: Remove filled trash can liner and twist tie top
Activity: Replace new trash can liner
Activity: Put dishes/cups away
Activity: Wash vegetables and fruit
Activity: Peel and section oranges
Activity: Peel banana
Activity: Prepare toast
Activity: Prepare cereal
Activity: Prepare sandwiches
Activity: Cook hot dogs
Activity: Prepare canned soup
Activity: Prepare juice from frozen concentrate
Activity: Prepare Kool-aide
Activity: Pour milk/Kool-aide/juice from pitcher into cup/glass
Sub-environment: *Eating area*
Activity: Set table
Activity: Remove items from table after meal
Activity: Wipe off table
Activity: Use fork to spear food
Activity: Cut food with knife
Activity: Use spoon to scoop appropriate solid/liquid foods
Activity: Drink liquid from cup
Activity: Use napkin to wipe hands/face
Activity: Get in/out of chair
Activity: Pass items on request
Activity: Pour beverage from container to glass
Activity: Ask for more food/beverage
Activity: Ask to be excused from table
Sub-environment: *Living room*
Activity: Put magazines in magazine basket
Activity: Dust furniture
Activity: Vacuum rug
Activity: Pick up trash/old newspapers
Activity: Water plants
Activity: Straighten couch cushions
Activity: Return coasters to container

Figure 3. The ecological inventory process: Domestic domain.

DOMAIN: *Community functioning*
Environment: *Supermarket*
Sub-environment: *Parking lot/entrance area*
Activity: Remove seat belt
Activity: Unlock and open car door from inside
Activity: Exit automobile
Activity: Lock and close door
Activity: Unlock with key and open door from outside
Activity: Enter automobile
Activity: Put on seatbelt
Activity: Walk to/from automobile from/to entrance
Activity: Use pop vending machine outside supermarket
Activity: Enter push door
Activity: Exit automatic opening door
Activity: Place groceries in automobile
Activity: Return cart to supermarket
Sub-environment: *Aisle area*
Activity: Obtain cart
Activity: Push carts up and down aisle
Activity: Select needed grocery items
Activity: Ask clerk to weigh produce
Activity: Ask clerk for particular cut/weight of meat product
Activity: Receive cash for returnable bottles/cans
Activity: Obtain frozen food items from pull open freezer door section
Sub-environment: *Check out area*
Activity: Select open/shorter check out line
Activity: Move cart forward as line progresses
Activity: Remove items from cart and place on conveyor belt
Activity: Pay cashier for groceries and receive change
Activity: Carry groceries/push cart out to automobile

Figure 4. The ecological inventory process: Community functioning domain.

that educators have not selected goals on the basis of family priorities. For this reason, it is suggested that instructional personnel develop a list of possible activities. Parents should then be encouraged to indicate the degree to which they perceive the activities as critical (e.g., high, medium, or low preference), and/or rank order the five to ten highest priority potential IEP targets. While parental input alone should not dictate IEP goals, it should be a major consideration in the IEP development process.

Student Preference/Reinforcement Value Goals should also be selected on the basis of activities enjoyed or likely to be reinforcing to the student. Assume that the recreation/leisure inventory depicted in Figure 5 has been developed for Laura described in Case History #1, above. If there is evidence to indicate that Laura has sufficient residual hearing to perceive music and that she, in fact, likes music, playing a record might be selected as an IEP goal, rather than looking at a book. Similarly, if the second student, James, has difficulty working in high temperature areas, where he becomes irritable, easily fatigued and quickly off-task, select instead an IEP goal

DOMAIN: *Recreation/leisure*
Environment: *Public library*
Sub-environment: *Desk/Entryway/Exit Area*
Activity: Enter push door
Activity: Enter turnstile
Activity: Return books
Activity: Check out books
Activity: Exit through push-bar electronic sensor
Sub-environment: *Book shelf area*
Activity: Scan shelf and select books
Activity: Look at books
Activity: Climb on ladder to reach book
Sub-environment: *Audio area*
Activity: Select record
Activity: Remove record from jacket and play
Activity: Attach headphone jack to record player or bank of headphone plugs and place headphones over ears
Activity: Select cassette tape/book
Activity: Play cassette tape and follow along in book
Activity: Return record or tape/book to shelf
Sub-environment: *Snack room*
Activity: Use pull-bottle pop vending machine
Activity: Open pop bottle
Activity: Use push-button snack vending machine
Activity: Open plastic wrappers
Activity: Find empty seat and consume snack
Activity: Look at newspaper
Activity: Operate dollar bill change machine
Activity: Obtain coffee from coffee pot
Sub-environment: *Parking lot*
Activity: Place books in book deposit box
Activity: Remove/put on seatbelt
Activity: Open/close door
Activity: Unlock door from inside
Activity: Unlock door from outside with key
Activity: Enter/exit automobile
Activity: Walk across parking lot to/from car

Figure 5. The ecological inventory process: Recreation/leisure domain.

such as cleaning tables in the eating area, rather than activities in the hot dishwasher area. While student preferences are not always easy to discern, efforts should be made to take this factor into consideration when selecting IEP goals.

Instructional Personnel Preference Professional judgments of teachers or therapists as to the most functional, meaningful, and appropriate goals for students should enter into the goal selection process. Teachers cannot totally abdicate decision making simply because increased efforts are being made to attend to parental and student concerns/interests. As the following example illustrates, teacher input regarding functional goals for students is critical.

At a recent IEP meeting for a 14-year-old female, who had severe handicaps, and who was visually and physically impaired, parents indicated that toileting was not a priority. They stated that, due to their daughter's size, it was easier for them to allow her to wear diapers and change her periodically, rather than attempt to transfer her to and from the toilet. The teacher, however, was aware that area group homes typically did not accept residents who could not toilet themselves. Because a possible subsequent environment for the student was a group home, the teacher felt it critical that the student be taught to toilet herself. Through their discussions, the parents and teacher reached a compromise: the parents would support the toileting IEP goal if the teacher included efforts to teach the student to assist in transferring from the wheelchair to the toilet seat and back. In this way, teacher input resulted in the inclusion of a potentially critical IEP goal activity.

In the above instance, teacher input to parents resulted in the IEP including a teacher preference goal. Not all negotiation attempts, however, are that successful. When families and practitioners disagree over IEP goals, staff members should first ask if family priorities are, perhaps, more appropriate than their own. If the teacher still feels strongly that a particular activity is functional and should be included on the IEP, negotiation efforts should be made to convince families of the objective need for such a goal. If this too fails, teachers are faced with two choices: 1) accede to parental requests that the goal be dropped; or 2) work toward the IEP goal at school, recognizing that it is not a priority at home. The latter action, of course, is quite drastic. At times, however, it is legitimate to take such action when staff members have a sound rationale for their position. While parental collaboration is preferred, it is possible for students to learn skills at school that are not reinforced/expected at home. At worst, students may learn to discriminate when such behavior is expected and perform it only in those situations. A better outcome, and one that is sometimes observed, is that student performance of an activity at school or in the community has prompted families to reconsider and make it a priority at home as well.

Frequency of Occurrence This refers either to the number of times an activity is required in a given environment or setting, or the number of environments or settings that require performance of a specified activity. In general, the more frequently an activity must be performed, the more functional it may be. Further, frequently occurring activities provide more natural practice opportunities, thus possibly promoting skill acquisition, maintenance, and generalization.

In the example inventories provided in Figures 2–5, it can be seen that walking to/from a car across a parking lot occurs in two inventories, as does the use of a vending machine, as well as scanning shelves to make a selection (supermarket and library). Thus, in considering only the above four inventories, these activities might be targeted as priorities. Further, activities such as setting the table, putting on/removing seatbelts, and entering/exiting automobiles might also be considered as possible priorities due to their frequent daily use.

Safety Concerns Setting activity priorities on the basis of the degree to which the activity will promote the safety of the student falls under the category of safety concerns. Obviously, activities such as riding in automobiles, crossing streets, traversing parking lots, climbing stairs, and using escalators can present potential dangers to students, especially those students whose visual and hearing impairments restrict their ability to attend to the typical warning signs (e.g., seeing approaching autos, hearing honking cars). Thus, practitioners might consider such safety concerns as priority IEP goals. While the severity of intellectual and sensory impairments might limit the extent to which students can perform the activities independently, adaptations (discussed below) might be considered that allow for partial participation and increased safety.

Social Significance As used here, social significance is a broad term that includes the extent to which an activity will enhance a student's social acceptability, promote interaction attempts from those near the student, or make the student appear less handicapped. This concern is of importance in that a major assumption of an ecological curricular approach is that students with severe handicaps should be prepared to function with nonhandicapped individuals in a wide variety of normalized environments. Thus, in a library setting, practitioners might target selecting and looking at books or listening to records. These are normal activities that would be socially acceptable and might, in fact, facilitate interactions with persons who are nonhandicapped.

The above six considerations, while not exhaustive, can provide practitioners with direction in determining IEP goal priorities. While no data exist to suggest whether the six considerations are equally important, or some more important than others, it may be possible to use a mathematical rating procedure to determine priority IEP goals. Table 1 presents such a priority ranking form. To use such a rating system, practitioners first generate a list of 10 to 15 possible priority activities. Instructional staff and parents then rate the activities according to the six priority considerations. Activities that are rated highest form IEP goals.

While such a procedure may assume incorrectly that all factors are of equal value, it does provide one means of setting activity priorities more objectively. Practitioners need to keep in mind, however, that if one or more criteria are particularly relevant in a given situation, the activity(ies) that best meet those criteria might be selected, despite a lower overall rating.

Step 6: Delineate the Skills Needed to Engage in a Targeted Activity

Once priority activities have been established, those activities need to be broken down into the component skills through a task analysis (TA) process. Task analyses represent a delineation of the skills necessary to perform any activity, arranged either in the order in which such skills would typically be performed by nonhandicapped individuals, or in a hierarchical (easy-to-difficult) order.

There are a number of ways in which tasks may be broken down. The simplest and most common form of task analysis (TA) is the sequential listing of steps. To employ this strategy, practitioners need only perform the activity themselves or observe others performing this activity. The task steps are then written down in the order

Table 1. Rating form for setting activity priorities

	Parent preference	Student preference	Practitioner preference	Frequency of occurrence	Safety concerns	Social significance	Total
Activity:							
1. Play records	2	3	1	2	1	3	12
2. Use seatbelt	3	1	3	3	3	1	14
3. Walk through parking lot	1	1	3	2	3	1	11
4. Use vending machine	1	3	2	2	1	2	11

(3 = high preference/frequency/safety/social; 2 = medium preference; 1 = low preference)

in which they occur. Figure 6 contains a sample task analysis in which the skills are delineated for using a vending machine.

An important consideration in any TA is the difficulty of a task "step." The nine phases or task steps in Figure 6 represent relatively large "chunks" of behavior. For many students, such steps would need to be reduced to smaller behavior samples. For example, the current Phase II, obtain two quarters, might be broken down further into the following skills:

IIa: Reach hand into pocket
IIb: Remove one quarter
IIc: Place quarter in other hand
IId: Reach into pocket again
IIe: Remove second quarter
IIf: Place second quarter in other hand

There are no empirically derived rules regarding the optimal task step size. However, a general rule of thumb is that the younger or more severely disabled the student, the smaller the recommended task step.

The "sequence of steps" task analysis can be taught as a total cycle, as indicated in Teaching Note 1 below Figure 6. A "total cycle" approach involves allowing students to attempt independently all skills during an instructional trial, providing the minimum level of corrective assistance required when students incorrectly perform any given task step. Again, a rule of thumb is that older and/or less severely disabled individuals (i.e., those likely to make more rapid progress) might benefit most from a total cycle approach (Sailor & Guess, 1983). Younger or more seriously disabled students (i.e., those likely to make slower progress) might require a strategy using a more structured variation of a sequential listing of steps.

Chaining approaches represent a variation upon the sequential listing of steps TA. Instructional personnel can employ either a forward or backward chain TA strat-

In the vending machine area of the library during free time, the student will:

Phase 1: Walk to vending machine
Phase 2: Obtain two quarters
Phase 3: Place two quarters in slot
Phase 4: Push selector button/panel
Phase 5: Obtain pop can from bin
Phase 6: Check coin return slot for change
Phase 7: Place any change in pocket
Phase 8: Walk away from vending machine

Teaching note 1 (If total cycle): This is a "sequence of steps" task analysis. Instruction should be in a total cycle format, with students given an opportunity to perform all task steps on each instructional trial.

Teaching note 2 (If forward chain): This is a forward chain TA. Therefore, allow the student to independently attempt all phases above, and including the targeted phase for a given session, assist the student to perform all phases below that targeted for a given session.

Teaching note 3 (If backward chain): This is a backward chain TA. Therefore, assist the student through all phases above the targeted phase, allowing him or her to attempt that phase and all subsequent phases independently.

Figure 6. Task analysis: Task steps in using a coin-operated vending machine.

egy. In a forward chain, the instructor allows a student to attempt the first task step independently and assists him or her through all remaining task steps (see Figure 6, Teaching Note 2). Once the first task step is independently performed to satisfy an established criterion, the student is allowed to attempt the first *two* steps, with assistance always provided on the remaining steps. In this manner, the response requirements are gradually increased until a student is able to perform all skills in a given activity.

A second variation is a backward chain TA strategy. In this approach, a staff member assists a student through all but the last phase, then all but the last two phases, and so forth, until the entire sequence is independently performed (see Figure 6, Teaching Note 3). Thus, the major difference between these two chaining variations is the part of the chain in which the assistance is provided.

As stated earlier, task analyses can reflect simply a logically ordered sequence of steps, or an easy-to-difficult hierarchy. In the latter case, practitioners must go beyond a simple sequence-of-steps TA strategy in developing a task analysis. Figure 7 provides a task analysis based on a presumed easy-to-difficult strategy. Each phase objective represents a gradually increased supermarket search skill.

Step 7: Conduct a Discrepancy Analysis

Once a task analysis of needed skills for a particular activity is delineated, practitioners should determine those skills currently performed by students who have severe handicaps. This process, referred to as pretesting or establishing a baseline, al-

When at a supermarket and given a heavily outlined pictorial representation of a grocery item, the student will find that item when:

Phase 1: No other items are on the shelf
Phase 2: Several other items are on the shelf
Phase 3: The item is among a 1′ × 3′ shelf full of different items
Phase 4: The item is on one of two presented 1′ × 3′ shelves of items
Phase 5: The item is anywhere within a 3′ wide six-shelf section
Phase 6: The item is anywhere within two adjacent 6′ × 3′ six-shelf sections
Phase 7: Gradual increase in number of sections until students can search an entire row/aisle.

Teaching notes: Begin at easiest phase not passed by a student. Take student to subsequent phase once criterion reached on prior phase.

Figure 7. Task analysis based on an easy-to-difficult strategy: Learning to locate items in a grocery store.

lows staff members to determine the discrepancies between required skills and those skills already in a student's repertoire.

Task analyses that involve hierarchically ordered enroutes can be baselined or pretested in one of two ways. Staff members can begin testing at the easiest task step or phase objective, and progress until the student fails a phase, thus suggesting the initial instructional target. Another strategy is to begin testing at the most difficult task step or phase objective and move back down the task analysis until the phase is revealed at which a student passes.

On a sequential listing-of-steps TAs, teachers should allow students to perform each step independently in order to determine both the specific skills needed and those already in the learner's repertoire. Another variation of this strategy would be to note the amount of assistance required to perform a task step, should it not be performed independently (e.g., verbal cuing, partial physical guidance, full physical assistance).

Typically, two or three baseline trials are provided, with the criterion for passing a phase being all trials correctly performed. Since baselining is not teaching, students should receive neither reinforcers for correct performance nor correction of errors. Students should, however, receive intermittent reinforcers for task attempts, attending, and compliance, in order to maintain responding.

Step 8: Determine Necessary Adaptations

Once a discrepancy analysis has been conducted, and skills missing from a student's repertoire have been identified, a decision should be made as to whether adaptations are necessary to allow the student to perform the activity independently or to allow for at least partial participation in the activity (Baumgart et al., 1982). Often, students with severe handicaps, in particular those students with physical and/or sensory impairments, are excluded from instruction on functional activities when it appears highly unlikely that they will be able to perform skills in the manner in which they are performed by nonhandicapped students. In that such instructional decisions unduly restrict students from participation in a wide variety of normalized activities, an alternative viewpoint is necessary.

Rather than exclude students from activities they might be unable to perform independently, instructional personnel serving students with severe and dual sensory impairments should adopt the principle of *partial participation* (Baumgart et al., 1982). This principle holds that, in cases where there is evidence to suggest that students may not be able to perform all required skills, adaptations should be considered that either compensate for skill deficits or allow for at least partial participation in functional, normalized activities.

There are a number of adaptations that can be made to either compensate for skill deficits or allow for partial participation (Baumgart et al., 1982; Brown, Branston et al., 1979). These include:

1. Creating adaptive/prosthetic aids
2. Adapting existing activity materials
3. Adapting skill sequences
4. Adapting rules
5. Utilizing personal assistance
6. Social/attitudinal adaptation

Each of these adaptations is discussed below.

Creating Adaptive/Prosthetic Aids This refers to the use of additional portable materials that compensate for skill deficits. There are numerous adaptive/prosthetic aids that creative staff members might develop. For example, in a situation where students with severe cognitive and dual sensory impairments are unlikely to acquire the coin discrimination skills necessary to use a vending machine, at least two adaptive/prosthetic aids could be considered. Imprints of quarters could be made of Brailon, a paper-like plastic material that is used with a heat forming process to produce raised materials. Students might be taught to place coins in the imprint in order to select the correct coins for use in the vending machine. Another adaptive aid would be to attach inside a wallet a slotted coin holder with all but the quarter-sized slots covered. Students might then be taught to compare coins to the slot size until two correctly sized coins (quarters) are selected and then inserted into the coin holder for use at the vending machine.

The number of adaptive/prosthetic aids is limited only by staff ingenuity. In an effort to provide several examples that might in turn spark staff members to develop even more creative alternatives, Table 2 is provided.

It should be noted that prosthetic/adaptive aids should be introduced only when it is clear that such additional materials are necessary. Because additional materials are required with these adaptations, portability can become a problem; thus, these aids should be employed only when judged necessary.

Adapting Existing Activity Materials Modifications of the materials typically used in the performance of an activity, although sometimes needed, may not always be nec-

Table 2. Sample adaptive/prosthetic aids

Problem skill/activity	Adaptive/prosthetic aid
1. Student's vision makes it difficult to look at a magazine.	1. Use a beam scope magnifier.
2. Required volume level for listening to radio/records/tape would disrupt others.	2. Use ear/head phones.
3. Nonverbal student with low vision and hearing impairments wishes to place an order at a fast food restaurant.	3. Use picture communication cards containing pictures with darkened, raised outline to place order.
4. Student with visual impairments and consequent lack of refined/precise upper extremity use often knocks equipment to the floor.	4. Dycem, a slip-resistant plastic material is placed between object (e.g. Simon game, plate) and surface.
5. Student is not able to determine which of two cards played in "War" wins the trick.	5. A number line is provided with which the student can compare cards played and determine higher value card.
6. Student "forgets" sequence of required vocational tasks.	6. Student carries a work-task sequence card with raised symbols for each job task to be accomplished. Student moves sliding tab down to next task as previous one is completed.

essary. Staff members occasionally have a choice of several materials and thus may be able to select materials that minimize difficulties for students. For example, in teaching pinball use, staff might select games that provide more auditory and/or visual input, (e.g., "fire power" versus "baseball" pinball games) that do not require movements that are as sophisticated (push one button versus move four-direction joystick while pushing another button), or that do not demand as quick a reaction (Space Invaders versus Defender). Other examples include low vision rather than standard sized playing cards, and selecting simple (one or two control button/knob) record players, TVs or other appliances rather than complex ones. It might not, however, always be possible to select simpler materials, and material adaptations are sometimes required.

The number of possible materials adaptations is virtually unlimited. In the tape player example discussed above, brightly colored, raised plastic tape could be attached to the end of the tape as a cue for its correct insertion by a student with residual vision (Hamre-Nietupski, Nietupski, Sandvig, Sandvig & Ayres, 1984). In that same example, color-coded tape might also be attached to the volume control knob as a cue.

In general, adaptations that provide additional tactile cues, or that make visual or auditory cues more salient, can be considered for materials adaptations. Table 3 provides examples of some possible materials adaptations.

Table 3. Sample material adaptations

Problem skill/activity	Materials adaptation
1. The student does not discriminate the inside from the outside of shirts or jackets.	1. Velcro or different textured material is sewn into the inside collar of the clothing item
2. The cassette tape player is frequently knocked off the shelf.	2. The cassette player is bolted to the shelf
3. The student is not able to locate the light switch in a dark/dimly lit room.	3. A lighted on/off switch is used in place of a standard light switch
4. The student does not place his or her clothes in the correct dresser drawer or section of the dresser drawer.	4a. Raised outlines of clothing items are attached to corresponding dresser drawers
	4b. Cardboard section dividers with raised outlines of corresponding clothing items are placed in each dresser drawer.
5. The student is not able to easily turn the magazine pages.	5. Pieces of tagboard or clear lamination are attached to the upper corners of each page; student wears rubber "thimble" on index finger.
6. The student cannot see the pitched softball to hit it.	6. A "beeper ball" is used in place of a standard softball.

Adapting Skill Sequences At times it is necessary to revise the typical order of performance of steps within an activity. Occasionally, simply rearranging the order of task step performance will compensate for student skill deficits. For example, students whose visual and motor impairments result in lengthy delays in obtaining their money from wallets, pockets or purses to pay for items at a fast food counter might be taught to have their money available prior to ordering. Within the same activity, if returning change to one's wallet, pocket or purse is time consuming, the student might be taught to place the change on their tray or into the bag containing their order, and then to return it to their pocket, purse or wallet once seated at their table. Staff members should carefully analyze where in the chain of skills students might be experiencing difficulties, and consider whether modifications in the sequence might ameliorate the problem.

Adapting Rules Modifying the guidelines that either formally or informally govern performance of an activity may be helpful. Many activities have such complex rules that they present insurmountable problems for students with severe handicaps. Rule adaptations may allow for at least partial participation, and are frequently possible in recreation/leisure activities where rules are somewhat more flexible.

Rule adaptations can take many forms. For example, in pinball, an informal rule followed by most pinball wizards is to press a flipper button only when the pinball approaches that particular flipper. Students with sensory impairments, however, might be taught the "rule" of constantly pushing/releasing both flipper buttons in order to increase the probability of hitting the pinball when it does, in fact, approach a flipper.

Several sample rule adaptations are contained in Table 4. As evidenced in these examples, such adaptations allow at least partial participation in the targeted activity.

Utilizing Personal Assistance This represents the most intrusive partial participation strategy. In essence, it involves another individual performing the problem skill for the student, or providing the student with considerable assistance in its performance. Because of its intrusiveness, use of this strategy should be restricted to those situations where less intrusive strategies are impossible or not feasible. For example, it is impossible to adapt all vending machines to highlight the location of the coin slot. Nor could a prosthetic aid conceivably assist in this situation. Thus, it might be the case that, when encountering novel vending machines, personal assistance may initially be required to complete this task step.

Baumgart et al. (1982) describe an example of personal assistance provided to an adolescent with severe handicaps who was totally deaf and blind. This student was receiving vocational training in a hospital setting where he was required to remove bandages from a perforated box and place them on a supply tray. The only problem step for this student was his inability to locate the materials. Personal assistance from a co-worker, who located materials and set up the work station, allowed this student to perform a valuable vocational task. Table 5 provides other examples of the use of this partial participation strategy.

Societal/Attitudinal Adaptations These involve efforts to improve the understanding, tolerance level, perceptions, and beliefs held by nonhandicapped persons toward

Table 4. Sample rule adaptations

Problem skill/activity	Rule adaptation
1. Student has difficulty discriminating between the king, queen and jack in a card game.	1. Size of deck is reduced by removing two of three types of face cards.
2. Student plays Uno out of turn.	2. "Pick Pile" is passed to student as cue to take turn.
3. The student cannot hit a pitched softball.	3. A "beeper ball" (material adaptation) placed on a batting "tee" rather than pitched.
4. The student is not able to complete the assigned vocational tasks in the time allotted.	4. Either the student is required only to perform *some* of the tasks or is allowed more time to perform all the typically required tasks.
5. The student is unable to find peers in a hide-and-seek game.	5. Peers are required to signal their location with a noisemaking object (e.g., a bell) as the student moves away from their hidden location.
6. The student cannot aim and hit the horseshoe post or dart ring from the customary distance.	6. The student is allowed to stand closer to the target.

their peers with severe handicaps. Often, nonhandicapped individuals either do too much for the person with severe handicaps whom they encounter, or are extremely intolerant or unaware of that individual's differences. In either case, a restricted degree of participation in normalized activities may result. Should these situations arise, staff members may need to provide information to nonhandicapped citizens that will enable them to interact in a more appropriate way with students who are severely disabled. Discussing more appropriate alternatives, demonstrating interaction attempts, providing written material, slide-shows, films or tapes often are necessary to improve attitudes of targeted groups. The reader is referred to Certo, Haring, and York (1984) for comprehensive information in this area.

To summarize, a variety of adaptations may be necessary to compensate for student disabilities and/or to allow at least partial participation in normalized, functional activities. Practitioners should consider the use of such adaptations when it is apparent that independent performance of activities in the "typical" manner is not reasonable or realistic for students with severe and dual sensory impairments.

Step 9: Develop An Instructional Program

Once steps 1–8 of the Ecological Curriculum Development Strategy have been completed, personnel are ready to develop instructional programs to teach the functional, age-appropriate, normalized activities targeted as IEP goals. An instructional program involves carefully developed responses to the following eight questions:

Table 5. Sample personal assistance strategies

Problem skill/activity	Personal assistance
1. The student is not able to move the record player arm to the correct location on a record.	1. A nonhandicapped peer, also listening to the records, physically assists the student to perform this skill.
2. The student is not able to determine when traffic permits starting to cross the street.	2. The student takes the arm of a companion and starts to cross as his or her companion does so.
3. The student is not able to discern when to get off the bus on the bus route.	3. The student informs the bus driver of his or her destination.
4. The student is unable to carry her lunch tray from the school cafeteria line to her table.	4. A nonhandicapped peer partner carries her tray or places it on her wheelchair lap tray.
5. The student is not able to determine when a sufficient amount of water is in the sink for dishwashing.	5. A sibling turns off the water when it reaches the necessary level.
6. The student is not able to find the bases or run fast enough in a softball game.	6. A nonhandicapped peer runs for the student, or pushes his or her wheelchair, once the student hits the beeper ball off the tee.

1. What activity will be taught?
2. Why teach this activity?
3. What materials and training task arrangements will be used?
4. How will this activity be taught?
5. How will progress be verified?
6. What are the expected criteria (including accuracy, fluency, latency)?
7. How will generalization be promoted?
8. How will self-initiated performance be facilitated?

In essence, an instructional program can be considered the "working" IEP. That is, it provides the specific information to carry out programming on IEP goals on an ongoing basis. The scope of this chapter does not allow for an indepth discussion of each instructional program component, but a sample program is provided in the appendix at the end of the chapter. The reader interested in this area is referred to Sailor and Guess (1983), Snell (1983), and any of the "Madison Volumes," a yearly collection of papers and programs related to teaching students with severe handicaps (address provided in reference list).

The nine steps in an Ecological Curriculum Development Strategy involve careful observation of natural environments, and of the activities of nonhandicapped individuals in those environments. Based upon the information gathered from such observations, activities are prioritized and IEP goals selected; activities are task analyzed into component skills; adaptations are considered; and instructional programs developed. An ecological approach offers a process for the provision of systematic instruction on community-referenced, individually determined, chronologically age-appropriate, functional curricular content. Such an approach is advocated so that students with severe and dual sensory impairments will be prepared to participate as fully as possible in activities in natural environments, with maximized opportunities to interact with nonhandicapped peers.

EMPIRICAL SUPPORT FOR AN ECOLOGICAL CURRICULUM APPROACH

An ecological approach to curriculum development for persons with severe handicaps has been advocated only recently. Numerous writers have provided cogent and persuasive arguments for an ecological approach. Empirical research has, nevertheless, lagged behind. Part of the difficulty in developing the data base for such an approach is that, in one sense, the task is enormous. To claim definitively the superiority of one curricular approach over another requires carefully monitored longitudinal studies in which the effects of different program models are studied. In that such studies are time consuming, costly, and affected by a variety of factors such as student drop-out and contamination, no definitive statements regarding the effectiveness of various approaches can be made. In this regard, the ecological approach is no different from any other approach, including the sensory developmental or other models.

Despite the lack of substantiation for claims of clear cut superiority of an ecological curricular approach, there is a growing body of research that, while conducted on a smaller scale, suggests that an ecological approach has considerable merit. The purpose of this section is to discuss the extant research in this area.

Research Findings

Several research investigations provide at least indirect evidence as to the effectiveness of an ecological curriculum development strategy. These studies are considered to be indirect indices in that certain aspects, rather than the entirety, of an ecological approach have been examined. Specifically, the research discussed below either has examined the effects of teaching skills within a natural context (as opposed to within artificial settings) or has examined the effects of programmed variations in stimulus and response characteristics, based upon careful environmental (i.e., ecological) analyses. While these studies were not conducted with learners with severe handicaps who had dual sensory impairments, they did involve students who would be considered severely disabled.

Oliver and Halle (1982) conducted a study designed to assess the effects of instruction in the natural environment on sign language skill acquisition and generalization. In this study, a 7-year-old male with moderate retardation served as the subject. Prior to determining specific signs to teach, the investigators conducted a careful analysis of the classroom routine. This analysis yielded nine normally occurring daily language opportunities (e.g., signing "help" when in the bathroom and about to unfasten pants; signing "push" when playing on a scooter during play time; signing "eat" in order to receive lunch; signing "more" in order to receive another food portion). A multiple baseline design was used to evaluate the effects of the training procedures used to teach sign use during normal daily activities. Generalization probes across different trainers and across similar but nonidentical opportunities (e.g., signing "help" when zipping or buttoning a coat) were administered periodically. The results indicated a dramatic increase in student self-initiated sign use and a reduction in required trainer prompts and student errors following naturalized instruction. Sign initiations also generalized to a second trainer and to novel opportunities. Based upon these results, the investigators concluded that teaching in the natural environment within the context of normal activities may be useful in promoting both sign language acquisition and generalization.

Similar findings are reported by Horner and Budd (1985). In this study, an 11-year-old male with autism was taught to communicate wants via the use of manual signs. Training in the corner of the classroom resulted in no generalization to natural settings. Only when instruction was extended to natural training times was generalization noted.

Freagon and Rotatori (1982) compared the effects of natural versus artificial environmental training on self-care skill acquisition, maintenance, and generalization of ten adolescents with severe handicaps. A small group, matched pairs design was employed with the data analyzed through use of the exact test for Wilcoxen matched pairs. The results indicated that subjects trained during natural times and in natural training settings made significantly greater skill gains than those trained at unnatural times and settings. No significant differences, however, were found between the two groups with respect to maintenance and generalization.

A number of investigations into the effects of what has been termed *general case instruction* on generalized responding have been reported recently. General case instruction involves teaching students to perform specific skills across a number of exemplars that represent the range of stimulus and response variations within the response class under investigation. For example, in teaching vending machine use, instructional personnel using a general case methodology would carefully examine the range of vending machines students might encounter. They then would select a sample of vending machines that represent the range of stimulus and response variations (e.g., location and orientation of coin slot, type of item display, cost of items, type of activation response), and teach students to operate a representative set of the various exemplars. By training in this manner, it is expected that generalized responding to the broader response class will be enhanced.

An ecological approach forms the core of general case instruction in that careful observation of the environment yields information as to appropriate instructional targets. Thus, the general case research discussed below relates to an ecological curriculum development approach.

Horner and McDonald (1982) conducted a study in which they compared the effects of general case versus single instance instruction on the generalized vocational skill performance of four adolescents with moderate/severe handicaps. The authors examined twenty different types of biaxle electronic capacitors that students were to crimp and cut as part of their vocational skill curriculum. The capacitors are formed by two wires which emanate from a metallic head. These capacitors differed in size, shape, color, and in a variety of other characteristics. The authors identified three capacitor variables that were logically associated with performance: head size, head shape, and distance between leads. General case instruction involved random presentations of any one of three capacitors that sampled the range of stimuli within the three variable clusters. In contrast, single case instruction involved training on only one capacitor exemplar. A multiple baseline mirror design across the four students indicated that general case instruction was vastly superior to single instance instruction in promoting generalized responding to untrained exemplars. Furthermore, their results suggested that errors made on untrained exemplars were functionally related to the restricted range of training stimuli students encountered in single instance training. Thus, the authors concluded that generalized responding can best be attained by carefully selecting training exemplars that sample the range of stimulus and response characteristics present in the general response class.

Sprague and Horner (1984) extended work in this area by comparing the effects of single instance versus multiple instance versus general case instruction on the generalized use of community vending machines. This program involved six adolescents with moderate to severe retardation, two of whom were legally blind. Single instance instruction involved training on one particular vending machine. Multiple instance instruction involved concurrent training on three different vending machines that did not sample the range of stimulus and response variations. General case instruction involved training on three vending machines that did, in fact, embody the full range of variations in stimulus features and response requirements. A single-subject, split multiple baseline design again yielded evidence as to the superiority of general case instruction in promoting a generalized response by all six students to unfamiliar vending machines. The results of this study further underscore the importance of careful environmental analysis in that only instruction on a representative sample of multiple instances resulted in generalized performance.

McDonnell, Horner, and Williams (1984) compared the effects of three instructional formats on the generalized purchasing skills of four adolescents with moderate to severe handicaps. In one condition, students role-played grocery purchasing skills in the classroom. The second instructional format involved classroom role-playing combined with slide training simulation based on general case analysis principles. In the third condition, students received general case slide training combined with training at an actual grocery store. The results indicated that the general case slide training combined with instruction in the natural environment was most effective in promoting generalized purchasing skills. These results not only suggest the effectiveness of ecological analysis, but also suggest the need for instruction in natural environments.

The results of studies conducted by Horner and his colleagues provide impressive evidence of the need for ecological observations in determining instructional targets. Their research, combined with that conducted by the other investigators cited above, would seem to suggest that practitioners need to identify and teach across the variations students might encounter in natural settings, and to provide instruction in natural environments at natural times if generalized responding is to be achieved. While the extant literature does not provide definitive evidence as to the superiority of an ecological approach over other curriculum development strategies, it does provide a firm foundation as to the utility of this approach. Further empirical investigations, along the lines discussed below, should yield more definitive conclusions.

FUTURE RESEARCH NEEDS

A number of research questions should be addressed in evaluating an ecological approach. On a large scale, a comparison of the post-school outcomes for students with severe handicaps on the basis of instructional approach should be conducted. Specifically, one might examine whether post-school vocational outcomes (sheltered versus nonsheltered employment, pay received), domestic outcomes (institutional versus nursing home versus group home versus sheltered apartment), community functioning outcomes (use versus nonuse of community stores, transportation, and other community services) and recreation/leisure outcomes (use of normalized versus handicapped-only recreation options) differ on the basis of instructional approach.

While it is perhaps unrealistic to believe it possible to randomly assign students to various approaches and track their outcomes after 18–21 years of instruction, it may be possible to capitalize upon the naturally occurring "studies" available. That is, much along the lines of the investigation of the effects of regular school integration (Brinker & Thorpe, 1984), a large scale study could compare outcomes in districts that have employed an ecological, community-based approach to outcomes in districts adopting other approaches. While such research efforts are fraught with logistical and methodological problems, they can provide partial evidence supporting or refuting the claims of various approaches.

On a slightly smaller scale, individual school districts should be encouraged to conduct their own follow-up evaluations of graduates. Brown (1984) has reported follow-up study results from the Madison, Wisconsin Metropolitan School District. He indicates that, from 1971–1978, only one of twenty graduates with moderate to severe/profound handicaps entered nonsheltered employment. From 1978 on, however, concurrent with the implementation of a community-based program based upon an ecological model, ever increasing percentages of graduates have entered nonsheltered post-school employment options. Such findings, while not derived from tightly controlled research efforts, provide supporting data on a program's effectiveness. Many more such descriptive research efforts are needed from the numerous programs in the nation utilizing an ecological approach.

A variety of areas should be addressed through more tightly controlled, single subject or small group designs. First, studies along the lines of those conducted by Horner and his colleagues should be conducted with students with severe handicaps and dual sensory impairments. Very little published research is available on functional skills training with this subgroup.

Second, the principle of partial participation, while frequently discussed, has seldom been demonstrated empirically. Studies are needed to document the effectiveness of the various partial participation strategies. This is particularly true in reference to students with dual sensory impairments. Examples of empirically verified adaptations in the four domains could greatly assist practitioners who may adhere to the approach, yet not know how to carry it out in particular situations.

Of additional interest would be a documentation of the *acceptability,* to parents and significant others, of such partial participation strategies as personal assistance. Social validity data would be useful on parental reaction to providing assistance and allowing a student to partially participate, as opposed to performing the entire activity for the student.

An additional area of inquiry might focus on the reaction of society in general to viewing persons with severe handicaps engaged in functional, community-referenced, age-appropriate activities. Bates, Morrow, Panscofar, and Sedlak (1984) have conducted a preliminary investigation into this area. They had members of a general education class for prospective teachers view a person with Down syndrome engaged in either functional or nonfunctional activities. The subjects then responded to a questionnaire regarding their views on estimated IQ, future earning capacity, best residential options, likely employment options, and best classroom location. The group that viewed the person with Down syndrome engaged in functional activities predicted significantly higher levels of competence than that viewing participation in nonfunctional activities. Similar research, conducted with nonhandicapped individuals who work, travel, recreate and live alongside persons wtih severe handicaps would be useful in order to document the social validity of an ecological approach.

Finally, research is needed to identify the most critical considerations in IEP goal selection. As stated above, ecological inventories generate an enormous number of potential teaching targets. To date, only suggestions regarding strategies for setting priorities and selecting IEP goals are available. Data-based decision rules would greatly assist teachers in selecting what would, in fact, constitute the most functional, critical activities for instruction.

SUMMARY

This chapter has discussed an ecological approach to curriculum development for students who are severely handicapped and have dual sensory impairments. This approach has been defined, a rationale for its use has been put forth and a nine-step process for its implementation has been presented and illustrated with examples. A review of related research and suggestions for further inquiry have been provided. In the authors' view, an ecological approach is extremely applicable to students with dual sensory impairments. Such a curriculum development strategy has great potential for preparing students to live, work, and recreate more independently in natural environments. The challenge facing educators is to convert that potential to reality.

REFERENCES

Alberto, P.A., & Troutman, A.C. (1982). *Applied behavior analysis for teachers.* Columbus, OH: Charles E. Merrill.

Bates, P., Morrow, S.A., Pancsofar, E.L., & Sedlak, R. (1984). The effect of functional vs non-functional activities on attitudes/expectations of non-handicapped college students: What they see is what they get. *The Journal of The Association for Persons with Severe Handicaps, 9*(2), 73–78.

Baumgart, D., Brown, L., Pumpian, I., Nisbet, J., Ford, A., Sweet, M., Mesina, R., & Schroeder, J. (1982). Principle of partial participation and individualized adaptations in educational programs for severely handicapped students. *The Journal of The Association for the Severely Handicapped, 7*(2), 17–27.

Brinker, R.P., & Thorpe, M.E. (1984). Integration of severely handicapped students and the proportion of IEP objectives achieved. *Exceptional Children, 51*(2), 168–175.

Brown, L. (1984). Preparing severely handicapped people to live, work, and play in the community. Presentation at the 31st Annual ARC/Iowa State Convention, Des Moines, IA.

Brown, L., Branston, M., Hamre-Nietupski, S., Pumpian, I., Certo, N., & Gruenewald, L. (1979). A strategy for developing chronologically age-appropriate and functional curricular content for severely handicapped adolescents and young adults. *Journal of Special Education, 13*(1), 81–90.

Brown, L., Branston-McLean, M.B., Baumgart, D., Vincent, L., Falvey, M., & Schroeder, J. (1979). Using the characteristics of current and subsequent least restrictive environments in the development of curricular content for severely handicapped students. *AAESPH Review, 4*(4), 407–424.

Certo, N., Haring, J., & York, R. (1984). *Public school integration of severely handicapped students: Rational issues and progressive alternatives*. Baltimore: Paul H. Brookes Publishing Co.

Ford, A., Brown, L., Pumpian, I., Baumgart, D., Nisbet, J., Schroeder, J., & Loomis, R. (1984). Strategies for developing individualized recreation and leisure programs for severely handicapped students. In N. Certo, N. Haring, & R. York (Eds.), *Public school integration of severely handicapped students: Rational issues and progressive alternatives* (pp. 245–276). Baltimore: Paul H. Brookes Publishing Co.

Freagon, S., & Rotatori, A.F. (1982). Comparing natural and artificial environments in training self-care skills to group home residents. *The Journal of The Association for the Severely Handicapped, 7*(3), 73–86.

Guess, D., Sailor, W., & Baer, D.M. (1977). A behavioral-remedial approach to language training for the severely handicapped. In E. Sontag, J. Smith, & N. Certo (Eds.), *Educational programming for the severely and profoundly handicapped* (pp. 360–377). Reston, VA: Division on Mental Retardation, The Council for Exceptional Children.

Hamre-Nietupski, S., Nietupski, J., Sandvig, R., Sandvig, M., & Ayres, B. (1984). Leisure skills instruction in a community residential setting with young adults who are deaf/blind severely handicapped. *The Journal of The Association for Persons with Severe Handicaps, 9*(1), 49–54.

Hawkins, R.P., & Hawkins, K.K. (1981). Parental observations on the education of severely retarded children: Can it be done in the classroom? *Analysis and Intervention in Developmental Disabilities, 1*, 13–22.

Holvoet, J., Guess, D., Mulligan, M., & Brown, F. (1980). The individualized curriculum sequencing model (II): A teaching strategy for severely handicapped students. *The Journal of The Association for the Severely Handicapped, 5*, 325–336.

Horner, R.H., & Budd, C.M. (1985). Acquisition of manual sign use: Collateral reduction of maladaptive behavior and factors limiting generalization. *Education and Training of the Mentally Retarded, 20*(1), 39–47.

Horner, R.H., & McDonald, R.S. (1982). Comparison of single instance and general case instruction in teaching a generalized vocational skill. *The Journal of The Association for the Severely Handicapped, 7*(3), 7–20.

Madison Volumes, Madison, WI: Metropolitan School District, 547 West Dayton Street, Madison, WI 53703.

McDonnell, J.J., Horner, R.H., & Williams, J.A. (1984). Comparison of three strategies for teaching generalized grocery purchasing to high school students with severe handicaps. *The Journal of The Association for Persons with Severe Handicaps, 9*(2), 123–133.

Oliver, C.B., & Halle, J.W. (1982). Language training in the everday environments: Teaching functional sign use to a retarded child. *The Journal of The Association for the Severely Handicapped, 7*(3), 50–62.

Sailor, W., & Guess, D. (1983). *Severely handicapped students: An instructional design.* Boston: Houghton Mifflin.

Snell, M.E. (Ed.). (1983). *Systematic instruction of the moderately and severely handicapped* (2nd ed.). Columbus, OH: Charles E. Merrill.

Sprague, J.R., & Horner, R.H. (1984). The effects of single instance, multiple instance and general case training on generalized vending machine use by moderately and severely handicapped students. *Journal of Applied Behavior Analysis, 17*(2), 273–278.

Wuerch, B.B., & Voeltz, L.M. (1982). *Longitudinal leisure skills for severely handicapped learners: The Ho'onanea curriculum component*. Baltimore: Paul H. Brookes Publishing Co.

Appendix

SAMPLE INSTRUCTIONAL PROGRAM

Student Description

Doug is a fourteen-year-old male who is severely retarded. He has no sight but does hear with amplification. He resides in a group home with three other residents who have moderate to severe disabilities.

What activity will be taught?

The terminal objective for the student is as follows: Given the following clothing items that have been washed and dried (pairs of socks, underpants and undershirts), the student, while in his bedroom in front of his dresser, will fold the items and place them in the correct dresser drawer in the divided drawer section marked with Velcro outlines of the corresponding clothing items, within 30 seconds per item on 5 consecutive occasions. The task analysis for this activity is as follows:

Phase I: The student will fold and put away socks using the following sequence of actions:

Part 1: Lay one sock flat on dresser top.
Part 2: Lay second sock on top of first sock.
Part 3: Fold socks in half from top to toe.
Part 4: Locate and open dresser drawer which is marked with Velcro outline of socks.
Part 5: Locate drawer section marked with Velcro sock outline.
Part 6: Place socks flat in corresponding drawer section.
Part 7: Repeat parts 1–3 and 5 and 6 with all remaining pairs of socks.
Part 8: Close dresser drawer.

Phase II: The student will fold and put away underpants using the following sequence of actions:

Part 1: Lay underpants flat on dresser, waist-band facing student.
Part 2: Fold underpants in half, right to left.
Part 3: Locate and open dresser drawer marked with Velcro outline of underpants.
Part 4: Locate drawer section marked with Velcro underpants outline.
Part 5: Place underpants flat in corresponding drawer section.
Part 6: Repeat parts 1 and 2, 4 and 5 with all remaining underpants.
Part 7: Close dresser drawer.

Phase III: The student will fold and put away undershirts using the following sequence of actions:

Part 1: Lay undershirt flat on dresser top, bottom toward student.
Part 2: Place palm of hand on middle of shirt, top half.

Part 3: Grasp right sleeve with right hand and fold to left until covering left sleeve.
Part 4: Slide left hand down to middle of shirt, bottom half.
Part 5: Grasp right edge of bottom half of shirt and fold to left until covering left bottom half.
Part 6: Place left hand on top half of folded shirt.
Part 7: Grasp bottom half with right hand and fold up until covering top half.
Part 8: Locate and open dresser drawer with Velcro undershirt outline.
Part 9: Locate drawer section with undershirt outline.
Part 10: Place undershirt flat in drawer section.
Part 11: Repeat parts 1–7 and 9 and 10 with all remaining undershirts.
Part 12: Close dresser drawer.

Teaching Notes: Teach one phase to criterion at a time, using a total cycle training format. Frequently review previously acquired phases when teaching new phases.

Why teach this activity?

This IEP goal was selected for several reasons. First, it is an age-appropriate skill performed by nonhandicapped adolescents. Second, it is a skill needed in semi-independent apartment living arrangements, a possible subsequent environment for the student. Third, the group home staff have stated this to be a priority. Doug needs considerable assistance or else his room is a mess and he is unable to find the clean clothes he needs each day. Fourth, if Doug acquires this skill, it will give him an opportunity to receive social reinforcement from his roommate, who likes to keep his section of the room neat and becomes upset when Doug does not do so.

What materials and training task arrangements will be used?

The materials are specified in the task analysis. As indicated, material adaptations have been made in order to compensate for Doug's visual impairment. Specifically, Velcro outlines on the dresser and on drawer dividers will serve as the cues for appropriate garmet storage areas. Personal assistance is provided for matching socks, since Doug's blindness prevents him from matching socks on the basis of color.

Training will be conducted three times per week in the simulated domestic living area of school. Once per week Doug will receive training in a community residential location, occasionally including his own group home.

How will this activity be taught?

A total cycle approach will be attempted. Doug will be given an initial verbal cue (e.g., "Doug, let's put away your laundry"). Doug will then attempt each task step. When errors occur, the following instructional hierarchy will be employed: 1) *Indirect cues* ("What do you do next?"); 2) if indirect cues fail to produce a correct response, a *direct verbal cue* will be used ("No, Doug, fold the socks in half"); 3) if direct verbal cues fail, the trainer will repeat the direct verbal cue and *partially physically assist* him to perform the task step; 4) *full physical guidance* will be provided if partial assistance fails. Completion of the cycle will result in verbal praise and access to reinforcing break time activities.

How will progress be verified?

A data sheet indicating each step in the task analysis will allow the charting of progress. Instructors will use a point system to record the level of assistance needed for the student to perform the task steps (4 points, independent; 3 points, indirect cue; 2 points, direct verbal cue; 1 point, partial physical assistance; 0 points, full assistance).

What is the expected criterion?

A fluency criterion of 30 seconds per item was targeted initally. This fluency level, while not similar to the time required by nonhandicapped adolescents (5–10 seconds), was considered acceptable to the group home staff.

To develop fluency, a timer will be used. Gradual approximations toward the 30-second fluency level will be reinforced with praise and access to preferred activities.

How will generalization be promoted?

Training will be conducted concurrently at school, in the group home and at other community residences. Verbal cues, materials, and trainers (school and group home staff) will be varied from trial to trial or session to session. Thus, a form of general case instruction will be provided.

How will self-initiated performance be facilitated?

Saturday is laundry day in the group home. Eventually, Doug will be given a tactile Velcro picture "schedule" of chores he is expected to complete. He will be taught to follow the schedule and thus put away the clothes he just washed and dried.

CHAPTER 10

Application of the Individualized Curriculum Sequencing Model to Learners with Severe Sensory Impairments

Edwin Helmstetter and Doug Guess

IN THE EDUCATION of persons with severe disabilities, attempts must be made to provide procedures and approaches that are applicable to a wide range of disabling conditions, and yet maintain the flexibility to accommodate individual and sub-group learning characteristics that include severe vision and hearing impairments. General educational approaches typically reflect varying theoretical perspectives on how learning occurs, as well as individual adaptations within these specific theoretical orientations. This chapter presents one of several educational approaches that have applicability to persons with severe sensory losses. This approach, referred to as the individualized curriculum sequencing (ICS) model, has evolved over the years and has been applied systematically to the teaching of a broad range of students with a variety of disabling conditions, including preschool children with multiple disabilities (Guess, Jones, & Lyon, 1981), adolescent learners with severe mental retardation (Holvoet, Mulligan, Schussler, Lacy, & Guess, 1985), and adolescent learners who demonstrate combined visual and hearing impairments (Helmstetter, Murphy-Herd, Roberts, & Guess, 1984).

The ICS model is prefaced on the theoretical and empirical assumption that learning is best achieved through the teaching of skill clusters that are meaningful for the learner. Learning, then, is perceived as the acquisition of combined skills that are related, one to the other, by their natural, functional, and environmental properties. The individual needs and motivations of the learner are also acknowledged. Within both the procedural guidelines and the underlying assumptions of the model, the learner is perceived as an active contributor in determining what is to be learned, and what the varying circumstances are under which skills are to be used and maintained.

The ICS model was developed also to address the problems of slow skill acquisition and poor generalization that are common to many learners with severe disabilities

Parts of this chapter appeared in Guess, D., & Helmstetter, E. (1986). Skill cluster instruction and the individualized curriculum sequencing model. In R. H. Horner, L. H. Meyer, H. D. B. Fredericks (Eds.), *Education of learners with severe handicaps: Exemplary service strategies*. Baltimore: Paul H. Brookes Publishing Co.

(Sailor & Guess, 1983). The model addresses these problems within the framework of current best practices that include community-based instruction, natural cues and correction procedures, and functional materials and activities. The model, in its most current form, provides additionally for the exercising of choice in the instructional environment (and elsewhere), and for including in the instructional program the opportunity to identify and expand appropriate, learner-initiated behavior.

Described below are the components of the ICS model that are utilized in the instructional process for learners with severe disabilities, including persons with dual sensory impairments:

1. Using distributed trial training
2. Relating skills to one another in clusters
3. Using multiple examples of materials, activities, locations, instructors, and learner responses
4. Providing learners with choices
5. Teaching in nonschool environments
6. Using functional materials and activities
7. Using natural cues and consequences
8. Scheduling learning at appropriate times
9. Incorporating learner-initiated behavior.

The first four components of the ICS are based upon research on the contribution of these factors to skill acquisition or generalization. The last five components lack an empirical base, but are considered either as current best practices or as possible critical variables in teaching learners with severe disabilities.

EMPIRICAL SUPPORT

Distributed Trial Training

When teaching a new behavior, the training trials can be presented to a learner in one of three ways. First, trials can be presented rapidly, one after the other, with no time interval between each trial. This is the *massed trial approach.* Second, trials can be presented one after the other with a brief pause between them. Typically, this pause is for the learner to rest or for the teacher to consequate the response, to record data, or to prepare materials for the next trial. This approach is called *spaced trial training.* Finally, training trials of one skill can be interspersed with training trials of one or more other skills. This is *distributed trial training,* and is the approach emphasized in the ICS model. These three methods for presenting training trials are shown in Figure 1, where A, B, and C represent three different skills (instructional objectives).

In a review of research on massed, spaced, and distributed training trial arrangements, Mulligan, Guess, Holvoet, and Brown (1980) conclude that faster learning occurs when trials are spaced or distributed. In addition, research in recent years with learners with severe disabilities has shown mild effects in favor of distributed trials

A, B, and C are different skills to be learned

Massed trials:	AAAAAAAAAA BBBBBBBBBB CCCCCCCCCC
Spaced trials:	A A A A A A A A A A A A B B B B B B B B B B C C C C C C C C C C
Distributed trials:	ABCABCBACACBCABABCBACBCABACABC

---> (Time)

Figure 1. Illustration of massed, spaced, and distributed training trials.

for spontaneous initiations of a response (Lacy, 1982), for generalization of a vocational task to other settings (Brewer, 1982), and for higher levels of correct responding and less resistance to instruction (Mulligan, Lacy, & Guess, 1982). Similar results have been found with learners with autism. Dunlap and Koegel (1980) found that with distributed trials, learners with autism responded correctly more often and displayed more enthusiasm, interest, and appropriate behavior. In conclusion, distributed trial training appears to lead some learners to faster skill acquisition, greater interest in learning, and better transfer of newly learned skills to nontraining conditions.

Relating Skills to One Another in Clusters

The traditional approach to teaching learners with severe disabilities is to concentrate on one skill at a time during short sessions throughout the day. For example, creeping is taught from 9:30 to 9:45 each morning, grasping materials is taught from 9:45 until 10:00, tactile search skills from 10:00 until 10:15, and so on. Rarely is the learner taught how to use these three skills together for a functional purpose, such as creeping closer to the shelves in the recreation room in order to locate and acquire a favorite videocassette.

Teaching learners to use skills together in functional ways makes good practical sense and is an important component of the ICS model. The empirical basis for this practice, however, remains to be developed. One study that does relate to this issue, by Janssen and Guess (1978), found that learners with severe disabilities learn more quickly to label objects when they also learn the function of the objects.

Using Multiple Examples of Materials, Activities, Locations, Instructors, and Learner Responses

The ICS model arranges instruction so that most skills are taught using two or more materials, activities, instructors, and locations. This use of multiple examples during training increases the likelihood that once skills are learned, they will be used with an even wider range of new materials, activities, persons, and locations (i.e., stimulus generalization) (Anderson & Spradlin, 1980; Dunlap, Koegel, & Koegel, 1984; Sprague & Horner, 1984; Stokes & Baer, 1977).

The ICS model also arranges instruction, whenever possible, so that a learner is required to use two or more variations of the response being taught. This use of variations of a response during training increases the likelihood that once a behavior is learned it will be used in an even greater variety of forms or for a greater number of purposes (i.e., response generalization) (Garcia, Baer, & Firestone, 1971; Guess & Baer, 1973). The type of problem that results when a learner fails to generalize to other forms of a response is illustrated by the following example. Allan, a learner with severe disabilities, has learned to use a pincer grasp to pick up from a table top such items as pens and coins. Because he was taught to use a pincer grasp with tasks that required his hand only to be positioned with the palm downward, he is unable to generalize the use of his pincer grasp to remove a pen attached by a magnet to the refrigerator door, or to grasp a string to pull a window shade. These new activities require Allan to use his grasp with his hand either raised or rotated; both of these positions are variations of the hand position used when grasping objects from a table top.

Providing Learners With Choices

Choice-making is not included in most programs for learners with severe disabilities (Gaylord-Ross & Holvoet, 1985; Guess & Siegel-Causey, 1985; Shevin & Klein, 1984). The orientation of the field has, in general, been to program for learners, not with them. This may reflect the attitude that persons with severe disabilities are unable to make choices, and that if they did choose, their choices would not reflect what attending adults and others would consider to be in the best interests of that person (Guess & Helmstetter, 1986).

Interest in choice is increasing and is focusing on its role in fostering independence and improving maintenance of behavior (Guess, Benson, & Siegel-Causey, 1985). Most research on choice has been with nondisabled persons. The studies indicate that the choice of reinforcers or instructional materials may result in better learning or performance (Berk, 1976; Monty & Perlmuter, 1975; Monty, Rosenberger, & Perlmuter, 1973; Perlmuter & Monty, 1973; Perlmuter, Monty, & Kimble, 1971).

Preliminary results from the limited number of studies of choice with persons with disabilities indicate that these learners are able to choose materials and reinforcers, but choice-making has an insignificant impact on learning (Alexander, 1974; Holvoet, Brewer, Mulligan, Guess, & Helmstetter, 1983; Newhard, 1984).

Based on the evidence that persons with disabilities can and do make choices, the ICS model uses this factor to increase learner involvement and to provide more individualized programming. This occurs as learners are provided opportunities to choose instructional materials, activities, and trainers.

RATIONALE FOR OTHER COMPONENTS OF THE ICS MODEL

Teaching in Nonschool Environments

Nonschool instruction is essential for learners with severe disabilities because these students learn fewer and less complex skills, often fail to generalize to nontraining settings, and forget skills they do not use (Brown et al., 1983; Sailor & Guess, 1983). In addition, learners sometimes fail to understand where they should display skills they have learned (Gaylord-Ross & Holvoet, 1985). One way to compensate for these characteristics is to teach, as emphasized in the ICS model, in the real life settings where learners will be required to use their skills, to teach only those skills that are most useful in those settings, and to provide repeated opportunities to use the skills (Brown et al., 1979, 1983; Brown, Nietupski, & Hamre-Nietupski, 1976; Wilcox & Bellamy, 1982; Williams, Vogelsberg, & Schutz, 1985). In addition, the ICS model emphasizes the clustering of skills in ways that resemble how they are used together for functional purposes in nonschool settings.

Using Functional Materials and Activities

The materials and activities used to teach skills must help the learner become more independent, must be appropriate for the learner's chronological age, and must increase the learner's chances of interacting with nondisabled peers (Brown et al., 1976; Wilcox & Bellamy, 1982). The ICS focuses on the use of materials and activities that occur in natural environments and that are used or engaged in by nondisabled peers or adults.

Using Natural Cues and Consequences

Learners with severe disabilities sometimes fail to display setting-appropriate behavior because they have not been taught to respond to the signals to act that exist in nontraining locations, and because teachers do not teach them to display responses in the presence of the consequences for behavior that exist in nontraining settings. The ICS model emphasizes natural cues and consequences by referencing those cues and consequences identified through environmental inventories or other procedures for examining settings (Falvey, Brown, Lyon, Baumgart, & Schroeder, 1980; Ford & Mirenda, 1984). Furthermore, the ICS reduces the dependency on artificial instructional cues through the use of skill clusters where completion of one skill is the signal to engage in the next behavior in the cluster.

Scheduling Learning at Appropriate Times

A learner may acquire the behavior of activating an electronic switch to turn on a cassette player, or learn how to roll to the bathroom, but never be taught when these behaviors should be displayed. The ICS model maximizes the teaching of skills at the times when they should occur. For example, turning on a cassette player is taught during breaks or other leisure times in the group home, job site, or classroom.

Incorporating Learner-Initiated Behavior

Learner-initiated responses are existing or emerging behaviors that reflect spontaneous attempts by the learner to interact with the environment (Guess & Siegel-Causey, 1985). These behaviors often cannot be responded to or even observed by teachers who use a more traditional and rigid instructional methodology. Furthermore, instructional goals and objectives for learners with severe disabilities often are not based upon learner-initiated behaviors. They focus, instead, on behaviors that adults identify for the learner. It may be that behaviors identified by others appear unimportant to the learner, and may actually interfere with the learner's expression of existing abilities and needs (Guess & Siegel-Causey, 1985).

According to Shevin and Klein (1984), the learner-initiated approach is primarily based upon two sources. First, research on child-adult interaction underscores the important role that adult responsiveness to child behavior plays in the development of the child's social, affective, and communicative skills. Second, environmental psychology provides theoretical models that describe how behavior occurs not in isolation, but in an interactive manner within the larger physical and social context that includes peers, teachers, and other adults.

The ICS model arranges instruction so that skills are taught within naturally occurring daily activities such as riding the bus, crossing the street, shopping, and ordering food in a restaurant. This is a looser programming format than the traditional model, in which a learner goes to an instructional area such as a table in the classroom or a work area in an industry, and then begins instruction, usually on one behavior at a time, for 10 to 20 trials each. Because the ICS is a less rigid programming format, and because instruction is continuous across daily activities instead of compartmentalized by behavior or location, there are more opportunities and conditions in which to observe and adapt to learner-initiated responses.

By accommodating learner-initiated behavior, it is hoped that (a) these behaviors will become more fully developed, and that once fully developed they will be more durable; (b) combining learner-initiated responses with other target behaviors will facilitate acquisition of the target behaviors; and (c) learners will increase their spontaneous behavior and, therefore, their role in the process of education.

APPLICATION TO EDUCATION

The ICS model is a procedure for organizing curriculum content. In other words, after one has determined what skills to teach a learner, the procedures that comprise the ICS model are used to arrange skills into clusters; to identify multiple examples of materials, activities, locations, and learner responses; to ensure that there are opportunities to exercise choice; and so on. In order to use the ICS procedures fully and effectively, the skills selected for teaching should be stated as a general description of the response, without specifying the materials, activities, locations, times, and instructors. For example, instead of saying that John will wait in line to be dismissed for recess, state only that he will wait in line. Instead of saying that Tina will sign "hello" when greeted during the "Good Morning" group, state only that she will give the sign for "hello." Instead of saying that Tony will wheel his wheelchair from the bus to the classroom, state only that he will wheel his wheelchair. Instead of saying Joy will grasp a cup, state only that she will grasp objects. By restating skills in general response terms, greater use can be made of the ICS procedures for programming for generalization, for teaching at appropriate times and in nonschool settings, for clustering skills, and for providing choices.

Developing an ICS provides specific program information that should be written on a learner's individualized education program (IEP). If the IEP is completed prior to ICS development, then it is suggested that one include in the IEP examples of materials, activities, locations, and so on that will be used in teaching skills, with the understanding that these factors may change. After the ICS is developed, it may be necessary to obtain approval for these additions from the IEP participants.

The following pages describe the steps for developing an ICS for an individual learner: a) complete the events/skills matrix, b) write the ICS, c) develop instructional programs, and d) adapt the ICS. Following the description of ICS development for an individual learner is a section on using the ICS with groups.

Complete the Events/Skills Matrix

The first step in developing the ICS involves completing the events/skills matrix (see Figure 2). The matrix, when completed, will contain lists of materials and activities for teaching each skill, and the location, time, and instructor for each skill. It also is a useful tool for assessing whether skills are scheduled to be taught with multiple examples of materials, activities, daily events, times, locations, instructors, and forms of the response.

Daily Events To complete the events/skills matrix, first list along the left side of the form the events the learner will engage in during the day. These daily events fall primarily into two categories:

1. Functional daily events that are part of most persons' lives. These consist of everyday occurrences such as travel to and from work, school, and community training sites; eating; working; toileting; and leisure/recreation.
2. School events that are necessary to the physical, social, and educational well-being of the learner. These events are limited usually to physical education classes, recess, school social events such as assemblies, and group or individual instructional time.

Traditional classroom activities such as perceptual development time, communication sessions, and fine motor group are not to be listed on the matrix. These activities describe what is taught rather than events that comprise a daily routine.

List the events in the order in which they occur during the day, with the first event at the top of the matrix. Ideally, the order of events would approximate the schedule in future living and working environments. For example, events for older learners might be ordered as follows: travel to work, check in, use the bathroom, get work materials, begin work, break time, work, eat lunch, use the bathroom, and so on. On days when the learner does not attend work sites, the schedule would be similar, except that locations would be at school where work, break, and other real life events are simulated for the purpose of obtaining additional training.

		Skill						
Event and Location	Time and Instructor	Strengthen neck muscles	Visual tracking	Toilet regulation	Reach 10 inches	Decrease screaming	Signal for attention	Hold onto stimulus
Arrival at school Bus	8:15 Chris	Head aligned while sitting	Teacher		Touch: teacher, lunchbox	Implement DRI program	To move wheelchair to class, to open door	Teacher's hand, lunchbox
Toileting Bathroom	8:30 Chris	Head aligned while sitting	Teacher	Toileting program	Teacher	Implement DRI program	To move wheelchair to bathroom	Teacher's hand
Cleanup/dressing Bathroom	8:45 Chris	Head aligned while sitting	Soap, towel		Teacher, soap, towel, bathroom door	Implement DRI program	For soap, towel, to open door	Teacher's hand, soap, towel, doorknob
Work group Worktable	9:15 Joan/Toni	Head aligned while sitting	Material as passed to peer		Teacher, work materials, reinforcers	Implement DRI program	For more materials	Teacher's hand, work materials, reinforcers

Depart for store Classroom door	9:45 Joan	Head aligned while sitting	Teacher		Teacher, doors	Implement DRI program	To open doors, to move wheelchair	Teacher's hand
Arrival at store Bus	10:10 Joan	Head aligned while sitting	Traffic	Pants check	Bus and store door	Implement DRI program	To move wheelchair, to open door	Teacher's hand
Shopping Merchandise area	10:20 Joan	Head aligned while sitting			Items on shelf; with money to pay for item	Implement DRI program	To indicate item desired, to go to cashier	Item from shelf; money
Leisure Store arcade	10:45 Joan	Head aligned while sitting	Arcade game piece		Arcade button or paddle	Implement DRI program	To move to arcade area, to get assistance with game	Arcade game paddle

Figure 2. An example of events/skills matrix for Mark, a learner with severe visual impairment. (DRI = differential reinforcement of incompatible behavior.)

A preschool child's schedule of events would reflect a more traditional school schedule: travel to school, use the bathroom, introductory group time, morning play group, cleanup, snack, use the bathroom, afternoon play group, and so on.

Two factors take precedence in scheduling daily events—toileting times and access to nonschool settings. Both of these factors are critical to the learner's educational program. Therefore, if a learner is being toilet trained, list the toileting times first in the daily events column of the matrix.

Access to nonschool settings (e.g., a group home or apartment) may be restricted to certain times of the day. Because participation in nonschool settings is an invaluable learning experience, arrange to use these settings whenever they can be accessed, even if the times they are available do not conform to a natural daily schedule of events.

Locations In the left column of the events/skills matrix, indicate the location where each event occurs. For example, the arrival event occurs on the bus; break time during work training at the retail department store occurs in the staff lounge; and cleanup after lunch in the group home occurs in the kitchen of the home. The purpose of specifying locations is to ensure that skills are taught in multiple environments. In addition, the structure of a location provides valuable information when writing the ICS (writing the ICS will be discussed later).

Time of Activity Write in the left column of the matrix the time that each event begins. Duration of events should approximate what is expected in future environments. For example, if potential supervised living programs provide for half-hour periods of independent leisure time, use this time criterion in schedule planning. Duration of events is useful also as a guide in writing skill clusters of the appropriate length.

Instructor Specify the instructor for each daily event. In doing so, consider allowing the learner to choose the instructor. For example, if a teacher and an assistant are teaming together to teach a group, then a learner could choose the preferred instructor who would then conduct the training.

Skills All of a learner's target behaviors are incorporated into the ICS. Therefore, across the top of the matrix write a brief description of each target behavior, with one behavior per column. These may be behaviors to be reduced, as well as those to be increased; they may be simple responses such as reaching, as well as more complex behaviors that can be task analyzed, such as putting on a coat or assembling a circuit board.

Fill Out the Matrix Cells Each cell in the events/skills matrix corresponds to one behavior and one event. Complete the matrix by asking, for each cell, "What functional materials or activities can be used to teach this behavior during this event?" For example, using Mark's events/skills matrix in Figure 2, how can the skill of visual tracking be taught during the event of arrival at school? The cell for this in Figure 2 is the first one below the skill of visual tracking. In the example, tracking will be taught during arrival by having Mark visually follow the teacher across the plane of vision.

During cleanup/dressing (in the third line of the "visual tracking" column), tracking will be taught by having Mark visually follow the soap or towel as he passes it across his plane of vision.

In most cases, many different materials or activities can be used to teach a skill. During arrival at school, for example, tracking could also be taught by having Mark visually follow a peer or the school bus. Select, however, the materials or activities that are most appropriate for the learner's abilities and needs, and that are feasible given the learner-teacher ratio and the conditions of instruction (e.g., managing of data sheets, wheelchairs, and instructional materials).

Whenever possible, utilize more than one material or activity, so the learner can be afforded opportunities to choose the one desired. The opportunity to choose should be provided to all learners, including those who are unable to verbally or physically select a material or activity. Some learners may have to be taught to choose if they have never been given the opportunity to do so, or if they have not developed a means for communicating their intentions. Other learners may indicate choice in subtle ways that are undetected by teachers who know only how to program for learners, not with them, or who are untrained as observers of behavior. A learner might, for example, display choice by being more attentive, cooperative, happy, or relaxed in the presence of preferred materials or activities.

Whatever materials and activities are selected, they should: a) be functional in that they help the learner to be more independent, b) be appropriate for the learner's chronological age, c) increase the chances for integration with nondisabled persons in community environments, d) be enjoyed by the learner, and e) be appropriate given the learner's sensory and motor development.

Check for Generalization and Choice After the matrix is completed, check that each behavior will be taught by two or more instructors, with at least two different materials or activities, and in multiple settings. Check also to see that, when appropriate, two or more variations of a response are required of the learner. In Figure 2, for example, the skill of "reach 10 inches" will consist of a class of responses in which Mark must reach with his hand and arm in different orientations—arm out and palm sideways to touch the teacher's hand, arm down and palm down to touch the soap, and so on. The skill of "strengthen neck muscles," on the other hand, is taught using only one activity—sitting in a chair. Other activities should be added so that the use of different muscle groups is required. For example, neck muscles could be strengthened by encouraging Mark to maintain head alignment when standing with support, when pulled to sitting from a supine position, and when being transferred from a desk to a wheelchair.

When the matrix is completed, check that choice-making will be incorporated into the ICS. This is possible if the matrix includes multiple materials or activities for some cells, and if multiple instructors will be involved in an event. In Figure 2, choice of materials will be possible by providing multiple work tasks for Mark to choose from. Choice of trainer will be possible during the work group because Joan and Toni will team up for group instruction. Change the matrix if there is insufficient generalization training for any skill, or if less than three opportunities for choice will be available during the day to the learner.

Write the ICS

A typical ICS comprises a variety of training formats, including massed trial arrangements, skill clusters, behavior checks, isolated trials of skills that cannot be related to other skills in clusters, and task analyses. All of these training formats are taught as they naturally occur within daily events and with functional materials and activities.

Massed Trials When writing the ICS, one way to arrange training trials is to mass them together so that the same skill is taught repeatedly with little time between trials. This arrangement is appropriate for those skills that are naturally repetitive, such as mobility skills (e.g., taking steps, moving a wheelchair, rolling), certain vocational tasks (e.g., sorting, placing one item after another on a counting jig), and some domestic tasks (e.g., placing one utensil at each place setting). It is inappropriate, on the other hand, to arrange in a massed trial format skills that do not naturally occur that way. For example, systematic tactile searching would, in most circumstances, be used to find an object that is then grasped and used. Rarely would one search to touch an object, then search to touch it again, search to touch it a third time, and so on.

Skill Clusters A second way to arrange training trials is to distribute trials of one skill among training trials of one or more other skills. In addition, skills should be distributed so that they relate in some functional way. One source for identifying how skills are functionally related is to observe how they are used together by nondisabled persons in the community. Another way to determine functional clusters is to arrange the skills as they would be used by a person typically interacting with the materials or activities.

The best length for clusters is 3–6 skills. When clusters are longer than this, it is difficult to remember the skills in the cluster, as well as the cues and correction procedures for each skill. In addition, longer clusters tend to appear, in practice, to be a drawn-out string of unrelated skills rather than a tightly knit, cohesive group of skills used to achieve a functional outcome.

To write a skill cluster, information is combined about the learner (e.g., capabilities, learning style); the event (e.g., arrives at school on a bus; gets off the bus at the front door of the school with other students present); the skills being taught (e.g., how they will be prompted or corrected, the degree of independence to expect); and the materials and activities used to teach the skills (e.g., adaptations needed, whether the materials and activities will be utilized by other learners). Each daily event is analyzed, to see how the skills being taught can be used naturally during the event, how they can be related to one another, and how the student's choice of teacher, materials, or activities can be incorporated into instruction.

Using the events/skills matrix for Mark in Figure 2, a teacher might work through the arrival event as follows: first, check that Mark's head is aligned; then call his name to get his attention; walk from Mark's side to the front of his wheelchair for the purpose of visual tracking; extend a hand which he must reach 10 inches to grasp; then shake his hand, measuring whether he holds on for at least five seconds. Finally, the teacher implements the behavior control program for screaming, reinforcing Mark for being silent or for vocalizing at a conversational level during his arrival at school.

This skill cluster for "arrival at school" is shown in Figure 3. The figure, which is for the first portion of Mark's school day, contains the cue to which Mark is to respond, the response required of him, and an area to collect data for five days. Mark's day, as shown in Figure 3, consists of a series of skill clusters. Three short clusters make up the arrival event. In addition to the first arrival cluster described above, a second cluster relates to acquiring his lunchbox to carry to the classroom. The third and final arrival cluster involves getting to the classroom.

Using again the information in Mark's events/skills matrix (Figure 2), the process of writing skill clusters for the group work event at 9:15 with Joan and Toni might proceed as follows. Since Joan and Toni are teaming together to instruct the work group, Mark can choose whom he wants as a teacher. He will do this by reaching 10 inches toward the instructor of choice. Once he selects the instructor, he will be taken to the shelves containing the work materials. Here he will be given a choice of work, making his selection by reaching 10 inches toward the materials of choice. At this point he will be reinforced if, since the last behavior check, he has either been silent or else vocalized at a conversational level.

He will be taken to the work area where his head alignment will be monitored and, if necessary, prompted by the instructor. After checking for head alignment, he will reach 10 inches to the instructor's hand and hold that hand for a minimum of five seconds while being transferred from the wheelchair to a chair at the table.

Both tasks performed during the work group require that Mark pick up an item from a box of unsorted parts and place it on a stand to be visually discriminated by Devin, who has no use of her arms and hands. After Devin visually discriminates the item and activates a light over the sorting bin to which it belongs, a third worker, Roy, will remove the item from the stand and deposit it in the lighted box.

Mark's role in the work trio will involve reaching 10 inches into the box of mixed parts, and holding the item for five seconds while moving it to the stand. In addition, he will be required to track the item as he moves it from the box of parts to the stand.

Mark is currently capable of working for one minute without reinforcement. He should be able to manage three work clusters in one minute. Therefore, he must complete three work clusters before he is reinforced. In addition, reinforcement for work is provided only if: a) the work is performed to the criterion of three items placed on the stand within one minute; and b) he has, since the last behavior check, either been silent or vocalized at a conversational level. Reinforcement will be part of a cluster that will consist of a behavior check and, if the conditions for work and behavior have been met, reaching 10 inches for a reinforcer. Two reinforcers will be presented each time in order to provide Mark a choice.

Most events will consist of one or more clusters. Typically, there is a cluster for entering and exiting a location, as well as one or more for engaging in the activities common to the location. A good example of this is found in the first cluster for Mark during toileting (Figure 3), when he signals to move to the bathroom. Once in the bathroom, a cluster is conducted for transferring to the toilet. Head alignment and a behavior check are monitored during toileting. The last toileting cluster is for transferring back to the wheelchair in preparation for exiting the area.

Cue	Response	Date				
8:15 Arrival at school	**Chris (Bus)**					
—	Head aligned					
V: Mark; walk	Visually tracks					
Extend hand	Reaches 10 inches					
—	Holds hand for 5 seconds					
Behavior check	Implement DRI					
—	Head aligned					
Extend lunchbox	Reaches 10 inches					
—	Holds box for 5 seconds					
Wait	Signal to move to CR					
Behavior check	Implement DRI					
Wait	Signal to open door					
8:30 Toileting	**Chris (BR)**					
—	Head aligned					
V: Mark; walk	Visually tracks					
Face toward BR, wait	Signals to move to BR					
Behavior check	Implement DRI					
Extend hand	Reaches 10 inches					
—	Holds hand for 5 seconds					
(Transfer from wheelchair to toilet.)		—	—	—	—	—

Figure 3. An example skill cluster for Mark that includes the events of arrival, toileting, cleanup/dressing, and work group. (V = verbal cue; DRI = differential reinforcement of incompatible behavior; CR = classroom; BR = bathroom.)

—	Head aligned					
Behavior check	Implement DRI					

—	Head aligned					
Extend hand	Reaches 10 inches					
—	Holds hand for 5 seconds					
(Transfer from toilet to wheelchair.)		—	—	—	—	—
Behavior check	Implement DRI					

8:45 Cleanup/dressing Chris (BR)

Move to sink, wait	Signals for soap					
Move soap	Visually tracks					
—	Reaches 10 inches					
—	Holds soap for 5 seconds					
(Assist with washing hands.)		—	—	—	—	—
Wait	Signals for towel					
Move towel	Visually tracks					
—	Reaches 10 inches					
—	Holds towel for 5 seconds					
(Assist with drying hands.)		—	—	—	—	—
Behavior check	Implement DRI					

—	Head aligned					
Extend hands	Reaches 10 inches					
—	Holds hand for 5 seconds					
(Transfer from chair to wheelchair.)		—	—	—	—	—
Face door, wait	Signal to open door					
—	Reaches 10 inches					
—	Holds doorknob 5 seconds					

(continued)

9:15 Work group Choose Joan/Toni (work table)

Choice of teachers	Reaches 10 inches for choice					
Place before shelf	Reaches 10 inches for choice					
—	Holds item for 5 seconds					
Behavior check	Implement DRI					
—	Head aligned					
Extend hand	Reaches 10 inches					
—	Holds hand for 5 seconds					
(Transfer from wheelchair to chair.)		—	—	—	—	—
—	Reaches 10 inches for item					
(Assist passing it.)	Visually tracks					
—	Holds 5 seconds while passing					
(Teach above cluster three times, then go to reinforcement cluster.)						
Behavior check	Implement DRI					
Offer two reinforcers	Reaches 10 inches for choice					
(Repeat above two clusters as often as necessary.)						
—	Head aligned					
Extend hand	Reaches 10 inches					
—	Holds hand for 5 seconds					
(Transfer from chair to wheelchair.)		—	—	—	—	—

Figure 3. *(continued)*

Skill clusters may be repeated consecutively during an event, or alternated with one or more other clusters. This occurs most often during events where the same tasks are completed over and over, such as during work. This occurs in Figure 3 during Mark's work group. Following the clusters for selecting the work task and transferring from the wheelchair to a chair, a cluster begins that relates to the work being performed. This cluster is repeated two additional times before a two-skill reinforcement cluster is conducted. The process of three work clusters to each reinforcement cluster continues for the remainder of the 30-minute work group. This work-to-reinforcement ratio may increase as Mark engages in sustained work for longer periods of time.

Behavior Checks All procedures for lessening excessive behaviors must include a plan for developing an alternative and more adaptive behavior. The ICS provides a ready means for building adaptive behavior through the use of behavior checks. Behavior checks are points in time during instructional programming when the teacher is reminded to observe for specified appropriate behavior and to implement at that time the plan for increasing it (Holvoet et al., 1985). For example, Figure 3 contains behavior check points where silence or appropriate vocalizations are reinforced as part of the procedure to decrease inappropriate screaming.

To incorporate behavior checks into the ICS, first determine the schedule of reinforcement (e.g., once a minute). Estimate how far into the ICS one would go in that length of time. Place the behavior check at that point. If the behavior check point falls within a skill cluster, place it, instead, at the end of the cluster. This avoids disrupting the meaningful flow of instruction of the cluster.

Isolated Skills Not all skills can be related in clusters or appropriately grouped in a massed trial fashion. For example, suppose that paying for food and locating the restroom are the only skills targeted for the learner that can be taught during visits to community fast food restaurants. These two skills do not flow together in a naturally occurring cluster. In other words, paying for food does not set the occasion for the immediate occurrence of locating the restroom. When skills cannot be clustered, teach them singly when they naturally occur during an event. At the fast food restaurant, for example, pay for the food after ordering it. Later, perhaps just prior to leaving the restaurant, provide instruction on locating the restroom.

Task Analyses Many learners will have in their ICS a task analysis of one or more complex behaviors, such as brushing teeth, making a bed, and setting a table. Task analyses occur in the sequence when and where they naturally occur. Skill clusters, massed trial segments, and isolated skills may, if appropriate, precede or follow a task analysis.

The ICS for Mark that is shown in Figure 3 includes skill clusters and behavior checks. To illustrate how massed trials, skill clusters, and task analyses might appear together in an ICS, a portion of an ICS for an adolescent who is deaf-blind is shown in Figure 4. At the top of the figure is a partial list of the target behaviors for the learner. Shown below the list of target behaviors are selected portions of the ICS for this learner. The first column in the ICS states the target behavior that is being taught. In the second column is the expected learner response.

The first portion of the partial ICS pictured in Figure 4 is a cleanup event that occurs in the bathroom area following toileting. Cleanup is taught using a skill cluster for moving from the toilet to the sink area. This cluster leads to a task analysis for handwashing. The ICS begins with the learner practicing a pincer grasp during zipping his pants. He then works on building strength in his arms by partially supporting himself while transferring from the toilet to the wheelchair. He must then signal for help, in this case for help in opening the bathroom door.

Arm strength once again is programmed as the learner pushes open the door, then wheels his chair to the sink. At the sink he learns handwashing, as is evident in the ICS by the task analysis for that behavior. Interjected into the task analysis for handwashing is a contrived opportunity for eliciting a signal for assistance. This oc-

Skills to be taught

Pincer grasp	Wash hands
Build strength in arms	Wait turn
Signal for assistance	One-to-one correspondence

Target behavior	Learner response
Cleanup (bathroom area following toileting)	
Pincer grasp	Pincer grasps zipper on pants
Strengthen arms	Transfers from toilet to wheelchair
Signal for assistance	Signals for help to open door
Strengthen arms	Opens door with assistance
Strengthen arms	Moves wheelchair to sink
Washes hands	Turns water on
	Wets hands
	Gets soap
	Lathers hands
	Scrubs hands
	Rinses hands
	Turns off water
Signal for assistance	Signals for towel that is missing
Washes hands	Replaces towel on towel rack
Cleanup (kitchen area of group home)	
Waits turn	Waits until all pots are dried
1–1 correspondence	Places pot on first hook
1–1 correspondence	Places pot on second hook
1–1 correspondence	Places pot on third hook
1–1 correspondence	Places pot on fourth hook

Figure 4. Selected portions of an ICS for a learner who is deaf-blind.

curs near the end of the task analysis where the towel that the learner needs in order to dry his hands is placed out of sight.

One precaution to take when incorporating communication skills, such as signaling for assistance, into the ICS is to frequently alter the conditions in which the communication skill must be displayed. This must be done so the learner truly acquires communication skills, instead of relying on irrelevant contextual cues to respond. Using the first portion of the ICS in Figure 4 as an example, if the towel is placed out of sight each time the learner is instructed in handwashing, he may learn merely to signal for help each time he reaches that point in the task. To prevent the use of such contextual cues, sometimes place the towel out of sight, other times remove the soap.

The next segment of the partial ICS shown in Figure 4 is a domestic event that involves hanging cooking pots on hooks on the wall. This occurs in a community group home that is a potential future residential setting and that is used during the school day for training purposes. This brief segment of the ICS illustrates the teaching of one-to-one correspondence using an activity that occurs naturally in a massed trial format. First, the learner practices waiting until all the pots are dried and ready to hang. Then, one-to-one correspondence is taught by having the learner hang one pot on each hook.

Develop Instructional Programs

An instructional program is a detailed description of how a skill will be taught. It specifies such components as the rationale for learning the skill, materials, activities, natural and instructional cues and consequences, task analysis, when to teach, data collection strategies, and so on. The development of an ICS for a student helps to outline some of these components (cues, materials, activities, location, when to teach). For this reason, it is suggested that completion of the written program be deferred until the ICS is developed.

The practicality of this is evident if one considers the difference in how instructional cues might be specified when the ICS model is used versus teaching one skill at a time. When teaching one skill at a time, it is usual to state for each skill a specific instructional cue. Using the ICS model, skills often fall within clusters of behaviors, so that one skill serves as a cue for the following skill. This approach is more natural in that responses are less tightly controlled by the instructor, and the learner must attend to how skills are used together for a functional purpose.

Theoretically, a number of different target behaviors might, for any given activity, serve as a cue for a specific skill. In reality, however, target behaviors usually cluster together in similar ways across the various daily events. Therefore, it is possible to specify in the instructional program which, if any, target behaviors will serve to cue other skills.

Adapt the ICS

When using the ICS, teachers must be careful not to be overly rigid in adhering to the sequence, nor to move so quickly through it that learners have no opportunity to display spontaneous behavior. Teachers should, instead, watch for at least three types of feedback from the learner.

First, look for additional situations in which learners might be able to display choice. Possible situations include choice of physical positioning during work or leisure (e.g., standing versus sitting), preference for the structure of work and leisure events (e.g., mobile, stationary, whole task, assembly line), location of events (inside, outside), and environmental variables (noise, illumination, crowdedness). With knowledge of these factors, teachers can adapt the ICS to provide additional choices. They can also match future work, residential, and other community settings to learners' preferences. This contrasts with the traditional approach of programming for learners that molds individuals to the environment or situation perceived by the teacher and others as being in the best interests of the learners.

A second type of feedback to watch for is the learners' attempts to use target skills with other materials or activities. Be flexible and use these opportunities in place of or in addition to those already included in the ICS.

Third, observe for non-target behaviors that exist or are emerging and that learners freely display or attempt to display. These may be very obvious behaviors, such as loud vocalizations to gain a peer's attention, or subtle attempts, such as tensing a muscle in an effort to reach for a toy, or slightly turning the upper body to try to initiate rolling. Freely emitted behaviors are meaningful to learners and should be incorporated into training in order either to develop that behavior more fully or to enhance the acquisition of targeted behaviors by combining the spontaneous behavior in clusters with target skills. For example, Dewayne was learning to follow the command signed in his hand for "come," followed by training in using a sighted guide. Each time the teacher indicated her presence by touching Dewayne's arm prior to giving the sign, Dewayne would grab her arm and pull it to his face. In doing this, he was attempting to identify the instructor through smell and touch. Although identification of persons was not targeted initially as an objective, it was adopted as one and incorporated into the ICS in order to provide Dewayne with a more appropriate method for identifying others in his environment. In addition, it provided an added opportunity for choice and, hopefully, enhanced his desire to participate in instruction.

Using the ICS with Groups

Group instruction using the ICS serves the same purpose as group instruction in general—to provide behavioral models by peers who are disabled or nondisabled, to teach group cooperation and interaction skills, and to manipulate motivational factors for learners who are reluctant to respond (Gaylord-Ross & Holvoet, 1985). Group instruction also provides additional opportunities for generalization training involving other persons (i.e., peers).

When to Teach in Groups Group instruction should be arranged for those events in which it occurs naturally—work, socialization, meals, and certain leisure activities. The first step in preparing a group cluster, then, is to identify those events during which group instruction will occur.

Select Materials or Activities The second step in constructing a group cluster is to select functional materials or activities with which to teach skills during the group event. Use the same criteria for material and activity selection that were outlined earlier—functionality, age appropriateness, enhancement of integration, enjoyability, and appropriateness for the learners' skill development.

Select Skills Pick for each learner two or three skills to teach during the group event using the materials or activities selected. Keep the number of skills small for each learner in order to move more quickly from learner to learner, providing a greater sense of involvement of each person in the group event. In addition, since it is necessary to remember the instructional cues and correction procedures for each skill, the fewer the number of skills taught in a group situation, the easier it is to implement accurately the instructional programs (Gaylord-Ross & Holvoet, 1985).

Write the Group Cluster There are two types of group ICSs—those with interaction between learners and those without (Brown, Holvoet, Guess, & Mulligan, 1980). In non-interactional sequences, the teacher constructs a brief cluster for each learner in the group, with no planned interaction between learners. During the group session, the teacher instructs the first learner with his or her brief cluster, then instructs the next learner with his or her cluster, and so on. Learners do not interact with one another or use materials cooperatively. Figure 5 contains an example of a noninteractional group sequence for mealtime. The skills to be taught to each learner are listed at the top of the figure. The teacher first instructs Gerald with his skill cluster; moves

---

Skills to be taught during mealtime

Gerald	David
Respond to gesture	Remain in seat
Signal for more	Reach and grasp
One-to-one correspondence	Drink from cup
	Use communication board

Michael	Laura
Receptively label cup, pop	Combine hands at midline
Pour	Drink from cup

Teacher's cue	Learner's response	Date				
Gerald						
Point to napkin	Picks up napkins					
—	Places one per place					
—	Signals for need one more					
Michael						
Allow him to feel milk or cup	Signs for milk or cup					
—	Signs for milk or cup					
	Pours milk in cup					
David						
Show juice/milk	Points to picture					
—	Reaches/grasps item					
	Drinks from cup					
Behavior check	DRI for being in seat					
Laura						
Give cup and milk	Brink to midline to pour					
—	Drinks from cup					

Figure 5. Example of a noninteractional group ICS for mealtime.

next to Michael using his cluster; then instructs, in turn, David and Laura. Figure 6 contains another non-interactional group sequence, this one for a leisure event. As in the last example, each learner is instructed using his or her individualized sequence. No interaction occurs between the learners.

Non-interactional sequences are written primarily when the learners' objectives differ so greatly that it is impossible to use the same materials or activities with two or more learners in the group. For example, if the only skill that can be taught to Janet during group time is grasping, but the functional material used with the remaining learners in the group is a small electronic wire that is beyond Janet's current ability to grasp, then different materials or activities must be used with Janet. This makes it more difficult to program for interaction between her and the other learners.

The use of different materials, activities, and skill clusters makes it more difficult to teach efficiently and effectively in group situations. It requires the teacher to

---

Skills to be taught during leisure time

Greg
Select leisure item (ball, puzzle) that is requested
Vocalize "ba" (for ball) or "pa" (for puzzle)
Use leisure items (roll ball, assemble puzzle)

Terri
Tactually scan
Find leisure item (doll, car) that is requested
Play with leisure items

Melinda
Localize to side when name is called
Visually track objects
Activate leisure item with a microswitch

Greg	Terri	Melinda
1. Select ball or puzzle upon verbal request		
2. Say "ba" or "pa"		
3. Roll ball or assemble puzzle		
	4. Tactually scan doll, car, and boat	
	5. Find doll or car when requested	
	6. Play with doll or car for at least one minute	
		7. Localize to name
		8. Visually track radio
		9. Activate radio using microswitch

Figure 6. Example of a noninteractional group ICS for a leisure event.

spend more time arranging different materials for the various learners and less time on instruction. In addition, the group is less cohesive and it is more difficult to keep the group focused on learning the task at hand.

The second type of group sequence involves interaction between the group's members. Interaction can occur as learners provide antecedents such as greeting one another, passing materials, and providing cues to respond; or consequating behavior by reinforcing correct responses or passing materials requested by another learner. Figure 7 repeats the sequence shown in Figure 5, but this time with interaction between the learners. At least one response in the learners' clusters represents a point of interaction. Interaction points are denoted in the figure by an asterisk. The response at this point may or may not be an instructional objective of the learner. The rationale for incorporating a nontarget behavior at this point is to promote the cohesive flow of instruction from one learner to the next and to facilitate incidental learning of group interaction behavior.

An interactional sequence has three major advantages. First, it provides more opportunities to program for generalization, because the learners can respond to one another as well as to the teacher. Second, it draws attention to peers in the group. Many learners, especially those with severe disabilities, spend a great portion of their time attending to adults, those who control instructional cues and consequences (Gaylord-Ross & Holvoet, 1985). By utilizing peers in these roles, more attention is directed to these group members. Third, interactional groups are more cohesive. There is a primary purpose for each learner's presence there as the group members work together toward a common outcome.

FUTURE PROGRAM AND RESEARCH DIRECTIONS

Over the years, the ICS model has evolved in a manner that acknowledges more extensively contributions from learners in the instructional process, and that attends more to individual needs in identifying instructional objectives. These components are reflected in programmed opportunities for learners to express choice and preferences (Guess & Helmstetter, 1986) and, recently, the perceived need to attend more closely to learner-initiated behavior during instructional periods. This orientation differs significantly from a more traditional ecological model that is based on intensive manipulation of environmental cues and consequences to teach skills and behaviors that have been identified by *others* to be important contributions to the student's level of adaptive behavior, and in preparing him or her for future environments. At issue is a growing divergence of both professional opinion and pedagogical practice on how, indeed, persons with severe handicaps—including learners with sensory impairments who are also mentally retarded—should be educated.

The need to balance existing instructional procedures and technology with an appreciation for a learner-centered expression of what should be taught and developed might well be the next most significant research direction for the ICS model and other instructional approaches. It is anticipated that future program and research directions

Skills to be taught during mealtime

Gerald

Respond to gesture
Signal for more
One-to-one correspondence

Michael

Receptively label cup, pop
Pour

David

Remain in seat
Reach and grasp
Drink from cup
Use communication board

Laura

Combine hands at midline
Drink from cup

Laura	Michael	Gerald	David
*1. Combine hands at midline to pick up pitcher (teacher assists in passing it to Michael)			
			2. Behavior check for in seat 3. Points to picture of cup
	4. Receptively labels cup 5. Pours 3 cups of milk		
		*6. Responds to point cue by Michael to cups *7. Passes one to each learner *8. Signals to Michael for 1 more for David	
	9. Pours 1 cup		
		*10. (Passes a cup to David)	
			11. Behavior check for in seat *12. Reaches & grasps cups 13. Drinks from cup
14. Combines hands at midline for cup 15. Drinks from cup			

Figure 7. Example of an interactional group ICS for mealtime.

for the ICS model will attend more closely to the identification of individual motivational factors and other organismic conditions (physiological and psychological) that determine the parameters under which the acquisition, generalization, and maintenance of skills are most likely to occur among learners with severe handicaps. In the area of language instruction, Goetz, Schuler, and Sailor (1983) for example, have pointed to an over-reliance on stimulus control teaching methods in relation to other motivational considerations. They also provide empirical support suggesting the role of organismic contributions to the learning process, which they refer to as functional competence.

The position of Goetz et al. (1983) has gained additional support in a recent study (Goetz, Gee, & Sailor, 1985) showing that inserting single trial communication responses in an interrupted sequence of behavior (e.g., washing dishes) increases correct responding on the communication task. Functional competence is again offered as one potential motivating factor for this finding.

> A single trial strategy, in addition to providing further indirect support for an individual curriculum sequencing model of instruction (Holvoet, Guess, Mulligan, & Brown, 1980), also appears to approximate real life language use: events are typically labeled, requested, and so forth only once, but this single trial or event has genuine meaning for the user. (Goetz et al., 1985, p. 28)

The functional competence motivational concept being explored by Goetz et al. (1983, 1985) offers an excellent example of how skill sequencing can be used as the basis for exploring motivational variables that influence response acquisition, and it provides for researchers the impetus to view behavior of persons with severe handicaps in a manner that deviates from traditional practices and theoretical assumptions that have dominated the field over the past two decades.

Research and program development efforts at the University of Kansas are following similar directions in attempts to include and combine other motivational theories and approaches dealing with skill cluster instruction and with variations of that model. In one research program (Bronicki, Houghton, & Guess, 1985), an observational code is being used to measure the extent to which classroom teachers and related service personnel provide opportunities for choice-making and expressions of preference in classrooms for learners with severe handicaps. These data will be used as the basis for researching methods and procedures for teaching choice-making skills to persons with severe handicaps, and, in particular, teaching these skills within the format of the ICS model.

A second ongoing research program (Siegel-Causey & Guess, 1985) is investigating movement-based procedures for accelerating prelinguistic skills among preschool children with visual and auditory impairment (see Siegel-Causey and Downing, Chapter 2, this volume). As part of this research, methods are being explored for instructing teachers and parents to respond more appropriately (and frequently) to learner-initiated behavior in classroom and home settings. Results of the research as well as the procedures being developed as part of this program will be applicable to that component of the ICS model that alerts teachers to the need to incorporate learner-initiated behavior into skill clusters. This research addresses also the perceived need to acknowledge internal motivating factors that contribute to successful response acquisition among persons with severe handicaps, and is considered a major new direction for the further development and refinement of the ICS model.

SUMMARY

The individualized curriculum sequencing (ICS) model represents an educational approach that uses skill clusters as the basis for organizing curriculum content among learners with visual and hearing impairments. This chapter reviews the rationale and supporting research literature for the conceptual underpinnings of the model. It points out that the ICS model has evolved over time as an instructional process, and that these changes reflect current best practice recommendations.

Specific guidelines for implementing the ICS model in classroom settings are provided for learners who have severe visual and auditory impairments. Procedures for application include arrangement for both individual and group instruction.

Future research and program development recommendations for the ICS model include provisions for acknowledging other organismic motivational factors as part of the instructional process and in the selection of skills to be trained. These considerations emphasize the need to more extensively involve the learner as an active participant in the instructional process. The need for teaching choice-making and for the recognition of learner preferences is stressed. Additional research recommendations address the need to identify and include learner-initiated behavior into the skill cluster sequences.

REFERENCES

Alexander, D. (1974). Comparison for mental retardates of non-choice, initial choice, and idiosyncratic-choice reward strategies. *Psychological Reports, 35*, 135–145.

Anderson, S.R., & Spradlin, J.E. (1980). The generalized effects of productive labeling training involving common object classes. *Journal of The Association for the Severely Handicapped, 5*(2), 143–157.

Berk, R.A. (1976). Effects of choice of instructional methods on verbal learning tasks. *Psychological Reports, 38*, 867–870.

Brewer, M. (1982). *The efficacy of distributed practice training on the facilitation of generalization skills of the severely retarded.* Unpublished master's thesis, University of Kansas, Lawrence.

Bronicki, G., Houghton, J., & Guess, D. (1985). *A classroom and home model for preparing students with severe and moderate handicaps to express preferences and display choice-making skills in their daily lives.* Unpublished manuscript, University of Kansas, Mental Retardation Research Center, Lawrence.

Brown, F., Holvoet, J., Guess, D., & Mulligan, M. (1980). The individualized curriculum sequencing model (III): Small group instruction. *Journal of The Association for the Severely Handicapped, 5*(4), 352–367.

Brown, L., Branston-McClean, M., Baumgart, D., Vincent, L., Falvey, M., & Schroeder, J. (1979). Using characteristics of current and subsequent least restrictive environments in the development of curricular content for severely handicapped students. *AAESPH Review, 4*(4), 407–424.

Brown, L., Nietupski, J., & Hamre-Nietupski, S. (1976). The criterion of ultimate functioning and public school services for the severely handicapped student. In A. Thomas (Ed.), *Hey, don't forget about me: Education's investment in the severely, profoundly, and multiply handicapped.* Reston, VA: The Council for Exceptional Children.

Brown, L., Nisbet, J., Ford, A., Sweet, M., Shiraga, B., York, J., & Loomis, R. (1983). The critical need for nonschool instruction in educational programs for severely handicapped students. *The Journal of The Association for the Severely Handicapped, 8*(3), 71–77.

Dunlap, G., & Koegel, R.L. (1980). Motivating autistic children through stimulus variation. *Journal of Applied Behavior Analysis,* 1980, *13,* 619–627.

Dunlap, G., Koegel, R.L., & Koegel, L.K. (1984). Continuity of treatment: Toilet training in multiple community settings. *The Journal of The Association for Persons With Severe Handicaps, 9*(2), 134–141.

Falvey, M., Brown, L., Lyon, S., Baumgart, D., & Schroeder, J. (1980). Strategies for using cues and corrections procedures. In W. Sailor, B. Wilcox, & L. Brown (Eds.), *Methods of instruction for severely handicapped students* (pp. 109–133). Baltimore: Paul H. Brookes Publishing Co.

Ford, A., & Mirenda, P. (1984). Community instruction: A natural cues and corrections decision model. *The Journal of The Association for Persons With Severe Handicaps, 9*(2), 79–87.

Garcia, E., Baer, D.M., & Firestone, I. (1971). The development of generalized imitation within topographically determined boundaries. *Journal of Applied Behavior Analysis 4*(2), 101–112.

Gaylord-Ross, R., & Holvoet, J. (1985). *Strategies for educating students with severe handicaps.* Boston: Little, Brown.

Goetz, L., Gee, K., & Sailor, W. (1985). Using a behavior chain interruption strategy to teach communication skills to students with severe disabilities. *The Journal of The Association for Persons With Severe Handicaps, 10,* 21–30.

Goetz, L., Schuler, A., & Sailor, W. (1983). Motivational considerations in teaching language to severely handicapped students. In M. Hersen, V. Van Hasselt, & J. Matson (Eds.), *Behavior therapy for the developmentally disabled.* NY: Academic Press.

Guess, D., & Baer, D.M. (1973). An analysis of individual differences in generalization between receptive and productive language in retarded children. *Journal of Applied Behavior Analysis, 6,* 311–329.

Guess, D., Benson, H., & Siegel-Causey, E. (1985). Concepts and issues related to choice making and autonomy among persons with severe disabilities. *The Journal of The Association for Persons With Severe Handicaps, 10*(2), 79–86.

Guess, D., & Helmstetter, E. (1986). Skill cluster instruction and the individualized curriculum sequencing model. In R.H. Horner, L.H. Meyer, & H.D.B. Fredericks (Eds.), *Education of learners with severe handicaps: Exemplary service strategies* (pp. 221–248). Baltimore: Paul H. Brookes Publishing Co.

Guess, D., Jones, C., & Lyon, S. (1981). *Combining a transdisciplinary team approach with an individualized curriculum sequencing model for severely/multiply handicapped children.* Unpublished manuscript, University of Kansas, Department of Special Education, Lawrence.

Guess, D., & Siegel-Causey, E. (1985). Behavioral control and education of severely handicapped students: Who's doing what to whom? and why? In D. Bricker & J. Filler (Eds.), *Severe mental retardation: From theory to practice.* Reston, VA: The Council for Exceptional Children.

Helmstetter, E., Murphy-Herd, M., Roberts, S., & Guess, D. (1984). *Individualized curriculum sequencing and extended classroom models for learners who are deaf and blind.* Unpublished manuscript, University of Kansas, Department of Special Education, Lawrence.

Holvoet, J., Brewer, M., Mulligan, M., Guess, D., & Helmstetter, E. (1983). Influence of activity choice among adolescent, severely multiply handicapped students. In J. Holvoet & D. Guess (Eds.), *The KICS model: Evaluation Studies.* Unpublished manuscript, University of Kansas, Department of Special Education, Lawrence.

Holvoet, J., Guess, D., Mulligan, M., & Brown, F. (1980). The individualized curriculum sequencing model (II): A teaching strategy for severely handicapped students. *Journal of The Association for the Severely Handicapped, 5*(4), 337–351.

Holvoet, J., Mulligan, M., Schussler, N., Lacy, L., & Guess, D. (1985). *The Kansas Individualized Curriculum Sequencing model.* Portland, OR: A.S.I.E.P. Education Co.

Janssen, C., & Guess, D. (1978). Use of function as a consequence in training receptive labeling to severely and profoundly retarded individuals. *AAESPH Review, 3*(4), 246–258.

Lacy, L. (1982). *The effect of functional scheduling on the initiation and latency responses of severely handicapped students.* Unpublished master's thesis, University of Kansas, Lawrence.

Monty, R.A., & Perlmuter, L.C. (1975). Persistence of the effects of choice on paired-associate learning: *Memory and Cognition, 3,* 183–187.

Monty, R.A., Rosenberger, M.A., & Perlmuter, L.C. (1973). Amount of locus of choice as source of motivation in paired-associate learning. *Journal of Experimental Psychology, 97,* 16–21.

Mulligan, M., Guess, D., Holvoet, J., & Brown, F. (1980). The individualized curriculum sequencing model (I): Implications from research on massed, distributed, and spaced trial training. *Journal of The Association for the Severely Handicapped, 5*(4), 325–336.

Mulligan, M., Lacy, L., & Guess, D. (1982). Effects of massed, distributed, and spaced trial sequencing on severely handicapped students' performance. *The Journal of The Association for the Severely Handicapped, 7*(2), 48–61.

Newhard, M.K. (1984). *Effects of student choice of materials on skill acquisition with deaf/blind adolescents.* Unpublished master's thesis, University of Kansas, Lawrence.

Perlmuter, L.C., & Monty, R.A. (1973). The effect of choice of stimulus on paired-associate learning. *Journal of Experimental Psychology, 99,* 120–123.

Perlmuter, L.C., Monty, R.A., & Kimble, G.A. (1971). The effects of choice on paired-associate learning. *Journal of Experimental Psychology, 91,* 47–53.

Sailor, W., & Guess, D. (1983). *Severely handicapped students: An instructional design.* Boston: Houghton Mifflin.

Shevin, M., & Klein, N.K. (1984). The importance of choice-making for students with severe disabilities. *The Journal of The Association for Persons With Severe Handicaps, 9*(3), 159–166.

Siegel-Causey, E., & Guess, D. (1985). *Language development in deaf-blind children.* Unpublished manuscript, University of Kansas, Department of Special Education, Lawrence.

Sprague, J.R., & Horner, R.H. (1984). The effects of single instance, multiple instance, and general case training on generalized vending machine use by moderately and severely handicapped students. *Journal of Applied Behavior Analysis, 17*(2), 273–278.

Stokes, T.F., & Baer, D.M. (1977). An implicit technology of generalization. *Journal of Applied Behavior Analysis, 10,* 349–367.

Wilcox, B., & Bellamy, G.T. (1982). *Design of high school programs for severely handicapped students.* Baltimore: Paul H. Brookes Publishing Co.

Williams, W., Vogelsberg, R.T., & Schutz, R.P. (1985). Programs for secondary-age severely handicapped youth. In D. Bricker & J. Filler (Eds.), *Severe mental retardation: From theory to practice.* Reston, Va: The Council for Exceptional Children.

CHAPTER 11

Some Innovative Educational Applications of Advanced Technologies

Steven F. Warren, Eva H. Horn, and Everett W. Hill

EXTRAORDINARILY RAPID ADVANCES in technology are revolutionizing many aspects of contemporary culture world wide. Massive changes are occurring in banking, retailing, communication, transportation, entertainment, warfare, education, and so on. Miniaturization based on the silicon chip now allows a technician to carry an entire recording studio on his or her back. Eskimos in remote arctic villages can direct their satellite receivers to receive live broadcasts of Atlanta Braves baseball. Issues such as the definition of life and death are being challenged by impressive advances in medical technology. In the midst of all this technological infusion and change, persons with sensorimotor handicaps are being directly affected, too, and generally in positive ways.

This chapter will discuss issues related to the development and application of advanced technologies for use by persons with severe sensorimotor handicaps. A full discussion of these developments would require several hundred pages. Instead, this chapter presents a discussion of basic issues in the application of technological advances, and provides two detailed examples of recent innovations: the use of direct, computer mediated instruction to teach basic gross motor skills; and the use of electronic aids to teach orientation and mobility skills to children with severe visual impairments.

SOME CURRENT TRENDS

Technological innovation is widespread in the field of special education. The Association of Retarded Citizens has recently embarked on a nationwide fund-raising drive to promote research to bring "space age developments" to bear on the lives of children with handicaps. New journals and associations are appearing. Concurrent with all this activity is the realization by many that technological breakthroughs in and of themselves will not solve the fundamental problems faced by persons with severe handicaps.

Some basic trends in technological innovation are likely to affect the field of special education for several years to come. Hardware continues to become cheaper, more sophisticated, and thus more widely available. Important breakthroughs will continue, particularly those involving further miniaturization, voice recognition, and natural language processing. In this field, as in many others, handware development will stay far ahead of software development (Stallard, 1982).

In recent years the field of special education has been flooded with new educational software, some of it of poor quality (Budoff & Hutten, 1982). For this reason, concern is now being focused on the need for software standards. As the field of special education technology gradually matures, it is to be expected that many useless and even silly tangents will be pursued, and that megabytes of flawed software will be produced, consumed, and angrily discarded. In the meantime, the field will steadily advance, and many of its important innovations will directly affect individuals with severe sensorimotor impairments.

TECHNOLOGICAL DEVELOPMENTS RELATED TO SENSORIMOTOR IMPAIRMENTS

Technological developments that directly affect persons with sensorimotor impairments can be divided into educational, prosthetic, recreational, and systems management categories. Educational applications include direct teaching of basic motor skills, electronic mobility aids, contingency awareness training (e.g., Brinker & Lewis, 1982), moisture monitors used in teaching bladder control (e.g., Watson, 1968), and switches and sophisticated communication boards that are used to teach language (e.g., Vanderheiden, 1976). All traditional curricula domains have been, and continue to be, affected, including sensorimotor development (e.g., direct teaching and mobility aids), communication development (e.g., augmentative communication systems), cognitive development (e.g., contingency awareness training), social development (e.g., the effects of having an efficient communication mode), self-help skills (e.g., moisture monitors), and vocational skills (e.g., ability to control tasks through switches).

Whether or not many of these educational applications actually enhance learning can only be determined by rigorous experimental analyses. To date very few of these analyses have been conducted. Thus the impact of many of these innovations on teaching and learning will probably not be clear for some time. In contrast, innovative prosthetic applications, designed to either permanently replace a basic function or to enhance its use, have appeared and their usefulness is already obvious. Among these innovations are environmental control systems to allow individuals to control lights, televisions, computers, sophisticated communication systems, robotics, wheelchairs, and a variety of electronic mobility and orientation aids. These prosthetic devices can allow persons with very severe sensorimotor handicaps to have some measure of independence and control of their environment—to socialize, travel, communicate, work and take care of their own basic needs. In some cases a single technological innovation (e.g., the microswitch) has revolutionized the lives of many persons with severe sensorimotor handicaps.

Much of the special education technological development has been in systems management. Software is now available to assist in IEP (individualized education program) development and monitoring; data collection, analysis and management; individualized scheduling; diagnostics and assessment; report generation and storage; and administrative systems management. These straightforward applications should benefit persons with sensorimotor handicaps by decreasing paperwork, increasing program accountability and communication, and streamlining the bureaucratic aspects of program management. The extent to which they result in better programs will probably remain an unanswered empirical question for some time.

Finally, technological innovation is also affecting how persons with severe sensorimotor handicaps recreate and socialize. Adaptive toys based on innovative applications of microswitches are now widely available. Although commercial products are generally expensive, this technology is so basic that with minimal training parents and teachers can modify toys and develop their own switches.

WHAT TECHNOLOGY CAN AND SHOULD DO

In the midst of all this technological innovation, the question of what technology can and should do for persons with severe sensorimotor impairments should be asked. Viewed as a form of prosthesis, technology may lead to greater independence, make previously difficult or impossible tasks easier or possible, facilitate normalization and social integration, and ultimately extend an individual's abilities. Technological innovations that fail along these dimensions are probably trivial and wasteful of time and money.

From an educational perspective, technological innovation can and should promote actual learning of new skills within the target domain, and increase and optimize teacher-learner contact. To date very few technological education innovations have been subjected to any type of empirical analysis of effectiveness along these dimensions.

There are many inherent limitations in terms of what technology can accomplish. One thing it cannot do is to make poor content better; that is, technology may dress up an ineffective educational approach, but it is not likely to actually make it effective. In fact technology might stimulate the use of ineffective educational approaches, such as over-reliance on massed trial teaching or use of reinforcers that learners easily satiate on, because the technology itself is so easily applied in these ways. Basic language, cognitive, and social functions are best learned in a wide variety of naturally occurring contexts and will probably never be teachable in any generalizable way with the direct assistance of microcomputers.

Many other variables can limit the impact and effectiveness of technology. These include problems with equipment reliability, effects of small markets on costs and basic maintenance of specialized equipment, insurance liability, and the difficulties of matching the capabilities of technology to the heterogenous and wide-ranging needs of persons with severe handicaps. Finally, sophisticated technologies require sophisticated consumers for appropriate, effective use.

PROMISES AND PITFALLS

So far, both the vast potential and impact of technological innovations on the lives of persons with severe handicaps, as well as some problems and limitations of these innovations, have been noted. Suggestions have been made about what technology must do to be useful. Given both the potential and the limitations, what characteristics will useful technological innovations likely have? Three basic characteristics seem essential. First, a useful technological innovation must either enhance the performance of an important behavior for the individual in question, or promote the acquisition and generalization of such a behavior. Applying this characteristic to management systems software (e.g., IEP software or data analysis and managment) suggests that these innovations must improve professional practice in ways that enhance the fundamental goals for program consumers. Second, useful technological applications must rely on simple, easy to use, reliable hardware. And third, to the extent it employs software, this technology must also be simple, easily used, and reliable. Innovations that fail to exhibit these characteristics and that are not cost-effective, flexible, and adaptable, are not likely to have any real impact no matter how attractive they are as abstract ideas.

OVERVIEW

The remainder of this chapter presents detailed discussions of two important areas of technological innovation.[1] First, the application of a microcomputer-based system for teaching basic gross motor skills to young children with severe sensorimotor impairments; next, a range of electronic mobility aids that have been developed and that are now being used experimentally to teach crucial orientation and mobility skills to young children with severe visual impairments. The chapter concludes with some predictions about the future of the field and a discussion of present research needs.

SENSORIMOTOR MICROCOMPUTER APPLICATIONS

Simple on/off microswitches in conjunction with battery operated toys are being used widely by teachers to facilitate learning within the sensorimotor domain. Additionally, a few researchers have used these switches in combination with a computer or other electromechanical devices to train children with severe sensorimotor delays. These devices offer a number of advantages. They can accurately record the occurrence of even minimal movements made by the child. Most can be programmed to monitor the frequency and duration of a child's movement, provide contingent reinforcers, and activate the presentation of a novel reinforcer for the child at any point that the movement falls below baseline rate. Lastly, some devices can summarize the data and present it to the trainer in graphed form.

[1]Technological innovations and advances have also been made for children who experience severe hearing impairments. Readers interested in this topic are referred to Niswander, Chapter 5, this volume.

Historical Perspective

Since the early sixties, a series of studies have addressed the use of automated equipment for training individuals with severe sensorimotor disabilities. One approach to the use of this technology has been termed "contingency awareness training" (Behrmann & Lahm, 1982; Bricker, 1976; Brinker & Lewis, 1982; Watson, 1966; Zuromski, 1978). This approach is based on the belief that children experiencing severe sensorimotor delays acquire secondary developmental delays because of their inability to interact with their environment (Goldenberg, 1979). By providing an environment that is responsive to movements that are in the child's behavioral repertoire, the child is given additional opportunities to explore and experience cause-and-effect relationships. A problem with the devices used in these early studies was that they had a relatively fixed response requirement and used a limited number of consequences as potential reinforcers (e.g., tape recorder and slide projectors). Watson (1968), for example, monitored postural status with a mercury switch that contingently activated a tape player. But no other contingency was provided regardless of the child. Zuromski (1978), while allowing for multiple contingencies, required only one motor response from the child, that of pressing a lever.

Later research used more sophisticated switching devices, and by incorporating the flexible monitoring made possible by a microcomputer, provided an array of consequence items based on child responses (Aeschleman & Tawney, 1978; Brinker & Lewis, 1982). These studies, however, were directed at a narrow set of skills. In each case, contingency awareness was the primary goal of the intervention. Body movements that the infant was already capable of making were used. While the children demonstrated inital "contingency awareness," their performance data were extremely variable and suggested that response generalization might be restricted. This may be attributed to a number of factors: 1) the context for teaching contingency awareness was very narrow and did not reflect the diverse opportunities for this response in the natural environment; 2) because of the unnatural context, it is unclear what a functional performance criterion should have been; and 3) when a cognitive hierarchy based on normal development was used, it was unclear what the next skill in the sequence should have been.

A few researchers have also been exploring the use of electromechanical devices for training specific gross and fine motor behaviors. In this application, instead of selecting a switch that is as easy as possible for the child to activate, one is selected that is activated only when the child correctly performs the movement being taught.

Using an applied behavioral analysis approach, the primary role of the device becomes one of presenting antecedent stimuli, providing a variety of automatic reinforcement options, and maintaining consistent detailed tracking of student performance. A few experimental investigations have been conducted using this model.

Herman (1974) targeted a child's decreased muscle tension; Woolridge and Russell (1976) targeted upright and midline head position in supported sitting; and Rugel, Mattingly, Eichenger, and May (1971) targeted weightbearing in a standing position in order to activate a toy or radio. In each of these studies, the child increased the use of the targeted behavior when the switch/toy feedback model was used. These investigations used a case study approach and therefore did not demonstrate experimental control, limiting the impact of the findings. Additionally, each study was conducted in a clinical rather than applied setting. While these experiments focused on functionally relevant instructional content, they still raise questions about the contrived stimuli, contrived contingencies, and the generalized use of the trained skills in the natural environment. Finally, empirical research in educational settings using readily available equipment is needed to provide information concerning the efficacy of this motor intervention technique.

The research reviewed have been limited in a number of ways: 1) Targeted tasks may have been irrelevant and nonfunctional, (e.g., Brinker & Lewis, 1982); 2) target skills have not always been selected on the basis of "individual" child needs, but rather on the basis of switch characteristics and design, (e.g., Zuromski, 1978); 3) consequences have not always been based on specific child preferences and sensory deficits, (e.g., Aeschleman & Tawney, 1978); and 4) generalization has not been assessed outside the training situation (e.g., Woolridge & Russell, 1976).

MICROCOMPUTER MEDIATED INSTRUCTION OF MOTOR SKILLS

A system for microcomputer mediated sensorimotor training has been developed and is currently being evaluated both in an empirical research setting and a field test classroom setting. The system combines the principles of dynamic positioning (Bobath & Bobath, 1972) with those of using simple on/off microelectric switches to teach movement behaviors. Specifically, the system combines the use of adaptive equipment for supporting the child, single switches to monitor the child's correct motor movements, battery operated stimuli (i.e., toys, tape recorder, etc.) for reinforcers, and the microcomputer for monitoring and delivery of reinforcement (see Figure 1).

To conduct a training session, the teacher positions the child, the switch, and the toy. For example, in a program designed for training trunk extension for sitting, the teacher places the child in an individually designed piece of adaptive equipment. The equipment provides a semi-supported sitting position in which children must extend their arms, extend their trunk, and lift their head and shoulders to attain and maintain a sitting position. The switch used in this program is a four-position mercury head switch. Four mercury switches are secured on a small cap in such a way that when the child's head and trunk are up, all four switches are closed, turning on the battery operated toy. If however, the child's head or trunk drop, one or more of the switches is opened, and the toy is turned off (see Figure 2). A pressure sensitive external pad (Powerpad, from Dunamis, Inc.) is used by the teacher for controlling the computer. The pad allows the teacher to stay close to the child or children during the training sessions by eliminating the need to interact with the computer keyboard. Pressing predefined squares on the Powerpad surface controls such functions as: 1) Recording of prompt levels; 2) momentarily pausing during a session; 3) ending a session;

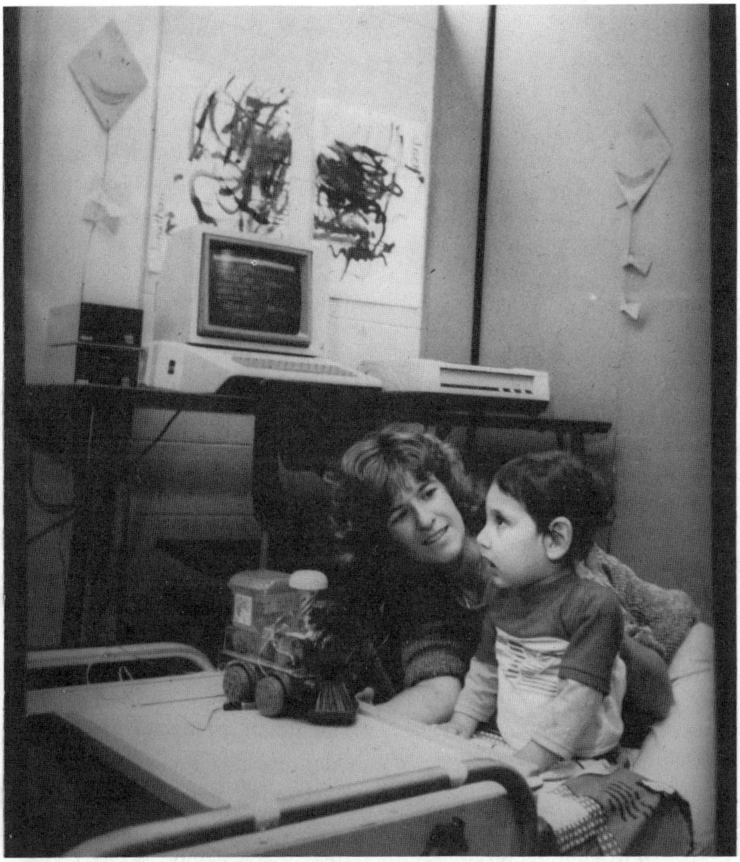

Figure 1. Microcomputers can both monitor behaviors and deliver reinforcement, by activating microswitches attached to battery-operated toys.

4) saving session data; 5) moving to the next child or skill to be trained; and 6) changing the order of training. At the end of a training day, log files can be printed that contain the child's name and program, date of session, toy used, total length of session, total number of switch closures, percentage of session time during which the switch was activated, and the total number of and type of trainer prompts provided for all sessions conducted.

Prior to implementing the system in the classroom, the following five tasks should be completed: 1) Selection of appropriate training goals based on the child's current motor programming in the classroom; 2) design, construction, and/or purchase of one or more microswitches for monitoring the target behavior; 3) design, construction and/or purchase of adaptive equipment that will provide stability and support to facilitate the child in performing the desired movement; 4) consultation with a physical or occupational therapist to assure that child positioning and task are

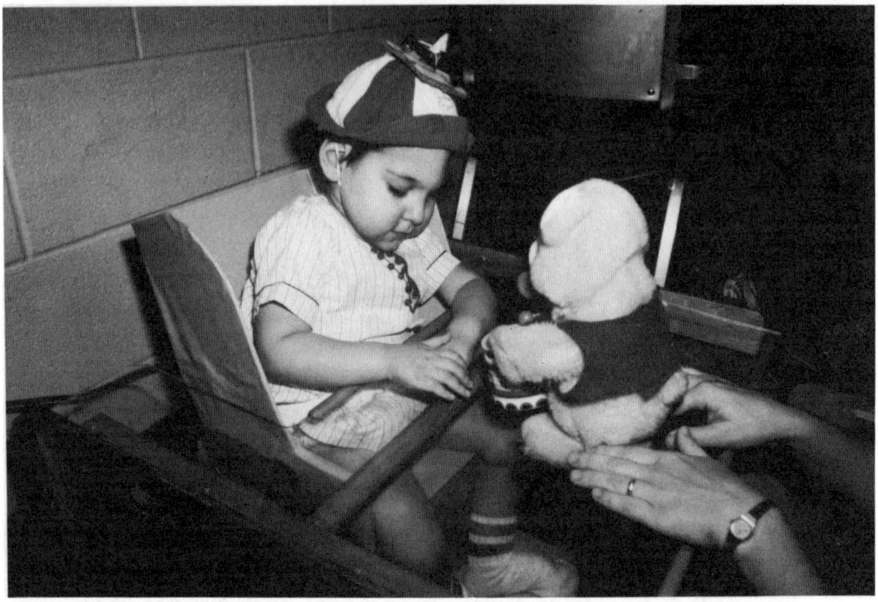

Figure 2. The use of a pressure-sensitive pad, rather than a keyboard, to control the microcomputer permits the teacher to remain close to the children during training sessions.

appropriate; and 5) selection of a variety of potential toys for reinforcement based on student preferences and optimal sensory modalities.

The primary hardware used is an Apple IIe computer with an OMNIBOX (Expert System Software Inc., 1985). The OMNIBOX is an external box attached to an interface board that plugs into one of the Apple's expansion slots. The box contains four subminiature plugs for accepting single switch input, (e.g., treadle switch, pressure switch) four miniature plugs for activating adapted battery operated external devices, (e.g., barking dog, flashing/siren fireman's hat, tape player), and a built-in programmable real-time timer.

The software, "The Switchmaster,"[2] is designed to be sufficiently flexible for research purposes, but simple enough for everyday classroom use. The primary purposes of the software are: 1) To activate the toys according to predetermined parameters; 2) to collect student response data; and 3) to allow for prompt cueing and recording. To use the Switchmaster, the teacher must specify a number of training

[2]The software and hardware applications described were developed in cooperation with Expert Systems Software, Inc., Suite 316, 2120 Crestmoon Rd., Nashville, Tennessee 37215. The research was supported by a Spencer Foundation Grant, "Facilitating the acquisition of sensorimotor behavior with a microcomputer based intervention system: An experimental analysis," 1984–1985, Steven Warren, principal investigator. Field testing was conducted as part of a demonstration grant, "Handicapped children's early education program model," Peabody College of Vanderbilt University (U.S. Department of Education, G008302259: "Optimal learning environments for handicapped infants"); Steven Warren, principal investigator.

parameters, including: 1) The behavioral objective(s) to be trained for each child; 2) the type of data (frequency, duration or accuracy) to be collected; and 3) the variety of possible toys to be used for reinforcers.

Thereafter, each morning before the children arrive the teacher specifies the students, their goal(s), and the student order and grouping in which training will occur throughout the day. This allows the sessions to be run with no further keyboard input. Additionally, the teacher has the option to specify and change daily the length of each individual seassion, the toy being used for reinforcement, and the minimum or maximum duration of reinforcement allowed for each switch closure. Duration of reinforcement is used when training for increases in the number of switch closures by requiring the child to reactivate the switch after a specified amount of time before receiving additional toy reinforcement. The minimum duration is important when a child is first acquiring a skill, since a switch closure may be so brief that the toy may barely start and then stop immediately.

Why Use the System

One of the major advantages of the microcomputer-based program is that it provides a convenient way of monitoring the child's progress by automatically collecting and recording data on the child's performance with very little effort from the teacher. While not viewed as a "stand alone system" (i.e., a totally independent activity for the child), it could be implemented in a small group or holding group. In this situation, the teacher or other adult could be working with several children simultaneously, providing prompting and assistance as needed. All children would be receiving direct and immediate reinforcement for appropriate movements as well as external physical support and stability, without requiring the full involvement of the teacher. These would be ideal situations in which to provide a student additional opportunities to practice a motor skill that is being trained during other activities and situations throughout the day.

The system may also be useful in one-to-one training for certain motor skills. In these situations the teacher frequently does not have enough hands to perform all the necessary tasks (i.e., holding and prompting the child, while monitoring and precisely recording the child's responses). The system could take over a number of these tasks for the teacher.

Finally, the system has the potential of being used by secondary trainers. In many classrooms, parent involvement is a critical component with parents working in the classroom on a regular basis. With minimal training these parents can conduct the sessions, as can practicum students, student teachers, or volunteers.

Two precautions for the appropriate use of this program need to be emphasized. First, devising a switch to measure a specific motor skill may be difficult. In fact, some motor movements may not be measurable by this method. Second, care must be taken to ensure that closure of the switch accurately reflects the child's performance of the target skill. Each switch arrangement needs to be carefully validated by a human observer to ensure that it is measuring the target skill as defined by the teacher.

Guidelines for Implementation

Successful applications of technology may prompt practitioners to embrace the approach indiscriminately. To avoid inappropriate use of microcomputer mediated sensorimotor training, applications must support good teaching practices, data collection, and the use of secondary trainers (Hooper & Hamlett, 1985).

Good Teaching It is crucial for software programs to facilitate what are known to be good teaching practices. For example, the first step in using microcomputer mediated sensorimotor teaching is to develop a clearly defined, measurable goal statement. The skill(s) selected for training should be relevant to the overall educational plan of the child. A skill should not be selected simply because it is easy to implement using the automated device. A good question to ask in determining the relevance and appropriateness of a targeted motor task is: Would the task be targeted if there were no special devices or computer systems available?

The appropriate role of microcomputer mediated training is a supplement to classroom training. The most relevant application is to select target motor skills based on current classroom programming and then to provide concurrent training using the automated device. The computer should be seen as an instructional aid that supports the training provided by the classroom staff, not as a replacement for the teacher.

It is also necessary to determine the level of instruction required for the skill; i.e., is the child currently working on acquisition, fluency building, or maintenance and generalization of the skill? Computers can be seen as a way to provide repeated practice on a skill to develop fluency. It is possible also to train new skills directly, thereby merging instruction and practice. Using the system, the teacher specifies whether prompts will be used during training. If the child does not perform the target behavior within a specified time period, the teacher provides a verbal prompt. If another specified period of time elapses without the demonstration of the target skill, the teacher physically assists the child in attaining the correct position. The computer signals the teacher visually when prompts should occur, and allows for easy recording of prompts administered.

Two other features of the program facilitate the incorporation of good teaching practices. Most special education teachers do not have the luxury of a one-to-one child-teacher ratio. When students-to-staff ratios are higher, children may experience a great deal of down time (McCormick, Cooper, & Goldman, 1979). Use of small groups, and the prior set-up of the material and content for instruction, may reduce some of this down time. The teacher should be able to do the majority of the set up, preparation, and organization of instruction at the beginning of the school day before the students arrive. This reduces the amount of time children wait on the teacher and increases the opportunity for teacher/child and child/material contact time. In many classrooms activities occur in a small group format using a cluster approach in which each student works on individual levels of similar but not necessarily identical tasks (Brown, Holvoet, Guess, & Mulligan, 1980). Microcomputer mediated motor skills training encourages this arrangement by allowing up to four students using four switch and toy configurations to be monitored at one time. The computer can collect continuous data on each child's movements based on their target skill, allowing the teacher to move to each child in turn, providing prompting and cuing as needed.

Data Collection An obvious advantage of a microcomputer mediated system is that data can easily be collected and graphed on each motor skill being trained. A microcomputer system can directly collect frequency and duration data, and automatically store it in files. At the same time it is important that this process not interfere with teaching. Data should be collected in a way that requires minimal teacher input and is appropriate to the goal(s) selected for training. The teacher must analyze the skill selected for training, determine the performance requirements, and determine what type of measurable data will reflect the teaching provided. Our program allows the teacher to select from a number of standard data types, (i.e., rate, frequency, percentage correct). Once the data type is selected, the computer will automatically record and graph the student performance data. Additionally, the teacher can directly record the number and levels of prompts during the training sessions. At the end of the session or school day, the teacher can print out data summaries and graphs of the training session.

Secondary Trainers A final aspect of this system is the use of secondary trainers. Classrooms frequently employ the services of a variety of individuals with a wide range of training knowledge and teaching competencies. Therefore, for a microcomputer mediated motor training program to be useful in the classroom, it should be operable by minimally trained individuals. Three aspects of the system facilitate this application: prior set-up, automatic data, and cuing of prompts.

As previously mentioned, the system allows for prior set-up. All sessions parameters for individual students and their various training goals (i.e., length of session, type of reinforcer, ratio of reinforcer to response, type of data collected) should be set up by the teacher prior to training. The trainer can then run sessions with each child and skill in the sequence determined by the teacher. Additionally, the system is easily used by nonprofessionals because the software automatically records appropriate data for the training sessions and reminds the trainer when to provide prompt cues for the child. At the end of the day the teacher can retrieve and print performance summaries for each child's specified skills.

Summary

The microcomputer mediated motor training application described is still undergoing development, systematic research, and field testing. The use of such a system may provide persons who have severe multiple disabilities with additional opportunities to practice important motor skills. As with all technology, applications should be appropriately integrated into educational programming in a manner that is consistent with functionally based curricular planning. The use of the guidelines provided above should allow practitioners to meet this objective.

ELECTRONIC TRAVEL AIDS APPLICATION

Orientation and mobility (O&M) are two separate but interrelated processes. *Orientation* is the process of using the senses to establish one's position and relationship to significant objects in the environment. *Mobility* is the capacity, readiness, and ability to move about in the environment (Hill & Ponder, 1976). Therefore, orientation provides meaning to movement. The ultimate goals of the O&M processes are to be able to move purposefully in any environment, familiar or unfamilar, and to move safely, efficiently, gracefully, and independently.

Over the years, persons with visual impairments have used many methods to satisfy their basic need and desire to move about. "From the earliest times, animals, sighted people and devices (such as sticks, or canes) have been used to achieve varying levels of mobilty" (Farmer, 1980, p. 357). The first formal system of orientation and mobility training in this country started in 1929 when the Seeing Eye, Inc. was founded (Whitsock, 1980). Shortly after World War II, a systematic method of traveling with a long white cane was developed at Valley Forge Army Hospital by Richard Hoover for veterans with acquired blindness (Bledsoe, 1980). According to Farmer (1980), the cane and the guide dog are the two most widely used, accepted, and proven systems of independent travel for persons with visual impairments. Another system, although unproven and not yet widely used, is the electronic travel aid (ETA).

Historical Perspective and Descriptions of ETAs

Electronic travelaids are devices that emit signals to sense the environment within a certain range or distance, convert the information received to an auditory and/or tactual display, and provide the user with relevant information about the immediate environment (Farmer, 1980). Electronic travel aids, sometimes referred to as electronic mobility devices or sensory aids, were experimented with as early as 1950 when the Veteran's Administration contracted to field test various models of a Signal Corps sensory aid. This early research and development effort by the Veteran's Administration has led to the development of several prototypical aids over the past several years.

During the 1970's, ETAs received a great deal of attention as supplemental O&M systems for adult travelers with visual impairments. For example, some cane travelers used ETAs to circumnavigate obstacles in the travel path in order to avoid physical contact with objects (Hill & Bradfield, 1983). Jacobson (1979) found an ETA to be useful with guide dog users to enhance their understanding of the environment, as a way for them to monitor the dog's performance. In recent years, however, attention has focused on using ETAs to teach spatial and environmental concepts to children with congenital blindness.

The four ETAs most used widely today are the: (a) Lindsay Russel Model E Pathsounder, (b) Mowat Sensor, (c) Sonicguide™, and (d) Laser Cane. All of these ETAs except the Laser Cane were originally designed for use by adults with blindness as supplemental O&M systems in conjunction with the cane or guide dog. Because of its size and weight, the current model of the Laser Cane does not appear to have much value for young children who are blind. Goldie (1977) trained four teenage students with blindness in the use of the Laser Cane and concluded that one must have excellent long cane techniques and understand the spatial layout structures of the environment in order to benefit from the device. A brief description of the Pathsounder, Mowat Sensor, and Sonicguide™ follows.

Pathsounder The Pathsounder is a box-like ultrasonic obstacle detector that was developed by Lindsay Russell at the Massachusetts Institute of Technology. The Pathsounder transmits and receives sonar waves to provide the user with information about obstacles in the travel path. The device weighs about 16 ounces, is chest mounted, supported by a neck strap, and is equipped with rechargeable batteries.

The Pathsounder has automatic auditory near-far range settings as well as manual tactile controls. To indicate the presence of obstacles on the far range (6 to 8 feet), the device buzzes (auditory mode) or provides chest vibrations (tactual mode). To indicate the presence of obstacles at near range (0 to 3 feet), the Pathsounder emits a beeping tone (auditory mode) or provides neck vibrations (tactual mode). The maximum area of coverage for the chest-mounted device is slightly below the waist to above the head and just outside the width of the shoulders.

Mowat Sensor The Mowat Sensor is a hand-held, ultrasonic obstacle detector developed by G. C. Mowat in New Zealand. The Mowat Sensor measures 6 inches × 2 inches × 1 inch, weighs about 6 ounces, and has a rechargeable battery. The Mowat Sensor has a manually operated (usually by the thumb) range setting (1 meter, near range; 4 meters, far range). Like the Pathsounder, the Mowat Sensor uses sonar waves to provide obstacle detection information. It can be used to locate signs, poles, pedestrians, and other objects on or off the travel path. The ultrasonic beam width of the device is approximately 15° wide and 30° high. When an object is in range, the entire device vibrates. Distance information is provided to the user when the device vibrates faster as the user approaches an object. An ear coupling that provides auditory information is also available for use by individuals who have difficulty with the tactual mode.

Sonicguide™ The Binaural Sensory Aid, later known as the Sonicguide™, was developed by Leslie Kay in New Zealand. Kay has also developed other versions of the present-day Sonicguide™, namely the Canterbury Babies and Child's Aid and the Trisensor (Ferrell, 1984). The Sonicguide™, like the Pathsounder and Mowat Sensor, uses ultrasonic waves that are transmitted and received, and then converted to auditory signals. The electronics are housed in spectacle frames with an accompanying power pack and rechargeable batteries.

The Sonicguide™ has a range of approximately 15–20 feet which is dependent upon the nature of the reflective target. It has a wide cone-line beam that provides protective coverage from above the head to just above the knees and approximately 45 degrees to either side of the body.

The Sonicguide™ differs from the Mowat Sensor and Pathsounder in that it may be used both as an obstacle detector and environmental sensor. According to Farmer

(1980), the signals of the Sonicguide™ enable the user to: a) estimate the distance from objects by relating the signals to changes in pitch; b) determine the direction/location of objects through perceiving amplitude differences in each ear; and c) identify object surfaces through the tonal differences of the signals received.

Small ear tubes are attached to the bottom of the eyeglass frame that allow the user to hear the ultrasonic signals. There is also a monitoring unit available for training purposes.

Research and General Use of ETAs

Pathsounder and Mowat Sensor There have been no empirical studies involving either the Pathsounder or Mowat Sensor with children with visual impairments. Although these devices were originally designed as supplemental aids for either cane or guide dog travelers, they appear to be potentially useful for teaching certain concepts and O&M skills to children with visual impairments. In fact, Baird (1977) described the Pathsounder as a concept development and mobility skill building tool for young children with visual impairments. She taught some elementary-age children with visual impairments to use the Pathsounder to locate independently playground equipment. Baird (1977) also used the Pathsounder to teach spatial concepts to children with visual impairments.

Because the Pathsounder and Mowat Sensor are simple to operate and have auditory and tactual options, they appear to be potentially useful as primary mobility aids for individuals with multiple handicapping conditions. Farmer (1980) reported the use of the Pathsounder with persons with blindness who use wheelchairs. Hill and Bradfield (1983) suggested that the Mowat Sensor has the same applications for use as the Pathsounder, but may be particularly useful with persons who are deaf and blind.

In another application, Farmer (1975) reported the use of the Mowat Sensor in adverse weather. Travelers who are blind were able to use the Mowat Sensor to locate landmarks that otherwise might have been masked with snow or located away from the travel path. Finally, Langbein, Blasch, and Chambers (1981) described the use of the Mowat Sensor during orienteering by travelers with blindness. Orienteering is an organized sport in which participants use a compass and follow maps through an outdoor course across different terrains. Travelers who are blind were able to use the Mowat Sensor on the course to locate landmarks noted on written braille instructions.

Sonicguide™ Since the development of the first binaural sensory aid, there have been several versions: Sonicguide™, Canterbury Aids, and Trisensor. These aids are very similar in appearance and function; therefore, in discussing this group of sensory aids, the term Sonicguide™ is used.

Historically, the Sonicguide™, like the Pathsounder and Mowat Sensor, has been primarily used by adult cane travelers. This narrow notion of use has caused some controversy (Jacobson, 1979, Kay, 1980), as well as interest in expanding its use for other populations.

In the later 1970s, there was a great deal of interest and activity directed toward expanding the use of the Sonicguide™ with children. The Sonicguide™ was used for concept development activities with children (Baird, 1977; Kay, Strelow, & Kay, 1977; Newcomer, 1977; Scione, 1978), as well as with infants and toddlers who are blind, to examine the effect of its use on development (Bower, 1977b; Ferrell, 1980; Strelow, Kay, & Kay, 1978). In its original form, however, the Sonicguide™ was not suitable for use with very young children with blindness. Its physical structure was too heavy and bulky, and the range was too long for practical use with infants; therefore, infant versions of the Sonicguide™ (Smith & Dailey, 1978; Strelow et al., 1978) were developed to make the device accessible to the young children with blindness.

Researchers have examined the use of the Infant Sonicguide™ as it affects such behaviors as reaching to sound, object/person location, locomotion, stereotypical mannerisms, and the development of residual vision. The first published report of research on the use of the Sonicguide™ with infants who are blind was by Bower (1977a, 1977b). Bower (1977b) stated:

> If the blind child is born with a perceptual system ready to seize on abstract information of a certain form, no matter what its method of presentation, the baby should be able to use a wholly artificial source of information, provided it had the same formal properties as natural functions. (p. 259)

Bower hypothesized that infants are sensitive to spatial information in general, regardless of sensory modality. Bower's reported observations of one 7-month-old subject using the aid supported his hypothesis. The child reportedly interposed his hand between his face and an approaching object; made converging movements with his eyes when objects were sensed through the aid; tracked objects as they were moved left to right; and "played peek-a-boo" by turning his head to and from his mother. Additionally, Bower reported on a second child who apparently explored with the aid in the first 20 minutes of wearing it. On the second day of using the device, the child reportedly reached for toys presented in a variety of locations. Details of what occurred between sessions and in subsequent sessions were not reported.

Strelow et al. (1978) reported a study on the use of the Infant Sonicguide™ with a 2½-year-old boy with developmental delays and little language, mobility or self-help skills, and a 6½-year-old girl. The boy was able to reach for objects signaled by the aid only after a conditioning procedure was used. There were also some small improvements in his listening and mobility skills as a result of using the aid. On the other hand, the girl was able to use the aid to move about her school environment and to identify simple object surfaces. Although the aid appeared to be successful primarily with the older child, the authors concluded that simple responses to sounds can be taught to a child with severe developmental delays, and that modest improvements in perception and mobility skills are possible with regular use of the aid.

Ferrell (1980) reported the use of the device with four children who were 6.0, 14.0, 14.5, and 20.5 months old. The major objective of Ferrell's study was to determine if the Infant Sonicguide™ was a useful intervention in attaining developmental milestones and reducing stereotypic behavior. Ferrell found that by 2–11 months after the start of the study, all four of the children were able to use the information from the device to reach accurately for objects. Three of the children were able to use the device to avoid objects during mobility tasks. Ferrell found also that stereotypic behavior was reduced when the children were wearing the aid. Stereotypic behavior increased when the subjects were not wearing the device. Although the Infant Sonicguide™ seemed to facilitate the acquisition of certain skills, the children exhibited overall the same proportionate developmental lag as they exhibited at the start of the study.

Aiken's and Bower's study (1982a, 1982b) involved a program of both short-term and long-term use of the Infant Sonicguide™ with subjects with congenital blindness who ranged in age from 4 to 20 months. The short-term children received 1½–7 hours of Sonicguide™ exposure over 2–3 days. No empirical data were offered but it was reported that reaching and tracking objects occurred with some frequency. For the long-term portion of the study, four of the children were followed-up for several months. During the study, the children wore the aid during meal- and play-time. The generalization resulting from long-term use of the infant aid was mixed. One child showed the use of the aid while moving around, two children showed modest use, while one child apparently did not use the Sonicguide™. One child, however, showed gains in development after using the aid. The authors stated that long-term studies do not permit easy generalization.

Strelow (1983) reported the use of the Sonicguide™ with four children ages 10, 21, 26 and 30 months. The youngest child learned to respond to the presence of objects at 10 months. The 21-month-old child learned to respond to objects in one training session. The two older children showed little use with the aid because of short attention spans and other competing behaviors.

Ferrell (1984) investigated the effects of the Infant Sonicguide™ on assisting infants to attend to visual information. She studied 18 subjects between the ages of 6 and 24 months, 10 of whom were classified as multiply handicapped. All subjects had light perception and were certified as being legally blind. The subjects' visual behavior was observed as they were exposed to four types of stimulus presentations—stationary visual, stationary visual-auditory, moving visual, and moving visual-auditory—under both Sonicguide™ and no Sonicguide™ conditions. The subjects with multiple handicaps seemed to maintain better visual attention when a combination of visual-auditory information was presented, irrespective of whether the information came from the Sonicguide™. Ferrell reported that the results with the children who were visually impaired only were not clear. Apparently the infants with visual impairments at times were searching with their eyes, and were deliberately avoiding the visual stimulus when the Sonicguide™ was on. Ferrell suggested that the sound of the Infant Sonicguide™, emitted as it is from the child's own head, may be a source of confusion.

Ferrell conducted a second experiment involving a cross-modal transfer task with the same children to obtain further information on their visual functioning. The method involved familiarizing the infants to a stimulus through the sense of touch.

Then the child's recognition memory was tested by pairing the touch stimulus with a novel visual stimulus under Sonicguide™ and no Sonicguide™ conditions. Typically, infants show a preference for the novel stimulus. Ferrell hypothesized that any change in cross-modal behavior over time might help to isolate Sonicguide™ effects from the normal developmental processes. She reported that all subjects improved their visual acuity scores over a 2–month period, but the Sonicguide™ did not help them in the process.

Finally, Harris, Humphrey, Muir and Dodwell (1985) reported on the most intensive case study to date. They studied a girl with visual impairments from age 6 months to 4 years. They examined the child's ability to use the aid in several areas, including reaching for objects, anticipating objects and surfaces while moving, and moving about and exploring novel environments. They reported that the chlid was able to use the aid quite proficiently in the above situations. The child, however, did not spontaneously use the aid to acquire a new skill. They found it necessary to have an ongoing auditory-motor intervention program along with the sensory aid training.

Potential Applications

In general, electronic travel aids appear to have potential for facilitating the development of several orientation and mobility concepts and skills in children who are visually impaired.

All three of the devices can be used as obstacle detectors. They have been used as supplementary systems in conjunction with primary mobility systems when the cane or guide dog were not feasible (e.g., with blind persons using wheelchairs, crutches, or walkers). Other applications of the devices, particularly the Sonicguide™, have been in training distance vision (Carter, 1975); engaging in recreation activities such as hiking, bowling, skating, and so forth (Carter & Hand, 1980); and improving posture and reducing stereotypic behavior (Ferrell, 1980). ETAs may have several useful applications with children who are visually impaired, including: a) stimulating exploratory behavior; b) teaching specific spatial and environmental concepts; c) facilitating alignment and maintaining a straight line of travel; d) judging distances; and e) establishing and utilizing landmarks.

Exploratory Behavior Children with visual impairments generally are not naturally curious about the environment (Garry & Ascarelli, 1960). Vision tends to motivate children to explore and interact with their environment. Consequently, many children with visual impairments have developmental delays in conceptual and motor development (Fraiberg, 1977).

Because ETAs stimulate the auditory and/or tactile senses, they may be intrinsically motivating for children with visual impairments. All three of the devices have ranges that extend beyond one's own reach. Having greater contact with the external world (other than what is within one's immediate reach) should potentially enhance exploratory behavior for several reasons. First, the notion of object permanence should be facilitated. Second, stress and fear of moving in the environment should be reduced because objects can be monitored and negotiated. Finally, sensory feedback is provided, which helps to organize the environment.

Spatial And Environmental Concepts Hill and Blasch (1980) describe and discuss several spatial concepts that are important for children with visual impairments to learn. Some of the important areas they mention are position (front, back, up, down, left, right, center, between, etc.), shape (round, circle, square, rectangle, etc.), and measurement (distances, size, and weight). Hill and Bradfield (1983) suggest that ETAs can be used to teach concepts of distance (such as near, far), specific units of measurement (inches, feet, yards), width, and height. Baird (1977) and Scione (1978) suggest that specific positional concepts such as left, right, up, down, center, between, parallel, and perpendicular can also be taught using the devices. Scione (1978) describes a training program using ETAs to facilitate the understanding of such environmental concepts as "intersection" and "corner."

Alignment Establishing and maintaining a straight line of travel are difficult tasks for individuals with visual impairments. Vision permits movement around obstacles and efficient re-establishment of the intended line of travel, as well as correction of errors in travel. Typically, persons with visual impairments use sound and tactile information for alignment and realignment purposes. Individuals with visual impairments use various methods of tactually traveling parallel surfaces with their hands, or through the use of the cane (Hill & Ponder, 1976). Travelers who are blind also use auditory information, particularly traffic cues, to establish and check their line of travel. Unfortunately, auditory cues and tactile surfaces used to "trail" are not always available. Electronic travel aids are useful in alignment tasks because constant auditory feedback can be maintained with objects. Additionally, ETAs can provide the user with more options for object use in alignment than guide dogs or the long cane. For example, hedges, fences, rows of poles or trees that are positioned away from the travel path can be easily used for alignment with an ETA. Scione (1978) also suggested the use of ETAs as a way of monitoring turns and the effects of moving in space.

Judging Distances All of the ETAs provide distance information feedback to the user. The Sonicguide™ accomplishes this through pitch changes (the closer one is to an object, the lower the pitch). The Mowat Sensory and the Pathsounder accomplish this through a ramp effect (the devices vibrate more strongly and/or produce a higher sound). Baird (1977), Newcomer (1977) and Scione (1978) have provided distance estimation training through the use of ETAs. Children with visual impairments have been trained with ETAs to judge distances in order to circumnavigate obstacles, establish object-to-object relationships, maintain a straight line of travel, and make decisions about when to turn or detour from a given route.

Landmarks Generally, children with visual impairments are limited in the range and variety of landmarks they can use. Because of the range capabilities of the ETAs, it is possible for children to establish and use landmarks overhead and away from the travel path. For example, a traveler who is visually impaired could make some contact with an overhead tree branch to locate a sidewalk leading to an objective. Without an

ETA, the traveler with visual impairment would have to use less reliable clues (i.e., sound of leaves rustling in the wind), or establish more concrete tactile landmarks.

Guidelines For Implementation

If ETAs are to be used as primary or complimentary systems of mobility for persons with visual impairment, instruction in their use should be done by certified orientation and mobility specialists. However, classroom teachers (with some ETA training) can develop and implement instructional programs using ETAs in such areas as motor development and the development of environmental concepts. The following steps should be considered by teachers when contemplating the use of ETAs as an intervention:

1. Secure training from a certified orientation and mobility specialist. The Association for the Education and Rehabilitation for the Blind and Visually Impaired (AER) is the certifying professional organization, and can provide a list of certified professionals (206 North Washington St., Suite 320, Alexandria, Virginia, 22314).
2. Try out device(s) in the training environment(s). If the ETA is to be used in an area of the school, it will be important to know exactly what information it will provide prior to using it with a particular child. For example, different objects will reflect varying amounts of ultrasound depending upon the nature of their surface and the angle of approach by the user. By checking out the physical environment in advance (with the aid), the teacher can anticipate potential problems that the children may have during the training phase.
3. Identify and select target children and behaviors; variables such as age, additional handicaps, prerequisite skills, and complexity and importance of behaviors should be considered. In using ETAs with children who have additional handicaps, the major concern is their ability to receive and interpret (at some level) ETA information. For example, children who have a severe hearing loss probably would not be good candidates for Sonicguide™ instruction. They may profit, however, from Pathsounder or Mowat Sensor instruction because of their tactile displays. On the other hand, children who are tactually defensive probably would not be good candidates for the Pathsounder or Mowat sensor. Of the three devices, the Sonicguide™ is the most complex to use and offers the most information.
4. Conduct a comparative analysis of ETA intervention to other interventions. Because ETAs are expensive and require the teacher to undergo some specialized training, there may be other intervention options that are more suitable. At any rate, the teacher should analyze the cost-benefits of ETA intervention relative to alternative interventions.
5. Identify specific target behavior(s). A number of specific motor and O&M behaviors applicable for Sonicguide™ intervention are listed and described in Carter, Carter, and Ferrell (1980). Examples range from such simple skills as "quiets

or smiles when the Sonicguide™ is turned on" or "reaches to a stationary object presented at midline" to more complex behaviors such as "walks down hallway without contacting walls" or identifies windows, poles, and bushes by their sonic signals."

6. Match child behavior and specific ETA to one another. For example, children who continually do not hold their heads up may not be candidates for Sonicguide™ instruction. In using Sonicguide™ it is imperative to keep one's head up in order to get clear signals and detect obstacles. The Sonicguide™ will emit "fuzzy," unclear signals if the head is continually kept down when using the device.
7. Familiarize child and significant others with the particular device. It is important that the child (if capable) understand basically how the device works, how to put it on and take it off, and how to care for it. Parents and significant others should have some working knowledge of the device in order to facilitate any planned home intervention.
8. Implement ETA intervention while concurrently monitoring the proper functioning of the device. It is important that the teacher carefully monitor the child's actual use of the ETA. This will not only assure that the device is functioning properly but also that the child is appropriately responding to the information received through the device.
9. Assess the impact of intervention. In evaluating the impact of ETA intervention, several factors should be considered. Obviously, time and cost are important. Other factors, however, such as mechanical breakdowns, social acceptance of the devices (by users, peers and significant others), and generalization of target behaviors when not using the devices should also be considered. Carter et al. (1980) have suggested several intervention activities with various ETAs. Selected samples of their Sonicguide™ intervention strategies that were designed for movement in near space, movement in a 6 foot area, and travel in an indoor area appear in Table 1.

Summary

Except for the infant version of the Sonicguide™, ETAs have changed very little since 1975, but their applications have. There will continue to be a need for some cane or guide dog users to utilize present-day ETAs as supplemental or complimentary aids. There also will be a continued need to use ETAs as primary mobility aids for certain children with visual and multiple handicaps. For example, Kitzhoffer (1983) used the Sonicguide™ with a child who was orthopaedically involved, blind, and in a wheelchair. ETAs may, however, have limited use with some children who are visually and multiply handicapped. While the Sonicguide™ provides a great deal of auditory information, it would probably not be useful with individuals with severe hearing losses. Additionally, Sonicguide™ information may be too complex or confusing for use by some persons with mental retardation and visual impairments. On the other hand, the Mowat Sensor and the Pathsounder (because of the simplicity of operation and infor-

Table 1. Intervention activities

Objectives	Suggested activities	Materials	Evaluation
	Movement in near space		
While seated at a desk and wearing the Sonicguide, the student will reach out and grasp an object placed on a desk within arms' reach of the student.	The teacher will alternate between placing and removing a small pole from the desk. The student is asked to verbally indicate when the pole is on the desk. The teacher places the pole on the desk and physically manipulates the student's head until he or she is looking directly at the pole thus centering the Sonicguide signal. Gradually, the physical manipulation is stopped and the student is asked to "look at the pole" by him- or herself. The teacher places the pole on the desk and the student is asked to "look at" it. Then the student and teacher co-actively bring the student's hand to his or her chin and then out to the pole. At first the pole is kept at midline and at a constant distance until the student can independently and consistently grasp the pole with both left and right hands. The distance is	Desk Small pole	The student will reach directly for and grasp a pole placed on a desk with 90% accuracy.

(continued)

Table 1. *(continued)*

Objectives	Suggested activities	Materials	Evaluation
	then changed and student and teacher work at this distance. Finally, the distances are alternated. The same procedure should be used for teaching horizontal displacement of the pole.		
While using the Sonicguide, the student will discriminate between two different objects placed on a desk, by grasping the object on the left or right as directed by the teacher.	The teacher will give the student experiences grasping different objects that yield different character signals from the Sonicguide. The teacher will set up two objects on a desk, and co-actively with the student reach for either the left or right object.	Desk Small toys Small poles	The student will reach directly for the correct object with 90% accuracy.
	Movement in a 6-foot area		
While using the Sonicguide, the student will walk to and locate the pole placed within a 6 foot area of the student.	After the student faces the pole have him describe the location of the pole. Then have the student stand and turn toward the pole before walking to it. In the beginning the student may be given physical or verbal assistance.	Student chair Large pole	The student will walk to the pole 90% of the time.

Travel in an indoor area with the Sonicguide			
While using the Sonicguide, the student will reach out and touch a wall he or she is walking to when he or she comes within hand-touching distances of the wall.	The teacher guides the student to the wall from a set distance and stops at hand-touching distance. The student is then asked to reach out and touch the wall. Gradually vary the starting distance from the wall. While the student is seated on a chair, the teacher rolls a 4 foot gym ball at the student. The student is asked to put his arms up and stop the ball when it gets to within hand-touching distance. Bring the student to a setting where corridor doors cut across a straight corridor. Ask the student to walk down the corridor without making contact with the wall.	A 4-foot gym ball	The student will stop at the correct distance 90% of the time.

From Carter, C., Carter, K., & Ferrell, K.A. (1980, May). *The implementation of Sonicguide™ with visually impaired infants and children* (pp. 77–82). Bensenville, IL: Wormald International Sensory Aids Corporation. Reprinted by permission.

mation afforded) may be very appropriate for children with mental retardation and visual impairments.

It is clear from the literature that a new trend is emerging, involving the use of ETAs to teach spatial and environmental concepts to children with visual impairments. In fact, a training manual describing several concept development activities with ETAs has been published (Carter et al., 1980). Empirical studies that would validate the effective use of ETAs for teaching spatial and environmental concepts are sorely needed.

This chapter has reviewed research studies of the Infant Sonicguide™ or infant Sonicguide™-line devices. There have been no reports of using the Pathsounder or Mowat Sensor with infants who are blind. Although there may be some potential benefits for using the aid with such infants, the results of most of these studies are inconclusive. Ferrell (1984), in referring to the research base, stated that "little attempt has been made to sort out individual differences in development, training, or sensory aid utilization, and conclusions appear to be based on personal or philosophical conviction more than on fact" (p. 56).

Using sensory aids with infants who are blind raises the question of what are the effects of sensory aids on the normal developmental process? It is clear that present infant sensory aids will not successfully serve as a substitute for vision. Although there have been some reports of generalization responses with these aids, the overwhelming evidence at this point is that infants need to be trained to respond (Ferrell, 1984; Harris et al., 1985). It appears rather that these devices, if carefully used, will serve as effective supplements to the sensory information that children who are blind gain through their senses by natural means (Warren, 1984). Warren has suggested that perhaps some unsuccessful attempts to use sensory aids with infants have been due to the limited exposure of the infant to the aids. Warren, however, cautions prospective researchers:

> Consider the impact on the child's overall development of devoting a large proportion of the child's energy to using the aid. . . . A particular concern, especially with younger infants, is the possible negative impact in such areas as the development of selective auditory attention and intermodality coordination. (p. 121)

FUTURE NEEDS AND DIRECTIONS

This chapter describes two specific technological applications that may be appropriate for training students with sensory handicaps. The purpose of these descriptions is not to promote their application per se. Rather, the intent is to both provide a rationale for applying and evaluating technological innovations in educational programs, and to stimulate further development, testing and applied research. From a training perspective, technology applications should be viewed as simply another teaching tool. These applications should promote learning of new skills and behaviors along a continuum of functional, appropriate skills. Empirical research is needed to produce evidence that technology applications with individuals with severe sensory impairments:

1. Are used in training relevant curricular content
2. Use effective training strategies
3. Result in the demonstration of new functional behaviors by the individual

To date, very few technological educational innovations have been subjected to any type of empirical analysis of effectiveness along these dimensions. This information is needed before the ultimate value of any technology for individuals with severe multiple impairments can be determined. Current and future developments must be guided by the need for relevant and appropriate training based on the general philosophy of preparing individuals for maximum independence in the larger community.

REFERENCES

Aeschleman, S., & Tawney, J. (1978, October). Interacting: A computer-based telecommunications system for educating severely handicapped preschoolers in their home. *Educational Technology, 18,* 30–35.

Aiken, S., & Bower, T.G.R. (1982a). Intersensory substitution in the blind. *Journal of Experimental Psychology, 33,* 309–323.

Aiken, S., & Bower, T.G.R. (1982b). The use of Sonicguide in infancy. *Journal of Visual Impairment and Blindness, 76*(3), 91–100.

Baird, A.S. (1977). Electronic aids: Can they help blind children? *Journal of Visual Impairment and Blindness, 71*(3), 97–101.

Behrmann, M., & Lahm, L. (1982). Critical learning: Multiply handicapped babies get online. In M. Behrmann and L. Lahm (Eds.), *Proceedings of the National Conference on the Use of Microcomputers in Special Education* (pp. 37–45). Reston, VA: Council for Exceptional Children.

Bledsoe, C.W. (1980). Originators of orientation and mobility training. In R.L. Welsh & B. Blasch (Eds.), *Foundations of orientation and mobility* (pp. 581–624). New York: American Foundation for the Blind.

Bobath, K., & Bobath, B. (1972). Cerebral palsy. In P. Pearson & C. Williams (Eds.) *Physical therapy services in the developmental disabilities* (pp. 31–185). Springfield, IL: Charles C Thomas.

Bower, T.G.R. (1977a). Blind babies are more important than machines. *New Scientist, 73,* 712–714.

Bower, T.G.R. (1977b). Blind babies see with their ears. *New Scientist, 73,* 255–257.

Bricker, W.A. (1976). Service of research. In M.A. Thomas (Ed.), *Hey, don't forget about me!* (pp. 162–179). Reston, VA: Council for Exceptional Children.

Brinker, R., & Lewis, M. (1982). Making the world work with microcomputers: A learning prosthesis for handicapped infants. *Exceptional Children, 49*(2), 163–170.

Brown, F., Holvoet, J., Guess, D., & Mulligan, M. (1980). The individualized curriculum sequencing model (III): Small group instruction. *Journal of the Association for the Severely Handicapped, 5*(4), 352–367.

Budoff, M., & Hutten, L.R. (1982). Microcomputers in special education: Premiums and pitfalls. *Exceptional Children, 49,* 123–130.

Carter, K. (1975). The Sonicguide and distance vision training. *Optometric Weekly,* 21–26.

Carter, C., Carter, K., & Ferrell, K.A. (1980). *The implementation of Sonicguide™ with visually impaired infants and children.* Bensenville, IL: Wormald International Sensory Aids Corporation.

Carter, C., & Hand, H. (1980). Potential use of electronic mobility aids in recreational activities. In C. Carter, K. Carter, & K.A. Ferrell (Eds.), *The implementation of Sonicguide™ with visually impaired infants and children* (pp. 83–86). Bensenville, IL: Wormald International Sensory Aids Corporation.

Farmer, L.W. (1975). Travel in adverse weather using electronic mobility guidance devices. *New Outlook for the Blind, 69,* 433–439.

Farmer, L.W. (1980). Mobility devices. In R. Welsh & B. Blasch (Eds.), *Foundations of orientation and mobility* (pp. 357–412). New York: American Foundation for the Blind.

Ferrell, K.A.(1980). Can infants use the Sonicguide™? Two years experience of Project VIEW! *Journal of Visual Impairment and Blindness, 74,* 209–220.

Ferrell, K.A. (1984). A second look at sensory aids in early childhood. *Education of the Visually Handicapped, 16*(3), 83–101.

Fraiberg, A. (1977). *Insights from the blind.* New York: Basic Books.

Garry, R., & Ascarelli, A. (1960). Teaching topographical orientation and spatial orientation to congenitally blind children. *Journal of Education, 143*(2), 23–30.

Goldenberg, E.P. (1979). *Special technology for Special Children.* Baltimore: University Park Press.

Goldie, D. (1977). Use of the C–5 laser cane by school age children. *Journal of Visual Impairment and Blindness, 71*(8), 345–348.

Harris, L., Humphrey, G.K., Muir, D.M., & Dodwell, P.C. (1985). Use of the Canterbury child's aid in infancy and early childhood: A case study. *Journal of Visual Impairment and Blindness, 79*(1), 4–11.

Herman, R. (1974). *Augmented sensory feedback for children with cerebral palsy.* Kryser Center for Research and Engineering, Philadelphia.

Hill, E.W., & Blasch, B. (1980). Concept development. In R.L. Welsh & B. Blasch (Eds.). *Foundations of orientation and mobility* (pp. 265–290). New York: American Foundation for the Blind.

Hill, E.W., & Bradfield, A.L. (1983). Electronic mobility aids for blind children and adults. *Exceptional Children Quarterly, 4*(4), 74–89.

Hill, E.W., & Ponder, P.E. (1976). *Orientation and mobility: A guide for the practitioner.* New York: The American Foundation for the Blind.

Hooper, E., & Hamlett, C. (1985, June). *Microcomputer applications for young children with severe handicaps.* Paper presented at the Council for Exceptional Children, Software Conference, Alexandria, VA.

Jacobson, W. (1979). Complementary travel aids for blind persons: The Sonicguide™ with a dog guide. *Journal of Visual Impairment and Blindness, 73,* 10–12.

Kay, L. (1980). The Sonicguide, long cane, and dog guide: Their compatibility. *Journal of Visual Impairment and Blindness, 74*(7), 277–279.

Kay, L., Strelow, E.R., & Kay, N. (1977). Electronic spatial sensors as training aids for blind children. *Journal of Visual Impairment and Blindness, 71,* 174–175.

Kitzhoffer, G.J. (1983). An adaptive approach to teaching the use of the Sonicguide™ with modifications for orthopedic involvement. *Journal of Visual Impairment and Blindness, 77*(3), 100–102.

Langbein, W.E., Blasch, B.B., & Chalmers, B.L. (1981). An orienteering program for blind and visually impaired persons. *Journal of Visual Impairment and Blindness, 75*(7), 273–80.

McCormick, L., Cooper, M., & Goldman, R. (1979). Training teachers to maximize instructional time provided to the severely and profoundly handicapped. *AAESPH, 4,* 301–310.

Newcomer, J. (1977). Sonicguide™ (1977). Electronic spatial sensors as training aids for blind children. *Journal of Visual Impairment and Blindness, 71,* 174–175.

Rugel, R.P., Mattingly, J., Eichenger, M., & May, J. (1971). The use of operant conditioning with a physically disabled child. *American Journal of Occupational Therapy, 25,* 247–279.

Scione, M.W. (1978). Electronic sensory aids in a concept development program for congenitally blind young adults. *Journal of Visual Impairment and Blindness, 72,* 88–93.

Smith, R.P., & Dailey, R.H. (1978). The Sonicguide™: A valuable aid for blind children and infants. *Journal of Visual Impairment and Blindness, 72,* 317–319.

Stallard, C.K. (1982). Computers and education for exceptional children: Emerging applications. *Exceptional Children, 49,* 102–105.

Strelow, E.R (1983). Use of binaural sensory aid by young children. *Journal of Visual Impairment and Blindness, 77,* 429–438.

Strelow, E.R., Kay, N., & Kay, L. (1978). Binaural sensory aid: Case studies of its use by two children. *Journal of Visual Impairment and Blindness, 72,* 1–8.

Vanderheiden, G. (1976). Providing the child with a means to indicate. In G. Vanderheiden and K. Grilley (Eds.), *Non-vocal communication techniques and aids for the severely handicapped.* (pp. 20–76). Baltimore: University Park Press.

Warren, D.H. (1984). *Blindness and early childhood development* (2nd ed.). New York: American Foundation for the Blind.

Watson, J.S. (1966). The development and generalization of "contingency awareness" in early infancy: Some hypotheses. *Merrill-Palmer Quarterly, 12,* 123–135.

Watson, J.S. (1968). Applications of behavior-shaping devices for training severely and profoundly mentally retarded children in an institutional setting. *Mental Retardation, 6,* 21–23.

Whitstock, R.H. (1980). Dog guides. In R.L. Walsh and B.B. Blasch (Eds.), *Foundations of orientation and mobility* (pp. 565–580). New York: American Foundation for the Blind.

Woolridge, C., & Russell, G. (1976). Head position training with a cerebral palsied child: An application of biofeedback techniques. Toronto: *Rehabilitation Engineering Research,* Crippled Children's Center.

Zuromski, E.S. (1978). Introduction to active stimulation. Warwick, RI: *Technical Newsletter #1,* Trudeau-Zambarano Active Stimulation Program.

SECTION IV

SUMMARY

CHAPTER 12

Program Evaluation in Support of Program Development

Needs, Strategies, and Future Directions

Luanna H. Meyer and Joanne Eichinger

EVALUATION HAS BEEN defined as "the process of providing information for decision-making" (Berk, 1981, p.4) and can vary in approach as a function of the particular decision which needs to be made. In special education, such decisions range from judgments regarding the overall effectiveness of a particular program or innovation to evidence as to how such an innovation can best be implemented in typical school programs. *Summative evaluation,* a terminal activity assessing the value of a program that has just been provided, is the most commonly used form of evaluation (Stufflebeam et al., 1971). Most typically, an experiment, designed to test an innovation or program component, uses established research design procedures to compare the effects of that component to a control or comparison group that is not exposed to the new techniques. This summative evaluation methodology is fundamentally based upon the procedures developed years ago by R.A. Fisher (1935), an agricultural researcher, and continues to be widely applied in studies evaluating the effects of early intervention, for example. The practical outcome of a summative evaluation is a decision as to whether or not the results of a given program justify its continued support. Thus, the ultimate goal of a summative evaluation of an educational innovation is to generate an empirical answer to the question of whether use of the innovation merits adoption. It is conceivable, from this perspective, that an entire program might be abandoned due to a failure to present convincing evidence of its positive effects.

In special education, various educational reforms have been promulgated, on behalf of students with severe disabilities, that are values-based rather than empirically-based (Peck & Semmel, 1982). Thus, concepts such as integration, community-based instruction, early intervention, and even individualized instruction have become widely recognized as desirable program components largely on the basis of

Preparation of this chapter was supported in part by Contract #300-82-0363, awarded to the University of Minnesota, and by Cooperative Agreement #G0084C3001, awarded to The Association for Persons with Severe Handicaps (TASH), with subcontracts to Syracuse University, by the Office of Special Education Programs, U.S. Department of Education. This material does not necessarily reflect the position or policies of the U.S. Department of Education, and no official endorsement should be inferred.

value judgments, and the evaluation activities that occur are unlikely to be summative in nature. That is, a comparison of the outcomes of integrated versus segregated schooling is not likely to be viewed as a legitimate evaluation direction unless this issue is viewed as exclusively empirical, for this is not generally regarded as a data-based issue, but is instead considered to be values-based. Thus, evaluation activities and applied research in this area have focused not upon whether children *should* attend integrated schools, but upon how to make integration *work best* for everyone involved (Voeltz, 1984). Ultimately, a summative evaluation of particular approaches to integration might be appropriate to test their relative effectiveness, and to assist program personnel who will select from among available program options. In the interim, ongoing educational decisions must be made on behalf of particular programs and individual children to produce continuing benefits and to prevent failure. A summative evaluation model is not well suited to the kinds of educational decisions that teachers must make, precisely because it is after the fact, and does not support the individualized instructional adaptations needed to ensure that every child learns.

From this perspective, the values-based goal of integration should result in the availability of integrated program options for individual children, *but at the same time* data must be gathered to support the effectiveness of particular strategies implemented to meet that goal. If such data are judged to show positive results for the individual child, all is well. If such data are judged to show negative results, program modifications to remediate this situation are required. A summative evaluation by definition does not allow for this kind of continuous program adjustment and modification, so that alternative proactive approaches to assist educational decision-making are needed for use by teachers, parents, and other clinicians who are attempting to maximize the development of individual children.

This chapter proposes a number of strategies to accomplish an alternative approach, *formative evaluation*. In formative evaluation, the emphasis is upon the ongoing collection of information throughout program implementation, in order to make continuous revisions to current efforts and to improve program quality based upon these collected data. Such formative or process evaluation efforts are directed toward making program changes before negative outcomes occur—rather than reporting either successes or failures after a program has ended (Posavac & Carey, 1980).

This chapter discusses strategies to address decision-making needs in three evaluation areas: a) staff development; b) program quality reflective of "most promising practices" in the field; and c) student performance and outcome data to support judgments regarding needed program modifications for individual students. Descriptions are provided of procedures and measures that can be adapted and applied in typical education programs serving students with severe disabilities that include dual sensory impairment. Each of the procedures and measures presented has been field-tested and validated in educational settings with students who have severe disabilities and sensory impairments. Throughout, suggestions for future program development efforts will be made based upon work conducted and data collected in school and community training environments.

STAFF DEVELOPMENT

The need for continuing education programs for teachers has been a recurring theme in recent efforts to define educational reform in America's schools (Boyer, 1983; Branscomb et al., 1986; National Commission on Excellence in Education, 1983). In a survey to determine those reforms likely to attract good candidates to the teaching profession, Harris, Kegay, and Leichenko (1985) report that 58% of the teachers surveyed (a total of 1,846) favored advanced study sabbaticals to support professional development. As of 1984, 20 states had enacted initiatives designed to foster the professional development of teachers, and initiatives of this nature have been proposed or were being considered by an additional 21 states (Goldberg et al., 1984). Specific proposals have included 11-month contracts, and summer study plans designed to ensure adequate time for curriculum and professional development (Boyer, 1983; National Commission on Excellence in Education, 1983). The Carnegie Forum on Education and the Economy (Branscomb et al., 1986) has most recently recommended a National Board for Professional Teaching Standards that would require periodical recertification and evaluation of teachers to ensure they remain current in their fields.

In special education, particularly with regard to learners who have dual sensory impairments and severe disabilities, the knowledge base of effective educational practices has expanded dramatically in the past few years. Many of these developments are summarized in this volume (see also Horner, Meyer, & Fredericks, 1986); others are projected as future efforts based upon current developments. Given this rapidly expanding data base, meeting staff development needs is critical to the provision of quality educational services that incorporate effective and innovative practices in the field. This section summarizes various procedures and measures that can be used to evaluate ongoing staff training needs as well as the effectiveness of any inservice training provided to meet such needs.

Needs Assessment

The administration of a needs assessment measure is a commonly used method to determine training needs for program staff, organizations, or an individual service provider. Items included in such a needs assessment should be statements of the knowledge, skills and/or competencies judged to represent "most promising educational practices." Based upon the items identified as "program quality indicators" (that is, considered to represent most promising practices; this component will be addressed below), a needs assessment was constructed for use in Connecticut and Massachusetts as the basis for planning inservice training activities for the academic year (Norman, Brookfield-Norman, & Meyer, 1985). Table 1 lists the dimensions surveyed in this needs assessment and includes selected item examples. Each respondent was asked to rate each item on two scales. First, the respondent was asked to assess the level of skill or knowledge he or she felt was required for a particular job. Second, he or she was to rate his or her own level of skill relative to that competency. By using this dual rating system, discrepancies between necessary and existing levels of skill

Table 1. Assessment of inservice personnel training needs (from Norman et al., 1985).

Dimension	Sample items[a]
Identification and referral for diagnosis	—Ability to collect data through a variety of observation techniques —Knowledge of a variety of diagnostic instruments which are appropriate for use with children who are deaf-blind and children who have other sensory impairments
Assessment/diagnosis for instructional planning	—Ability to do an ecological inventory in order to identify possible instructional goals for: —domestic living —leisure/recreation —vocational —community participation —Ability to collect and use data to modify instruction based on student performance and behavior
Creating and arranging opportunities for learning	—Knowledge and use of strategies to develop social interactions between students with disabilities and their nonhandicapped peers —Ability to schedule the school day to maximize instructional time
Instructional design (IEP development) and instructional strategies	—Ability to write IEP objectives which reflect a concern for acquisition, generalization and maintenance of new skills —Knowledge and use of strategies to incorporate augmentative systems and adaptive equipment into instructional procedures
Team cooperation, family collaboration, and use of community resources	—Ability to train and supervise paraprofessional personnel in the classroom and in community settings —Knowledge of relevant agency resources available to families (e.g., medical, respite, adaptive equipment, vocational rehabilitation services, protection and advocacy)
Long range planning, transitions and use of resources	—Knowledge of long-range planning procedures and techniques —Knowledge of postsecondary vocational opportunities

[a]Respondents rate each item for the extent to which it is required, and whether he or she has the particular competency, on the following scale: 1 = none, 2 = minimal, 3 = moderate, 4 = considerable, and 5 = extensive.

or knowlege can be identified. Such discrepancies between the level of skill actually needed and the level that exists are, of course, a more accurate reflection of training needs than a simple rating of current skill level without regard to the applicability of the item to a particular job. (The complete needs assessment is included as an appendix to this chapter.)

Inservice Training Approaches

Training activities designed to address identified needs should be based upon a proactive approach to staff development. Such an approach communicates an expectation of the potential for the positive growth of teachers as they meet the challenges they will face within their organizations. In contrast, the traditional deficit model emphasizes the staff's lack of certain skills and competencies. Several factors are commonly espoused as characteristic of successful staff development efforts. First, teachers assume an active role as professionals in articulating their needs, directing the focus of the inservice training, and being involved in the staff development activities. Second, a collegial atmosphere exists wherein teachers have time to address the practice of teaching, and to mutually assist one another. This assistance might take the form of teachers observing each other and providing useful evaluations of these observations. Third, programs are individualized rather than including the same activities for all participants. Fourth, the inservice training involves the demonstration of materials or an instructional technique, combined with a supervised practice session, followed by feedback. This format differs greatly from an inservice training activity that provides information which is to be stored for (possible) future application. Examples of staff development activities include professional reading, programmed instructional modules, staff-to-staff instruction, staff exchanges or visits across programs and schools, workshops, consultation and technical assistance, coursework, lectures, and conferences (Brookfield, 1981).

One effective inservice training model—the Teaching Research Inservice Model (Stile, Peters, & Piazza Templeman, 1986)—embodies these attributes of success. There are six components of this model: the identification of training needs, identification of inservice training outcomes, design of objectives, development of the training activities, design of a follow-up plan, and development of an evaluation system. Four "success markers" are incorporated into the model. Individual teachers can shape the inservice training through the needs assessment process. Mutual assistance among teaching staff can occur during the training activities through discussions and role playing sessions. Within the Teaching Research Model, technical assistance activities are individualized to accommodate the needs of the learners. This is accomplished primarily through the practica sessions and through the follow-up provided to trainees on site. The fourth success marker represents the actual Teaching Research Model, which will be elaborated upon in the next section.

Levels of Inservice Training

Stile et al. (1986) identify three levels of inservice training: (1) awareness level; (2) knowledge level; and (3) skill implementation level. Each of these levels of inservice training will be discussed using a hypothetical example of a need identified from items listed in Table 1. When given the needs assessment listed at the end of the chapter (see Appendix 1), 15 teachers indicated that they had minimal ability to conduct an ecological inventory in order to identify possible instructional goals for domestic living, leisure/recreation, vocational training, and community participation, while at the same time these teachers indicated that considerable ability in this area is required in their present positions. Therefore, inservice instruction on procedures for community-based instruction would be a feasible professional staff development topic.

Awareness Level Training An inservice training session that focuses upon the awareness level would typically last from 1 to 2 hours and would include general information. Regarding the area targeted for instruction in the above example, an awareness level workshop might focus on the rationale behind providing community-based instruction, the importance of assessing skills in natural contexts, and the sites in the community which might be appropriate for such training.

Knowledge Level Training Knowledge level training moves beyond general awareness of a topic or a curricular component, and includes more specific and concrete information. For the previous example, knowledge level training would include information on how to conduct an ecological inventory to provide teachers with the skills needed to carry out such an inventory in a community site, in order to target an appropriate instructional objective. Since this level of training lasts for one-half to a full day, a demonstration of how to conduct an ecological inventory would probably be provided. After being exposed to this knowledge level training activity, a teacher would be equipped to return to his or her setting and conduct an ecological inventory in a potential training site in the community.

Skill Implementation Level Training Skill implementation level training enables the participants to practice the skills that are the focus of the session. This level of training incorporates both awareness level and knowledge level training. Thus, short lectures or demonstrations are typically followed by an opportunity to actually apply the skill which has been described. For example, within the third level of training, participants would actually carry out an ecological inventory in an actual community site (e.g., a McDonald's restaurant).

As indicated previously, the most successful types of inservice instruction allow participants to use the skills being taught, and to receive feedback from the trainers regarding their performance. Ideally, participants can use the techniques they have learned through inservice training activities with their own students, while being observed by one or more of the trainers. This enables the participants to receive immediate feedback on their performance and to obtain clarification or additional modeling and demonstrations by the trainer, if needed. One or several of these "on-site" observations and consultations can be incorporated into an inservice training model. This type of inservice may be structured so that it occurs on an ongoing basis. For example, a group of 5–10 teachers might come together at a training site where they receive skill implementation level training on how to conduct ecological inventories. During the training session, each teacher would practice the assessment strategy in the training site. At that point, the teachers have acquired the knowledge and skills needed to go back to their own community and conduct the inventories at sites where their own students might receive instruction. To ensure that these assessments are done correctly, an inservice trainer would observe each of the teachers conducting the ecological inventory. This would assure the trainers that the participants had acquired the skills needed for assessment of community settings at a predetermined mastery criterion level.

Evaluation of Inservice Training Activities

There are five levels of evaluation that measure whether positive outcomes have occurred as a function of inservice training. The first level of evaluation measures whether the participants were satisfied with the training provided. Following an inservice session, participants would typically be asked to respond to questions about several aspects of the inservice activities, using a Likert Scale rating or answering open-ended questions. Because responses reflect how well the consultant and the information presented by that consultant were received, this technique provides rather subjective data. To use the same example from the needs assessment, after a workshop or lecture on conducting ecological assessments, participants could rate how satisfied they were with regard to such factors as the scope, organization, clarity, and utility of the presentation.

A second level of evaluation determines whether knowledge and skills have been acquired or whether changes in attitudes have occurred. Usually this type of data is collected through pretest and posttest measures. For example, participants at a workshop on conducting assessments in natural settings could be tested prior to and after the workshop on specific issues (why an ecological inventory is important, how to conduct the assessment, and so forth). A better indicator of whether knowledge on this subject has been acquired could be obtained by observing the participants actually demonstrate how to conduct an ecological inventory immediately after the workshop.

The third level of evaluation examines whether the trainees are able to use the acquired skill or knowledge in their own work environment. Therefore, a teacher who has received instruction on conducting ecological inventories would be asked to select a community-based instructional site appropriate for one of his or her students, and demonstrate that he or she could adequately assess the skills needed for that activity in that environment.

Program change constitutes the fourth level of evaluation. How has the inservice training had an impact upon the instructional program? Regarding the discrete example of instruction centered around conducting ecological inventories, evidence could be collected to document that a program change has occurred by looking at length of time spent per week in community-based instruction. Given that the inservice training session should increase the teacher's skills in assessing community settings, it should follow, if the training has been effective, that the teacher is now more able to teach students in community settings and thus will increase the amount of instruction occurring in this environment. Other discrete and measurable areas of program change that might be observed as a result of professional staff development activities include: the amount of "down time" which occurs each day; the amount of time spent by members of a transdisciplinary team in planning and implementing integrated programs; the types (natural versus artificial) and frequency of instructional cues used by teachers; and the mechanisms used by school personnel to communicate with parents (frequency and types of communication). These types of data would be collected over time to document whether program change has taken place.

The fifth level of evaluation involves child-change data. Have children acquired skills or made progress as a result of staff development activities? With the examples used throughout the chapter, it would be impossible to document child change as a result of inservice instruction solely by conducting ecological inventories, since this is only one step in delivering effective community-based instruction. However, it seems logical that inservice training on related strategies—such as conducting a discrepancy analysis, targeting skills for instruction in the community, and providing systematic instruction of those skills in community settings—would naturally complement the initial inservice training activity. After this larger inservice training package had been delivered, child-change data could then be collected. This could take the form of weekly progress noted for IEP (individualized education program) goals involving instruction in the community. For example, as a result of the inservice training, a teacher may decide to teach students to purchase and eat a snack at a local fast food restaurant. The teacher targets 10 out of the 17 steps involved in the task, and provides intensive, systematic instruction. Data are collected twice weekly on these 10 steps. Progress can then be evaluated by noting the number of steps completed with less assistance than during the previous week. Child-change data could also be collected on other discrete behaviors. In one successful demonstration of child-change as a function of staff training activities, following direct technical assistance and other training activities provided to staff, Durand and Kishi (1987) were able to document improvements in serious behavior problems of students who were deaf-blind.

Measuring Long-Term Outcomes

Sometimes change evolves slowly, as in inservice training efforts directed to systems change. In these instances, data collection techniques are not always sensitive to the changes that actually occur. A more global pictorial representation can often highlight child-change and program change data. An example of such a tool is found in Figure 1. This grid can be used by individual classroom teachers, by district personnel, or by state personnel to reflect movement of students to less restrictive educational environments. The markers on the horizontal axis represent actual placement sites that students attend for instruction. Movement from left to right involves increasingly less restrictive instructional environments. The markers on the vertical axis reflect the belief that mere physical proximity to nondisabled individuals is not sufficient; planned efforts must take place if persons with severe disabilities are to be socially integrated into school and community environments (Meyer & Putnam, in press). Moving from bottom to top, the markers designate less restrictive options. To use the grid, each student's current level of integration can be assessed by examining his or her present placement and the extent to which social interactions occur with

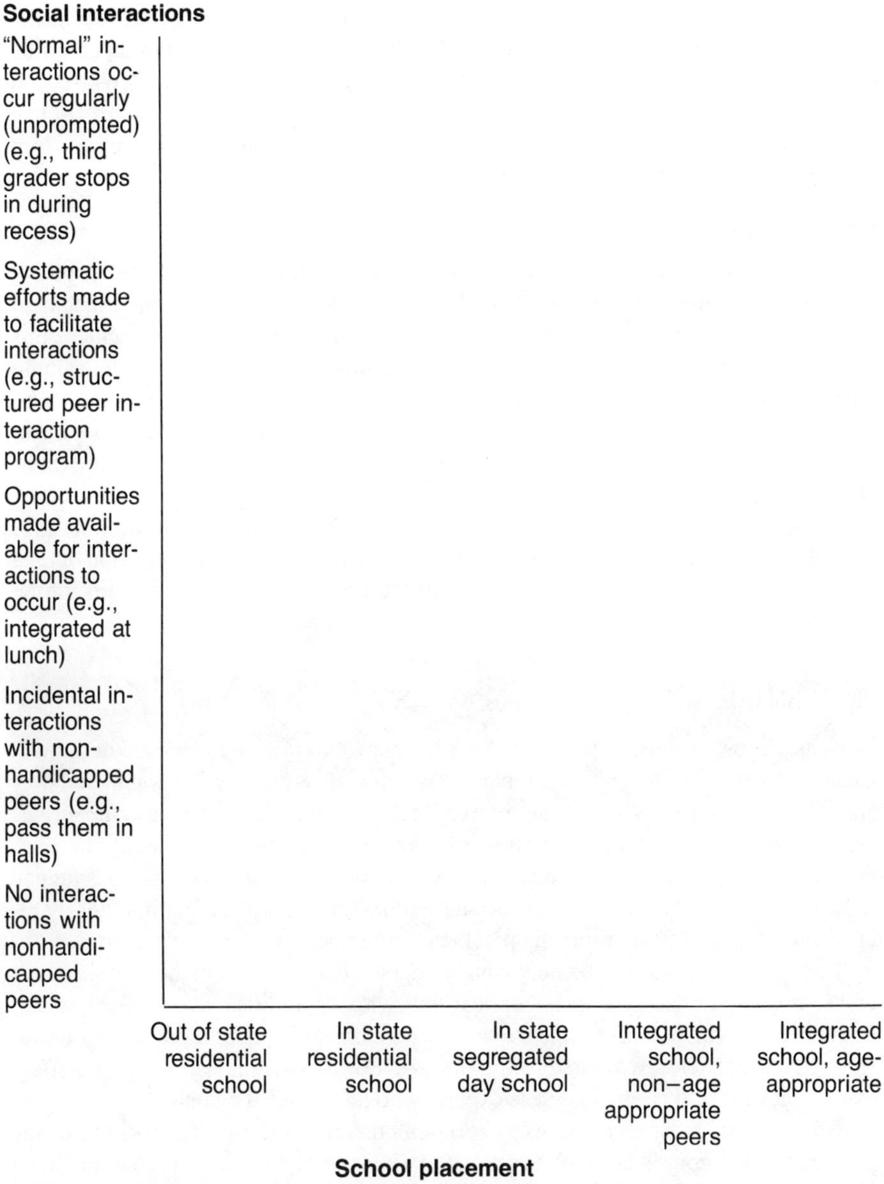
Social interactions
"Normal" interactions occur regularly (unprompted) (e.g., third grader stops in during recess)
Systematic efforts made to facilitate interactions (e.g., structured peer interaction program)
Opportunities made available for interactions to occur (e.g., integrated at lunch)
Incidental interactions with nonhandicapped peers (e.g., pass them in halls)
No interactions with nonhandicapped peers
Out of state residential school
In state residential school
In state segregated day school
Integrated school, non–age appropriate peers
Integrated school, age-appropriate
School placement

Figure 1. School involvement (life space). Based upon a process described and recommended in Galloway and O'Brien [1981]. Adapted with permission.

nondisabled student peers. Color-coded indicators (numbers, letters) could designate where information about each student is located on the grid. An analysis could be done on an annual basis—and then every few years—using the same color-coded indicators as before. Movement toward increasingly integrated and less restrictive environments at the systems level could be clearly seen by indicators that move from the bottom left corner toward the upper right corner.

Developing Local Expertise

It is imperative that change occurring as a result of professional staff development activities be maintained over time, and that staff continue to seek out and implement new educational innovations as they are made available. One strategy to achieve this goal is to train someone on staff sufficiently so that he or she can provide training reflective of ongoing developments in the field. It is particularly critical that local expertise be developed to continue training efforts in settings such as group homes, for example, that currently experience extremely high staff turnover rates. The training of the future on-site trainer should be incorporated into an inservice training model. One technique used successfully to support the development of this expertise is to have an on-site supervisor assume shared responsibility for the collection of data to evaluate any training activities, in order to promote feelings of "ownership" of the training.

PROGRAM QUALITY

What are "most promising practices"? As the phrase has come to be used in the vernacular, it generally refers to exemplary and innovative developments generated by applied research efforts to validate more effective instructional strategies or service delivery patterns. Thus, these practices may be defined as "most promising" because their use has been empirically related to the achievement of certain outcomes judged to be important or meaningful. At the same time, a slightly different but closely related definition of "most promising practices" might be those practices recommended by the experts or leaders in the field who "understand and represent the leading edges of exemplary service strategies for learners with disabilities . . . " (Baer, 1986, p. 145). The contribution of expert recommendations to the definition of most promising practices is closely related to the first—innovations demonstrated to be effective—since in most cases it is these experts who have done the applied research and program development work necessary to demonstrate the empirical validity of the practices they recommend. (Incidentally, Public Law 94-142, which refers to "most promising practices," at one point also explicitly states that experts in the field define "appropriate" services.) Yet, asking experts what they think should be done can differ from the first criterion. Their recommendations can be different for several reasons: a) There may be no empirical data to support one or another recommendation, and the recommendation might be purely values-based and/or based upon a "best guess" by the expert. As such, professionals are free to agree or not agree with the expert for many reasons. Also, experts can and often do disagree with one another. b) There may be some or even a great deal of empirical data to support a recommendation, but there is sufficient ambiguity in its interpretation that experts will disagree and each claim—with absolute conviction—that the data support recommendations that are diametrically opposed to one another. The Missouri court case [(*St. Louis v. Mallory,* 1985),] in which experts called by both sides gave contradictory interpretations of the data on integration, is a perfect example of this situation. c) Ultimately, someone has to decide what makes someone an "expert"!

Thus, the problem regarding a definition of "most promising practices" is not really solved by stating that it will be what the expert recommends, because then it becomes necessary to define what makes someone an expert. Is it someone who is well-known (does a journalist qualify?), respected as a leader in the field (does someone who published most of his or her work long ago qualify?), prominent among a particular constituency (does the president of a major professional organization qualify?), responsible for major service delivery systems (do U.S. Department of Education or State Department of Special Education administrators qualify?), or publishes research in peer-refereed journals (does someone who does all of his or her work in a university-based laboratory setting qualify?)? And at what point does this definition allow for input from direct service personnel who do the teaching, therapy, and so forth? Where do parents and consumers of services enter into the picture? Are they ever experts and, if not, what is the *survival value* (to use Baer's term) of a recommendation that does not reflect meaningful input of some kind from those who provide and participate in the consequences of the most promising practices? In his review of the recent book supported by The Association for Persons with Severe Handicaps (TASH) on exemplary practices (Horner, Meyer, & Fredericks, 1986), Baer (1986) observed:

> This book is a picture of a few professions and a few citizens leading their society into new practices, rather than following their society's earlier mandate to deal with an old long-standing problem in the old long-standing ways. . . . [But] the book does not say strongly enough and often enough that much of what it displays as exemplary is at some risk of being repudiated by its society in favor of the old ways, and so had better be exemplary, not as a point of merit but as a point of survival . . .
>
> The book is written . . . as if exemplary service were knowledgeable, conscientious, and careful service based as much as possible on exemplary science. If the essence of good service was that it accomplished what is set out to do in the most efficient and effective way that our knowledge base allows, then this book would indeed represent exemplary service. But the essence of good service, *from the point of view of survival,* is not that at all: It is instead that the service is *liked* by almost everyone who needs or wants to have an opinion about it. . . .
>
> The book is so devoted to the rightness of its adventure that it does not attend to the survival of that adventure, which morally is the most important outcome variable of all . . . The name of that class of outcome variables is social validity, or consumer satisfaction (Wolf, 1978). . . . If the survival figures are good, then these adventures must have social validity . . . [But] These exemplars . . . are meant to represent a class that is brought into existence on an enduring social basis, not as one-time experiments in the research program of some agency or university. Exemplars, in their littleness, are easy to

> tolerate . . . the truly crucial outcome variable is survival when the exemplar fulfills its purpose by becoming widespread practice. (Baer, 1986, pp. 145–146)

The remainder of this section summarizes the results of efforts to define and to assess the social validity of the most promising educational practices for students with severe disabilities and/or dual sensory impairments.

Indicators of Program Quality

In the area of severe disabilities, there is an apparent consensus that educational best practices are referenced to the "criterion of ultimate functioning" (Brown, Nietupski, & Hamre-Nietupski, 1976). Numerous position papers, journal articles, and books have been published that both describe what these promising practices should look like and report empirical evidence that supports various components of these recommendations (see Horner et al., 1986, and this volume itself for examples and references to previous work). In addition, at least one package of inservice training modules has been developed, by several experts in their respective areas, for use in staff development to support program changes (Meyer Voeltz, 1983). Donnellan (1984) and Donnellan and Neel (1986) point out that while data are rapidly accumulating to support many of these innovations, other recommended changes have not yet had an empirical demonstration of their effectiveness and meaningfulness. Educators, of course, cannot necessarily wait until "the data are in" when confronted with daily and continuous educational decision-making situations. In cases where the data are not available or clearly interpretable, Donnellan (1984) has recommended application of a "criterion of the least dangerous assumption." This criterion holds that when data are absent, educational decisions should be directed to practices that, if ultimately in error, would have the least dangerous effect on the potential for students to function independently as adults. While this too fails to resolve the dilemma, and judgment must still be made, some combination of a concern for ultimate functioning and an attempt to avoid educational components that, if ineffective, would have serious negative consequences for independence as an adult, could assist in making choices among program options.

Nevertheless, there have been several efforts to identify most promising practices—whether supported by data or expert opinion—that could provide criteria for the evaluation of given programs. The settlement agreement in Philadelphia regarding the right of students with severe disabilities to attend appropriate public school programs included a listing of components of "best practices" which the school district was ordered to incorporate (McGregor, Janssen, Larsen, & Tillery, 1986). Fox and his colleagues developed a "best practices" manual which school personnel might use to self-evaluate the extent to which their program was consistent with recent developments. The items in their manual were initially based upon a literature search, and the final listing reflected input from various professionals both in Vermont and from across the country who were asked to review and edit the original listing (Fox et al., 1986). This strategy is typically referred to as a Delphi approach, in which polling experts in the field is viewed as similar to seeking advice from the oracle, though the usual application of the approach would involve methodological rigor in the use of established survey research strategies (see, e.g., Putnam & Bruininks, 1986).

The *Program Quality Indicators* (PQI) checklist was developed through a series of steps and studies designed to establish both its validity and its usefulness as a measure of "most promising practices" (Meyer, 1985). A literature search was the source of the original listing of items, including indicators supported by empirical data as well as those recommended according to general principles of "quality" and expert professional opinion. The listing was revised based upon input from a dozen national "experts," from a small group of master teachers, and from the six coordinators of the TASH Technical Assistance Project in the area of persons who are deaf-blind. The revised list was then rated by a large national sample representing six relevant respondent groups: a) behavior therapists experts; b) TASH/severe disability experts; c) experts in working with persons who are deaf-blind; d) mental retardation researchers; e) state department directors of special education; and f) parents of individuals with disabilities. (For more detail regarding the development and validation of the PQI, see Meyer, Eichinger, & Park-Lee, 1987). Table 2 lists the indicators, organized into seven program components, and the ratings and relative ranking assigned to each indicator by the sample (250 individuals, representing a 67% return rate overall). From the information on the table, one can derive a general impression of the relative value assigned to each indicator by persons who are in a position to care about and have an impact upon educational programs for this population. Thus, it is interesting that long standing principles of special education do indeed enjoy general agreement about their importance: The two top-ranked items refer to *individualized instruction* and the availability of *instructional alternatives and adaptations*. Others which might be viewed as more recent recommendations were ranked much lower; for example, the indicator regarding attendance at the same school the student would attend if not handicapped was rated slightly above the "undecided" mean point, and ranked 116th out of a total of 122 items. Alternatively, certain indicators that have been controversial were also among the most highly rated items. The indicator stating the philosophy that every child is educable *and* that the program was accountable for student gains was ranked sixth, and an emphasis upon preparation for living in the least restrictive adult environment was ranked eighth.

This effort represents a social validation of these program components by some experts and consumers of services. The majority of the items were highly rated, and thus were judged to be socially valid by the sample as a whole (other studies are underway to investigate other aspects of the social and empirical validity of the PQI). The PQI is intended to be used for self-evaluation by program personnel, and these results support its use in this way. The directions for using this measure describe an assessment process designed to identify program development goals based upon both obvious discrepancies between the existing program and PQI items, and upon the priorities established by the program for the modification of existing practices.

Table 2. Ranking and ratings of Program Quality Indicators individual items by program components[a]

Component	Program quality indicator	Rating[b]	Overall ranking[c]
Program philosophy	Does the program:		
	View every child as educable and program accountable for student gains?	18.09	6
	Emphasize preparation for living in least restrictive adult environment?	18.03	8
	Emphasize goal of individual independence?	17.66	18
	Support family needs and emphasize responsiveness to families?	17.52	21
	Emphasize continuous upgrading of services by actively seeking information on new curricular developments?	17.31	24
	Emphasize goal of maximum participation in integrated community environments?	17.11	29
	Emphasize goal of competitive/ supported employment in integrated, community work environments?	17.08	32
	Emphasize development of both autonomy and individual responsibility by individual learners?	16.92	37
	Emphasize goal of social acceptance/ adjustment?	16.87	41
	Support staff inservice training on a regular basis?	16.67	53
	Support an "open door" policy regarding visits by parents and others?	16.60	54
	Emphasize an integrated therapy model (rather than "pull out" direct service model)?	16.16	65
	Emphasize continuous upgrading of services by actively seeking collegial interactions with "experts"?	15.79	73
	Emphasize sharing own innovative and effective efforts with other services in the region?	15.04	86
Student opportunities for learning	Does the student:		
	Spend increasing amount of time in the community for training as graduation approaches?	17.01	34
	Participate in competitive job or job training for part of the school day (at secondary school age level)?	16.43	59

Table 2. *(continued)*

Component	Program quality indicator	Rating[b]	Overall ranking[c]
	Spend most time engaged in active learning activities, with "down time" comprising no more than a few minutes between activities?	16.24	64
	Attend a school which is appropriate for his or her chronological age?	16.00	69
	Eat lunch in the cafeteria with same-age, nonhandicapped peers?	15.12	83
	Access the school's enrichment areas (e.g., library) on a regularly scheduled basis?	15.12	84
	Participate in leisure and social interaction activities with same-age nonhandicapped peers on a daily basis (recess, school sporting events, etc.)?	15.09	85
	Participate with other students (including nonhandicapped) in extra-curricular activities at school that are typical for age range?	14.99	87
	Receive instruction in the community, outside school setting, at least twice monthly (for ages 3–8), twice weekly (ages 9–12), or 3–4 times weekly (ages 13 and up)?	14.84	90
	Participate in small group instruction with students who have similar needs on regular basis (at least 3 times weekly)?	14.22	100
	Receive 1:1 instruction, by certified personnel, according to individual needs?	13.77	107
	Participate in heterogeneously grouped instruction (with nonhandicapped peers) on a regular basis (at least 3 times weekly)?	13.61	109
	Participate in heterogeneously grouped instruction (with peers having different levels of handicapping conditions) on a regular basis (at least 3 times weekly)?	13.14	112
	Travel to and from school using the general education transportation system?	12.94	113

(continued)

Table 2. *(continued)*

Component	Program quality indicator	Rating[b]	Overall ranking[c]
	Attend different "subject area" classes throughout the day according to patterns typical for age in regular education (rather than remaining in one room, with same teacher and student peer group)?	12.80	115
	Attend the same school he or she would attend if not handicapped?	12.78	116
IEP features	Does the IEP:		
	Include objectives for functional skills that will be used in community settings in the future (e.g., when employed)?	17.94	11
	Include objectives to develop social skills?	17.94	12
	Specify measurable criteria to determine skill mastery by the learner?	17.53	20
	Clearly reflect active family involvement in assessing student needs and designing the IEP?	17.49	22
	Primarily include objectives for functional skills that can be used immediately by the learner in community settings (e.g., at home, in a store, etc.)?	17.22	26
	Include vocational training objectives for every student 14 or older?	16.99	35
	Include objectives to develop leisure activity skills which reflect personal preferences of the learner?	16.76	46
	Specify present levels of functioning referenced to environmental activities rather than IQ scores, mental age, or norm-referenced achievement test scores?	16.70	49
	Include objectives to develop domestic living skills (e.g., household chores)?	16.69	51
	Include personal management objectives, reflecting a concern for teaching decision-making, choice-making, and autonomy?	16.69	52
	State objectives that describe what the learner will do, not what he or she will stop doing, or what staff will do?	16.31	60

Table 2. *(continued)*

Component	Program quality indicator	Rating[b]	Overall ranking[c]
	Require performance in criterion situations in actual environments, without teacher assistance, to indicate mastery?	16.29	62
	Include objectives to teach the learner to interact with and help others?	16.15	66
	Include at least one measurable behavioral objective involving interactions with peers who are not handicapped?	15.37	82
	Require performance in the presence of nonhandicapped persons in actual situations in the community, either independently or with help from another person in the environment (not the teacher), to indicate mastery?	14.89	88
Instructional strategies	Are instructional strategies individualized (rather than being nearly indentical across students)?	18.31	1
	Are alternate communication models and adaptive equipment devices used in instruction, for learners who need them, across all program areas?	18.29	2
	Are instructional objectives practiced throughout the day, in addition to during scheduled program sessions, whenever natural opportunities occur (e.g., a communication skill would also be practiced at lunchtime if relevant, and not only during language instruction sessions)?	17.83	16
	Are behavior problems viewed as instructional needs, indicating areas where skills for more appropriate behaviors are not adequate and need development and practice?	17.45	23
	Are instructional cues designed to be closely related to available natural cues in criterion environments?	17.15	27
	Are students physically positioned according to their individualized needs throughout the school day and the various instructional programs?	17.12	28

(continued)

Table 2. *(continued)*

Component	Program quality indicator	Rating[b]	Overall ranking[c]
	Are schedules of instruction evident that provide sufficient time scheduled to meet individual learner goals?	17.03	33
	Does scheduled time reflect a variety of situations, including independent work, small group, large group, 1:1 instruction, socialization, and free-time for each learner?	16.83	43
	Are new skills taught in the context of naturally occurring activities and daily routines (e.g., skill clusters rather than massed trial practice of an isolated skill)?	16.81	44
	Are instructional corrections and consequences designed to be closely related to available natural corrections and consequences in criterion environments?	16.70	50
	Do instructional programs specify procedures for fading teacher assistance, including instructional cues, corrections, and consequences?	16.44	58
	Are data on student performance for each IEP objective collected at least once weekly, and those data used to modify programs?	16.29	61
	Are instructional programs written so that substitute personnel would understand how to teach them?	16.28	63
	Have individualized task analyses and discrepancy analyses been done as the basis of individual instructional programs?	16.14	67
	Do student performance data include information on levels of assistance being provided?	16.02	68
	Is the body position of any student with a physical disability changed at least once every half-hour?	15.78	74
	Are new skills instructed in actual community environments?	15.44	80
	Are at least 3 postural (stationary) positions incorporated into program for any student with a physical disability	14.76	92

Table 2. *(continued)*

Component	Program quality indicator	Rating[b]	Overall ranking[c]
	(e.g., who has cerebral palsy and/or is nonambulatory)?		
Program characteristics	Does the program:		
	Offer training to parents who are interested and/or ask for assistance in working on skills with their child at home?	18.23	4
	Provide for direct training in actual situations and environments where skills are to be used whenever needed for generalization?	18.12	5
	Maintain up-to-date medical records, including information on any medications, and monitoring of effects for any student on medication?	17.94	13
	Encourage input from parents in identifying individually effective instructional strategies (e.g., effective reinforcers)?	17.77	17
	Share information on each student's record with the family, while maintaining confidentiality of all records?	17.65	19
	Maintain regular contact with "feeder" program/school and the "next" program/school to facilitate student transitions (including community college and/or rehabilitation agency for secondary students)?	17.24	25
	Show evidence of longitudinal planning for the demands of subsequent environments?	17.09	31
	Require team collaboration in both planning and delivery of instruction?	16.92	38
	Share a formal report on pupil progress with parents on a quarterly basis?	16.86	42
	Utilize an educative approach and "least intrusive means" guidelines to intervene with behavior problems?	16.72	47
	Reflect age-appropriateness in instructional arrangements, materials, and activities?	16.53	55

(continued)

Table 2. *(continued)*

Component	Program quality indicator	Rating[b]	Overall ranking[c]
	Use ecological inventories as input in the design of individualized programs (that is, assessing environmental domains)?	15.48	78
	Communicate at least weekly with each student's care-givers, including sharing information about skill generalization to relevant nonschool environments?	15.48	79
	Utilize an outside consultant (with recognized expertise) to provide program technical assistance and/or training at least once yearly?	14.67	94
	Include planned daily interactions with same-age nonhandicapped peers?	14.52	96
	Maintain a collaborative research, development, and/or training relationship with an institution of higher learning?	14.39	98
	Use a standardized measure of student progress or functioning level (with use of alternative response modes as needed by individual students) to evaluate overall program accomplishments at least once annually?	14.17	101
	Provide for nonschool, community-based instruction at least twice weekly?	13.92	104
	Reflect the natural proportion in school placement arrangements (i.e., according to the approximate prevalence of a disability in the general population)?	12.08	118
Staff qualifications	Are paraprofessional personnel required to receive formal training relevant to the disability area served?	15.87	70
	Do all team members working with an individual student meet at least once a month to discuss student progress and program changes?	15.86	71
	Do special education staff attend general faculty meetings and regularly interact with all staff (i.e., not only other special education staff) at the school?	15.80	72

Table 2. *(continued)*

Component	Program quality indicator	Rating[b]	Overall ranking[c]
	Do staff meet formally and consult with one another at least once a month regarding special education issues?	15.64	75
	Are all personnel observed during instruction by the building principal or program supervisor at least quarterly, and provided with written feedback on performance at least annually?	15.59	76
	Has the school principal received training directly relevant to disability areas served in the school?	14.82	91
	Do teaching staff alternate observing one another during instruction to both monitor programs and problem-solve when needed?	14.71	93
	Are all professional personnel certified by the state in the disability area served?	14.26	99
	Does each professional maintain at least one professional contact outside the home school for advice and sharing on educational and therapy concerns?	13.88	105
	Do all special education staff (including therapists) participate in generic, professional, and extra-curricular activities at their school along with regular education staff?	13.80	106
	Does each professional maintain collegial interactions with at least one colleague in his or her discipline working with similar students in another school?	13.16	111
	Does each staff member attend at least four inservice training workshop days each year?	12.92	114
	Have all professional staff attended a professional conference (regional or national) within the past year?	12.20	120
	Do all staff participate in at least one community service activity annually	11.01	120

(continued)

Table 2. *(continued)*

Component	Program quality indicator	Rating[b]	Overall ranking[c]
	that is relevant to that person's role (e.g., speak at PTO meeting, present a paper at a conference)?		
	Have all professional staff completed at least two credits of university coursework in a directly relevant area within the past year?	10.65	121
	Do all professional personnel have a master's degree in the disability area served?	9.84	122
Facility resources	Is/does the facility:		
	Have the adaptive equipment needed for each individual child?	18.01	9
	Accessible for persons with disabilities?	17.99	10
	Keep all equipment and individual prosthetic devices in good working order?	17.87	14
	Reflect adequate and appropriate pupil-teacher staffing ratios?	17.71	15
	Offer a cheerful environment? (That is, if visitors walked into this facility, would they find the environment pleasant and positive; or would they find it barren, depressing and/or unpleasant)?	16.89	40
	Include adequate space provisions for program needs?	16.49	56
	Use general school classrooms (computer room, shop, home economics room, etc.) which are accessible and/or include an adapted area for students with multiple disabilities?	16.47	57
	Appear normalized for students' chronological ages (e.g., decor and decorations, furniture, wall displays, etc.)?	15.42	81
	Use state-of-the-art technology for instruction and evaluation (e.g., VCR, computers, optacon, laser cane, etc.)?	14.89	89
	Include adapted equipment on the playground that is also used by nonhandicapped peers?	14.52	95

Table 2. *(continued)*

Component	Program quality indicator	Rating[b]	Overall ranking[c]
	Locate classrooms for students with severe disabilities close by those for same-age nondisabled peers?	14.42	97
	Operate one school calendar for all programs (rather than separate ones for special programs)?	14.17	102
	Accessible to potential community training environments?	14.06	103
	Provide each classroom with a "per student" budget for instructional materials purchases of at least $30 per child per year?	13.74	108
	Have access to a gymnasium?	13.48	110
	Have access to a swimming pool?	11.04	119
General issues	Do staff utilize "caregiving" interactions and natural routines (e.g., eating, going to the bathroom, etc.) as opportunities for instruction?	18.25	3
	Do the teachers, therapists, and other staff talk with (and about) students in a manner that communicates respect (i.e., not yelling at or making fun of, or talking about someone as if he or she were not present)?	18.08	7
	Are students given opportunities to make choices, provide input, and so forth, where appropriate (e.g., asking a student where in the room he or she would like to sit, etc.)?	17.11	30
	Do the teachers, therapists, and other staff explain changes in activity/place to students (rather than just pushing the wheelchair to another location, etc.)?	16.98	36
	Does each student receive appropriate positive reinforcement and feedback (i.e., at least 75% positive to 25% corrections in the classroom)?	16.90	39
	Does the program reflect a balance between safety concerns and normalized risk taking for the ages of the students?	16.79	45

(continued)

Table 2. *(continued)*

Component	Program quality indicator	Rating[b]	Overall ranking[c]
	Would a nonhandicapped student of the same age as students in this class feel that his/her privacy and dignity are being respected?	16.71	48
	Do nonhandicapped peers spontaneously interact with students with disabilities when passing them in the hall or meeting them in central areas such as the lunchroom or playground?	15.49	77

[a]Based upon the responses of 250 individual experts representing six respondent group categories: (a) Behavior therapy; (b) TASH; (c) deaf-blind; (d) mental retardation research; (e) state department directors of special education; and (f) parents.

[b]On a scale from 1 to 20, where 1 = Not a consideration, 10 = Undecided, and 20 = Very important consideration.

[c]Of a total of 122 items, which were presented to each respondent in random order (generated by a computer program so that no more than approximately 15 respondents would receive the same ordering).

Dimensions of Program Quality: A Social Validation

The PQI is organized according to seven program components (see Table 2) that reflect practical and administrative realities, but may not necessarily coincide with consistent value ratings within each of the various components. For example, the "IEP Features" category on the PQI lists quality indicators that relate to the IEP process, a discrete and identifiable event in educational settings. Thus, program personnel can efficiently self-evaluate their program on this one component. However, the program components may not reflect attitudinal dimensions; that is, there may be attitudinal dimensions that affect one's ratings across categories of the PQI, so that an individual rater might view certain items within the "IEP Features" category as being more important than others as a function of his or her attitudes on a particular issue. Differences in ratings as a function of such dimensions would indicate areas where consensus has not been reached regarding the value of particular aspects of program quality that have been recommended. Where such differences can be systematically related to particular expert groups and constituencies, this may reveal important information that could explain why certain PQI items may be less likely to be accepted into current practices than others. Furthermore, where there are clear group differences, and the groups involved are each in a position to have an impact upon the survival value of an innovation, these disagreements reveal areas where change may not occur over the long run unless the issues are resolved constructively.

To test for the existence of such attitudinal dimensions across the PQI items, a factor analysis was conducted based upon the responses of the 250 individuals in the 6 groups mentioned earlier. In addition, an analysis of variance and tests of mean differences were performed to identify respondent group differences on the dimensions emerging from the factor analysis. A detailed discussion of the study and findings is available in Meyer et al. (1987), but a brief overview of certain issues will be provided here. Table 3 summarizes the preliminary results of the factor analysis and differences in group ratings which emerged for those dimensions of "most promising practices." Factor 1 (integration) clearly consists of those items which included references to interactions with nonhandicapped peers and participation in various generic environments shared with nondisabled persons. Factor 2 includes items that referred to home-school interactions, family input, parent training, the development of social skills, and the maintenance of medical records; other items loading on this factor referred to team involvement and individualized instruction as well as upgrading services with new curriculum developments. Thus, this factor is more difficult to label, but is referred to here as "Home-School and Professional Practices." Factor 3 consists of items involving data-based instruction, such as measurement of student performance, task analysis, application of behavioral procedures, and recommended ratios of positive to negative feedback; this factor is referred to as "Systematic Instruction." Factor 4 is clearly made up of items related to "Professional Training and Staff Development," while Factor 5 (with only two items loading extremely high on this dimension) has been labeled "Criterion of Ultimate Functioning"; the items included in this factor relate to the development of functional skills for criterion environments, such as vocational and domestic living settings.

There were significant group differences on all five factors. On the "Integration" dimension, the TASH experts and parents were significantly higher than all other groups, while the deaf-blind experts and behavior therapists were significantly lower than all other groups. For the "Home-School" and "Professional Practices" dimension, parents were significantly higher than all other groups, while the behavior therapists rated these items lower than any other group. Thus, TASH experts, deaf-blind experts, mental retardation researchers, and state directors rated "Home-School" and "Professional Practices" lower than did parents, and higher than behavior therapists. The items that made up the "Systematic Instruction" factor were rated significantly higher by the TASH experts and the behavior therapists in comparison to all other groups. For "Professional Training and Staff Development," parents were significantly higher than all other groups and TASH experts significantly lower than all others. Finally, the only significant group difference for the "Criterion of Ultimate Functioning" dimension was that the behavior therapists rated these items lower than did the other five groups (see also Table 3).

The differences in ratings which emerged for these five respondent groups raises a number of interesting issues. First, the group of nationally recognized applied behavior analysts rated all items relatively low with the exception of the "Systematic Instruction" dimension. A closer look at the literature in this area does show a recent trend toward research that reflects the kinds of educational best practices included in the PQI (McGregor & Meyer, 1986), but the obvious lack of agreement by these individuals about the value of integration, a criterion of ultimate functioning, and the

Table 3. Dimension ratings by six expert/constituent groups on the PQI[a]

	Level of overall group rating on each dimension (relative ranking on dimension across groups)[b]				
Respondent group:	Integration	Home-school and professional practices	Systematic instruction	Professional training and staff development	Criterion of ultimate functioning
A) Behavior therapist experts	Low (6)	Low (6)	High (2)	Middle (3)	Low (6)
B) TASH/severe disabilities experts	High (2)	Middle (5)	High (1)	Low (6)	Middle (2)
C) Deaf/blind experts	Low (5)	Middle (2)	Middle (3)	Middle (4)	Middle (3)
D) Mental retardation researchers	Low (4)	Middle (3)	Low (6)	Middle (2)	Middle (4)
E) State department directors of special education	Middle (3)	Middle (4)	Low (5)	Middle (5)	Middle (4)
F) Parents	High (1)	High (1)	Middle (4)	High (1)	High (1)

[a]This is a preliminary summary of these data. For more information see Meyer et al. (1987).

[b]For each group, "High" indicates above the mean; "middle" indicates near the mean; and "low" indicates below the mean. The ranking in parentheses after these designations refers to how this group rated the particular dimension in comparison to other groups. One indicates that the group rated the dimension as being more important than did the other groups; 6 indicates that the group rated the dimension lowest across all groups.

involvement of the family should be disturbing to those who recognize the pioneering contributions of these professionals to serving persons with severe disabilities. Experts in the area of dual impairment not only rated the "Integration" dimension nearly as low as did the behavior therapists, but generally regarded the other four dimensions with only slightly more enthusiasm. This group did not rate any dimension highly, and was only occasionally higher in ratings than the lowest group on a particular dimension (though this reflected a median rating rather than a high one). Apparently, these professionals do not embrace many of the dimensions cited as most promising practices. Again, the implications for services for students with dual sensory impairment are clear, if these professionals do indeed play a significant role in defining and maintaining those services.

Certain patterns in the responses of the parents are also most interesting. First, parents invariably rated all dimensions except the "Systematic Instruction" factor highest or higher than other groups. This includes the "Professional Training and Staff Development" dimension, for which the parents were significantly higher than all other groups, and the TASH experts significantly lower. Given the obvious efforts of TASH as an organization and the emphasis upon involving parent input to professionals who work with children having severe disabilities, this difference of opinion is intriguing. Why do TASH experts consider this dimension to be less important in their ratings and in comparison to the other dimensions? Finally, the mental retardation researchers rated the "Integration" and "Systematic Instruction" dimensions lower than they did the other three dimensions, and the state directors of special education rated "Systematic Instruction" lower than they did all four other factors; neither of these groups rated any of the dimensions high, either with reference to the mean of the scale or the other groups.

What are the implications of these findings for the kinds of practices included in the PQI as they reflect recommendations regarding most promising practices in educational services for students with severe disabilities? Will these practices make the transition from "exemplary" to "typical" in current service delivery? If these respondent groups do have influence upon current thinking in their disciplines and among their constituencies, then the lack of consensus regarding the value of these innovative developments is disturbing. One interpretation of such findings that is common in social validity studies is to conclude that because certain groups fail to value a strategy or an outcome, it does indeed lack validity and should not be implemented or function as a goal. A more proactive interpretation, one reflecting the reality that social practices and current societal attitudes generally lag behind the recommendations made by social reformers, is to conclude that these findings do indeed reveal an absence of social validity, say nothing regarding the empirical validity of the recommended practices, but do indicate a critical need to enter into a dialogue with fellow professionals and the public regarding future practices. What is necessary in the way of data, theory, or programs to adapt or expand these exemplary practices toward common adoption and social acceptance in services for persons with severe disabilities?

STUDENT PERFORMANCE AND OUTCOME DATA

The ultimate purpose of an educational program is not, of course, to demonstrate either that its staff are well trained or that its program components represent best practices. The true test of the *educational validity* of a program is its impact upon the students: Are students learning important new skills and behaviors which will improve their quality of life? Voeltz and Evans (1983) identified three essential questions which must be addressed in the evaluation of child-change data which are attributed to an educational intervention:

1. Is the change in the child's behavior meaningful (empirical and social validity)?
2. Has this change occurred as a function of the planned intervention (internal validity)?
3. Did the educational intervention occur as specified in the educational intervention plan (procedural reliability or educational integrity)?

Taken as a whole, these issues provide an assessment of the educational validity of the educational program (Voeltz & Evans, 1983), and Evans and Meyer (1985) detail evaluation strategies and specific measures to address each question. This section reviews only the first of these criteria (interested readers are referred to Evans and Meyer [1985] Chapter 6, for more information on the second and third criteria and strategies).

The purpose of education for students who have severe disabilities and dual sensory impairments is the same as it is for other children; with appropriate educational programming, all of these students should be able to acquire a repertoire that enables them to function as independently as possible across their lifespans. Educational programs should also take into account the normalized interdependencies available to each person, so that children with disabilities learn to participate in these interdependencies as well as be independent in various activities. All adults depend upon others (friends, spouses, roommates, fellow employees, paid services, family members, employers, and so forth) on a daily and continuous basis according to various voluntary agreements that are negotiated either formally (paid and contractual arrangement outside family and friendship networks) or informally (understandings among peers and family members). This means that, in some cases, an individual need not be completely independent in a particular activity if another person is available to assist according to normalized and socially acceptable social interaction patterns. In other cases, the individual must learn constructive interdependent interactions in order to use skills in ways that are both effective and likely to be viewed as socially acceptable by others. Many, if not most, community participation skills fall into this category (e.g., shopping, using public transportation, working on the job). By applying both of these outcome goals to an approach to evaluating program accomplishments, it should be obvious that simply demonstrating that a child has changed his or her behavior is not enough. The changes which have occurred must be meaningful. What makes behavior change meaningful? In order to demonstrate that a program has a meaningful outcome, any measure of the degree of behavior change must be preceded by a decision that the behavior that has been increased or decreased is critically related to that child's daily life, both now and in the future, after graduation.

Identifying Meaningful Skill and Behavior Change Goals

Many years ago, Risley (1969) called for the evaluation of programs according to a "therapeutic criterion"—the extent to which the changes brought about by the program have resulted in general improvements for the child's well-being and overall social adaptation. Brown et al.'s (1976) "criterion of ultimate function" reflects a similar focus upon meaningful outcomes as the crucial test of the effectiveness of an educational program. In order to accomplish maximum independence and socially appropriate patterns of interdependence for young people with severe disabilities, decisions must be made each year on the IEP (and in other, less formal contexts) to set goals that have lasting value for the child.

Voeltz and Evans (1983) listed several considerations which might help to identify such goals: a) the behavior should have functional value now and/or in the future; b) the behavior might set the stage for many positive changes in the child's repertoire; c) the behavior change desired by others will not result in significant "cost" to the child (such as might occur by taking away a functional behavior or activity without replacing it with a positive alternative); and d) the behavior is valued by the child and/or significant persons in the child's environment (peers, friends, family members, teachers, employers, and so forth). Measuring changes in the frequency, intensity, or duration of behavior is secondary to providing evidence that the behavior-change goal is important or meaningful. This is particularly critical for persons with severe disabilities, who by definition will take longer to learn fewer skills and have more difficulties maintaining and generalizing those skills unless they are used regularly. Unlike a nondisabled child who perhaps can afford the time spent learning a variety of skills, some of which may never be used, an individual with severe disabilities has less time available to participate in activities with little to no future value. Thus, for these students, instruction should be closely matched to the development of a minimum set of criterion skills and behaviors known to be functional in current and future environments.

The assessment and curricular strategies delineated by Brown and others require that student performance be evaluated with reference to natural activities in criterion environments. What specific skills are needed for home, the workplace, leisure time and the community (Brown et al., 1979)? In principle, these ideas are similar to the notion of "minimum competencies" in regular education (Evans & Meyer, 1984). Yet there have been few efforts to identify what these skills might be. Vincent and her colleagues (1980) approached the task by observing the daily routines of regular education kindergarten and first grade classrooms, and by asking teachers in those settings what their expectations really are. Based upon this information, Vincent et al. listed a minimal set of "survival skills" that might become priority goals for instruction in early education programs. Most recently, Ford et al. (1986) listed a limited set of curricular goal areas in each of four environmental domains—domestic living, vocational, leisure/recreation, and community—including essential and negotiable activities for each area. Within the goal areas, specific essential and negotiable activity objectives are delineated for targeted transition ages, based upon expectations for children who are not handicapped. Thus, within the domestic living goal area of "Budgeting and Planning/Scheduling," children would be expected to "prepare for an outing" by age 5 (with assistance) and "schedule daily/weekly events" by age 16 (independently). These listings were based upon a search of the literature and upon feedback from teachers in one school district as part of an ongoing major curriculum revision effort; thus far the targeted transition goals (and expectations) are unvalidated.

Further Measurement of Student Outcomes

Evans and Brown (1986) noted that the emphasis of evaluation efforts by states and local educational agencies appears to be shifting from compliance monitoring to the measurement of student outcomes. During the first ten years of PL 94-142, it was necessary to document that the states were meeting their obligation to provide an appropriate education to students with disabilities. Following this decade of implementation, more recent federal funding initiatives have focused upon the " . . . need to develop widely accepted criteria for measuring general student progress . . . towards more universally desired outcomes" (Evans, Brown, Weed, Spry, & Owen, 1986, p. 5). One heuristic strategy for doing so is to simply document the cumulative mastery of the IEP goals and instructional objectives included on each year's IEP. If these skills are meaningful (as discussed earlier), it should follow that their mastery is a desirable achievement. However, there are as yet no generally accepted student measures that allow teachers and program administrators, parents, and policy makers to confidently judge the successive attainment of critical skills for universally valued outcomes upon graduation. Evans et al. (1986) describe the Assessment of Functional Life Routines (AFLR) measure being developed which attempts to delineate this cumulative mastery process. This instrument is currently undergoing a systematic psychometric validation that includes normative referencing (i.e., sequences are based upon ages at which nonhandicapped children master particular routines) and information on levels of independence (by further analyzing skill performance according to its content, extension, and enrichment components). This measure is promising, but has not yet been extensively field tested with students with severe disabilities and dual sensory impairment.

SUMMARY

It should be obvious from the preceding discussion that a great deal of progress has been made in the area of staff development, moderate progress is evidenced by the work to establish the indicators of program quality, and a great deal of work needs to be done toward the evaluation of meaningful student outcomes. A discussion of student outcomes such as employment and community living has been purposely avoided, as these are as yet primarily tied to the availability of such opportunities for adults with disabilities, rather than being offered through the educational system, or being considered totally or even primarily a function of a graduate's actual skill level. If adult opportunities after graduation were equivalent, programs could obviously be held accountable for concrete outcomes like employment. Yet, even then, it would not do to wait until after graduation to judge whether the previous 15–20 years of a student's public education had been appropriate and beneficial. Clearly, benchmarks of progress toward meaningful outcomes must be established and organized into student outcome evaluation measures for use at successive school levels, to allow professionals, parents, consumers, and policy makers to evaluate the accomplishments of their educational programs. This chapter briefly describes some efforts in this direction, but primarily emphasizes the work that needs to be done. Two final recommendations are offered. First, research and development activities in the area of severe disabilities have tended to focus almost exclusively upon curricular and instructional strategies. This work should of course continue, but needs to be accompanied by an equal emphasis upon the evaluation of student outcomes that result from these instructional strategies. Finally, professionals in this field tend to proceed as if everyone agrees with and is willing to enthusiastically adopt the latest innovation or recommended best practice in education. This is undoubtedly naive and, as the results of the PQI study indicate, probably incorrect as well. If it is desirable that these innovations and best practices receive widespread support and implementation, establishing a data base is only the first step. Sometime soon, it will also be necessary to communicate with fellow professionals, consumers, and the public as to why these changes are desirable. If this is not done, it is easy enough for systems to remain as they are, and most students with severe disabilities will find their school careers little changed, regardless of exciting developments in books, journals, and a few model projects.

REFERENCES

Baer, D.M. (1986). Exemplary service to what outcome? Review of *Education of learners with severe handicaps: Exemplary service strategies*, in *Journal of The Association for Persons with Severe Handicaps, 11*, 145–147.

Berk, R.A. (1981). Introduction, In R.A. Berk (Ed.), *Educational evaluation methodology: The state of the art* (pp. 1–10). Baltimore: Johns Hopkins University Press.

Boyer, E.L. (1983). *High school: A report on secondary education in America.* New York: Harper & Row.

Branscomb, L.M., Campbell, A.K., Futrell, M.H., Gardner, J.W., Hechinger, F.M., Honig, B., Hunt, J.B., Katz, V., Keon, T.H., Lanier, J.E., Madrid, A., Malcolm, S.M., Randall, R.E., & Shanker, A. (1986). *A nation prepared: Teachers for the 21st Century.* New York: Carnegie Forum on Education and the Economy.

Brookfield, J. (1981). *Staff development: A systematic process.* Western States Technical Assistance Resource.

Brown, L., Branston-McClean, M.B., Baumgart, D., Vincent, L., Falvey, M., & Schroeder, J. (1979). Using the characteristics of current and subsequent least restrictive environments in the development of curricular content for severely handicapped students. *AAESPH Review, 4*(4), 407–424.

Brown, L., Nietupski, J., & Hamre-Nietupski, S. (1976). The criterion of ultimate functioning and public school services for severely handicapped students. In M.A. Thomas (Ed.), *Hey, don't forget about me: Education's investment in the severely, profoundly and multiply handicapped* (pp. 2–15). Reston, VA: The Council for Exceptional Children.

Bryk, A.S., & Light, R.J. (1981). Designing evaluations for different program environments. In R.A. Berk (Ed.), *Educational evaluation methodology: The state of the art* (pp. 11–31). Baltimore: Johns Hopkins University Press.

Donnellan, A.M. (1984). The criterion of the least dangerous assumption. *Behavioral Disorders, 9,* 141–150.

Donnellan, A.M., & Neel, R.S. (1986). New directions in educating students with autism. In R.H. Horner, L.H. Meyer, & H.D.B. Fredericks (Eds.), *Education of learners with severe handicaps: Exemplary service strategies* (pp. 99–126). Baltimore: Paul H. Brookes Publishing Co.

Durand, V.M., & Kishi, G.S. (1987). Reducing severe behavior problems among persons with dual sensory impairments: An evaluation of a technical assistance model. *Journal of The Association for Persons with Severe Handicaps, 12,* 2–10.

Evans, I.M. & Brown, F.A. (1986). Outcome assessment of student competence: Issues and implications. *Special services in the schools, 2*(4), 41–62.

Evans, I.M., Brown, F.A., Weed, K.A., Spry, K.M., & Owen, V.E. (1986). The assessment of functional competencies: A behavioral approach to the evaluation of programs for children with disabilities. In R.J. Prinz (Ed.), *Advances in behavioral assessment of children and families: A research annual* (Vol. 3). Greenwich, CT: JAI Press.

Evans, I.M., & Meyer, L.H. (1984). Basic life skills. In J.E. Ysseldyke (Ed.), *School psychology: The state of the art* (pp. 37–56). Minneapolis: National School Psychology Inservice Training Network.

Evans, I.M., & Meyer, L.H. (1985). *An educative approach to behavior problems: A practical decision model for interventions with severely handicapped learners.* Baltimore: Paul H. Brookes Publishing Co.

Fisher, R.A. (1935). *The design of experiments* (1st ed.). London: Oliver and Boyd.

Ford, A., Dempsey, P., Black, J., Davern, L., Schnorr, R., & Meyer, L. (1986). *The Syracuse Community-referenced curriculum guide for students with moderate and severe handicaps.* Syracuse, NY: Syracuse City School District.

Fox, W., Thousand, J., Williams, W., Fox, T., Towne, P., Reid, R., Conn-Powers, C., & Calcagni, L. (1986). *Best educational practices '86: Educating learners with severe handicaps, 6*(1).

Galloway, C., & O'Brien, J. (1981). *Mapping vocational services accomplishments.* Unpublished paper (Available from Charles Galloway, Department of Mental Retardation, Office of the Deputy Commissioner, State of Connecticut, 90 Pitkin Street, East Hartford, CT 06108).

Goldberg, M., Baten, B., Foley, C., Gerber, P., Harvey, J., Haslam, B., Jenkins, J., Longworth, A., Lykes, I., MacAdams, M., Mayberry, C., Sam, S., Selden, R., Tomlinson, T., Traiman, S., & Welch, P. (1984). *The nation responds: Recent efforts to improve education.* Washington, DC: U.S. Government Printing Office.

Harris, L., Kegay, M., & Leichenko, S. (1985). *The Metropolitan Life Survey of the American teacher. 1985: Strengthening the profession* (Report No. T238883). Metropolitan Life Insurance Company.

Horner, R.H., Meyer, L.H., & Fredericks, H.D. (Eds.). (1986). *Education of learners with severe handicaps: Exemplary service strategies.* Baltimore: Paul H. Brookes Publishing Co.

McGregor, G., Janssen, C.M., Larsen, L.A., & Tillery, W.L. (1986). Philadelphia's Urban Model Project: A system-wide effort to integrate students with severe handicaps. *Journal of the Association for Persons with Severe Handicaps, 11,* 61–67.

McGregor, G., & Meyer, L.H. (1986, May). *The social validity of behavioral interventions: An analysis of three years of research reports.* Paper presented at the 12th annual convention of the Association for Behavior Analysis, Milwaukee.

Meyer Voeltz, L.H. (1983). *A series of professional training modules on the education of severely handicapped learners: An update on educational best practices.* Minneapolis: University of Minnesota Upper Midwest Regional Resource Center.

Meyer, L.H. (1985). *Program quality indicators: A checklist of most promising practices in educational programs for students with severe disabilities.* Syracuse, NY: Syracuse University Division of Special Education and Rehabilitation.

Meyer, L.H., Eichinger, J., & Park-Lee, S. (1987). *A validation of program quality indicators in educational services for students with severe disabilities.* Paper submitted for publication.

Meyer, L.H., & Putnam, J. (in press). Social integration. In V.B. Van Hasselt, P.S. Strain, & M. Hersen (Eds.), *Handbook of developmental and physical disabilities.* New York: Pergamon.

National Commission on Excellence in Education. (1983). *A nation at risk* (Publication No. 065-000-00177-2). Washington, DC: U.S. Government Printing Office.

Norman, M.E., Brookfield-Norman, J., & Meyer, L.H. (1985). *A professional development needs assessment: A discrepancy model.* Syracuse, NY: Syracuse University Division of Special Education and Rehabilitation.

Peck, C.A., & Semmel, M.I. (1982). Identifying the least restrictive environment (LRE) for children with handicaps: Toward an empirical analysis. *Journal of The Association for the Severely Handicapped, 7*(1), 56–63.

Posavac, E.J., & Carey, R.G. (1980). *Program evaluation: Methods and case studies.* Englewood Cliffs, NJ: Prentice-Hall.

Putnam, J., & Bruininks, R.H. (1986). Future directions in deinstitutionalization and education: A Delphi investigation. *Exceptional Children, 53*(1), 55–62.

Risley, T.R. (1969). Behavior modification: An experimental–therapeutic endeavor. In L.A. Hamerlynck, P.O. Davison, & L.E. Acker (Eds.), *Behavior modification and ideal mental health services* (pp. 103–127). Calgary, Alberta: University of Calgary Press.

St. Louis Developmental Disabilities Treatment Center Parents Association v. Mallory, 767 F. 2d 518 (8th Cir. 1985).

Stile, S., Peters, J., & Piazza Templeman, T. (1986). Improving performance of school personnel: The teaching research inservice training model. *The Performance and Instruction Journal, 25*(9), 22–24.

Strain, P.S., & Odom, S.L. (1986). Innovations in the education of preschool children with severe handicaps. In R.H. Horner, L.H. Meyer, & H.D.B. Fredericks (Eds.), *Education of learners with severe handicaps: Exemplary service strategies* (pp. 61–98). Baltimore: Paul H. Brookes Publishing Co.

Stufflebeam, D.I., Foley, W.J., Gephart, W.J., Guba, E.G., Hammond, R.L., Merriman, H.O., & Provus, M.M. (1971). *Educational evaluation and decision making.* Itasca, IL: F. E. Peacock.

Vincent, L.J., Salisbury, C., Walter, G., Brown, P., Gruenewald, L.J., & Powers, M. (1980). Program evaluation and curriculum development in early childhood/special education: Criteria of the next environment. In W. Sailor, B. Wilcox, & L. Brown (Eds.), *Methods of instruction for severely handicapped students* (pp. 303–328). Baltimore: Paul H. Brookes Publishing Co.

Voeltz, L.M. (1984). Program and curriculum innovations to prepare children for integration.

In N. Certo, N. Haring, & R. York (Eds.), *Public school integration of severely handicapped students: Rational issues and progressive alternatives* (pp. 155–183). Baltimore: Paul H. Brookes Publishing Co.

Voeltz, L.M., & Evans, I.M. (1983). Educational validity: Procedures to evaluate outcomes in programs for severely handicapped learners. *Journal of The Association for the Severely Handicapped, 8*(1), 3–15.

Wolf, M.M. (1978). Social validity: The case for subjective measurement, or how applied behavior analysis is finding its heart. *Journal of Applied Behavior Analysis, 11,* 203–214.

APPENDIX

A Professional Development Needs Assessment Instrument: A Discrepancy Model

M.E. Norman, J. Brookfield-Norman, and L.H. Meyer 1985

1.0 Demographic information

1.1 Name:

1.2 Organization or agency

1.3 Brief description of services provided by your organization or agency

1.4 Population served by your organization or agency

1.5 Your current position:

1.6 How many deaf-blind students do you serve?

1.6.1 Age range of deaf-blind students

1.7 Training

1.7.1 Undergraduate major:

1.7.2 Graduate major:

1.7.3 Additional courses/training:

Please review each of the following items. Using the scale provided below, in the first column, indicate for each item the level of skill or knowledge required for your job performance. In the second column, indicate your existing *level relative to that skill or knowledge.*

At the end of each section, space is provided for you to include other areas that may be a target area for professional development.

Scale
1 = None, 2 = Minimal, 3 = Moderate, 4 = Considerable, 5 = Extensive

2.0 Identification and referral for diagnosis

		Re-quired	Exist-ing
2.1	Knowledge of early signs of potential sensory impairment		
2.2	Knowledge of referral procedures and resources for appropriate diagnosis		
2.3	Knowledge of a variety of observation techniques to record needed information for child's files		
2.4	Ability to collect child data through a variety of observation techniques		
2.5	Knowledge of available consultative resources in the region for assistance with instructional adaptations, behavior problems, etc.		
2.6	Ability to provide comprehensive data reports to the diagnostic team		
2.7	Strategies to develop and utilize professional and home-school collaboration to support children's programs		
2.8	Knowledge of a variety of diagnostic instruments which are appropriate for use with deaf-blind and other sensory impaired children		

2.9 List any other concerns you have about identifications and referral or any training you feel you need.

3.0 Assessment/diagnosis for instructional planning

		Re-quired	Exist-ing
3.1	Ability to do an ecological inventory in order to identify possible instructional goals for:		
	3.1.1 Domestic living		
	3.1.2 Leisure/recreation		
	3.1.3 Vocational training		
	3.1.4 Community participation		

3.2 Ability to make training/instructional decisions for a student once priority instructional objectives have been identified

3.3 Knowledge of strategies to identify priority instructional goals and objectives for individual students based upon environmental needs, student level of functioning, parent priorities, and empirical information on skill acquisition sequences

3.4 Ability to construct task analysis

3.5 Ability to identify and use functional assessments in the following areas for instructional planning:
- 3.5.1 Cognitive skills
- 3.5.2 Personal management
- 3.5.3 Social skills
- 3.5.4 Communication
- 3.5.5 Motor

3.6 Ability to collect and use data to modify instruction based on student performance and behavior

3.7 Knowledge of observation and procedures and data sheets available to monitor the effects on student performance and behavior

3.8 Knowledge of procedures to adapt assessments to accommodate students who use augmentative communication systems, have motor impairments, are sensorily impaired, etc.

3.9 Ability to analyze and summarize assessment information into a clear statement of present level of performance in relevant areas for a student's IEP

3.10 Ability to explain assessment results to parents and, when appropriate, the child

3.11 Knowledge of strategies to assess functional vision

3.12 Knowledge of strategies to assess functional hearing

3.13 List any other concerns you may have in the area of assessment for instructional planning or any training you feel you may need.

4.0 Creating and arranging opportunities for learning

	Required	Existing
4.1 Knowledge of community resources, facilities and programs that are available after school, on weekends, etc., that would support a child's school program and provide community participation opportunities (e.g., a recreation program)		
4.2 Knowledge and use of strategies to develop social interactions between students and their peers who are also disabled		

4.3	Knowledge and use of strategies to develop social interactions between students and their nonhandicapped peers		
4.4	Ability to appropriately group students for instruction		
4.5	Knowledge of enrichment areas and extracurricular opportunities available for students in school and community		
4.6	Knowledge and use of strategies to enable students to participate in generic school environments (such as the lunchroom, library, recess, etc.) along with nonhandicapped peers		
4.7	Knowledge and use of strategies to conduct instruction directly in the community in relevant areas (e.g., how to shop at a grocery store)		
4.8	Knowledge of vocational training resources and opportunities available to students		
4.9	Ability to schedule the school day to maximize instructional time		

5.0 Instructional design (IEP development) and instructional strategies

		Re-quired	Exist-ing
5.1	Ability to write IEP objectives that address student needs as indicated in the statement of present level of performance		
5.2	Ability to write IEP objectives for functional skills the student will need for daily life		
5.3	Ability to design an IEP that reflects an appropriate balance of objectives in the various skill domains based upon the student's skills, chronological age, and parent priorities		
5.4	Ability to specify measurable criteria to determine mastery by the student		
5.5	Knowledge of strategies to involve families actively and positively in IEP development and instructional planning		
5.6	Ability to write IEP objectives which reflect a concern for acquisition, generalization, and maintenance of new skills		
5.7	Knowledge and use of strategies to conduct instruction in community environments		
5.8	Knowledge of strategies to identify effective instructional cues, corrections and reinforcers		
5.9	Ability to design procedures to fade instructional prompts and consequences		
5.10	Ability to schedule a variety of appropriate instructional arrangements, including one-to-one, small and large group, independent work, and free time		
5.11	Knowledge and use of strategies to incorporate augmentative systems and adaptive equipment into instructional procedures		
5.12	Knowledge of different positioning and transfer strategies for students with motor disabilities		
5.13	Knowledge of available adaptive devices and alternative systems for students with sensory impairments		

5.14 Ability to design a transitional plan to prepare a student to move to the next environment (e.g., from elementary school to secondary school or from high school to postsecondary training opportunities)

5.15 Knowledge and use of strategies of reinforcement to strengthen positive behavior

5.16 Knowledge and use of strategies to remediate behavior problems (excess behavior) and design an instructional program to teach a positive alternative behavior or skill

5.17 Knowledge and use of strategies to rearrange the environment to prevent behavior problems from occurring

5.18 Knowledge and use of strategies to design effective programs for classroom and community training environments to deal with problem behavior when it occurs

5.19 List any other concerns you may have in the area of instructional design and instructional strategies or any training you feel you need:

6.0 Team cooperation, family collaboration, and use of community resources

	Required	**Existing**
6.1 Knowledge and use of effective instructional team cooperation in assessment and programming for students		
6.2 Ability to develop positive relationships between home and school		
6.3 Ability to train and supervise paraprofessional personnel in the classroom and in community settings		
6.4 Ability to train and supervise volunteers and special friends–peers in school and community settings		
6.5 Knowledge of relevant agency resources available to families (e.g., medical, respite, adaptive equipment, vocational-rehabilitative services, protection and advocacy, etc.		

6.6 List any other concerns you may have in the areas of team cooperation, family collaboration, and use of community resources:

7.0 Long-range planning, transitions, and use of resources

		Re-quired	Exist-ing
7.1	Knowledge of long-range planning procedures and techniques		
7.2	Knowledge of postsecondary vocational opportunities		
7.3	Knowledge of postsecondary residential opportunities		
7.4	Knowledge of procedure for providing the child's future financial security		
7.5	Knowledge of how to access the following resources at the *state/regional* level:		
	— medical care		
	— respite care		
	— adaptive equipment		
	— financial aid/assistance		
	— recreation		
	— protection and advocacy		
7.6	Knowledge of how to access the following resources at the *community* level:		
	— medical care		
	— respite care		
	— adaptive equipment		
	— financial aid/assistance		
	— recreation		
	— protection and advocacy		

7.7 Indicate any other concerns you may have about long-range planning, transitions, and use of resources:

8.0 Priority training needs

Directions: Please review your responses to sections 2.0–7.0.

8.1 Are there areas in which you feel you have training needs that are not covered by the instrument? Please list them.

8.2 Below, list your 5 priority training (professional development) needs and how they could best be met (e.g., workshops, print material or information, available media, etc.).

Training needs	Appropriate process

INDEX

Page numbers followed by *n* indicate footnotes.

ABR, *see* Auditory brainstem response
Acoustic immittance measurements, 109–111
Activities
  delineation of, in ecological curriculum approach, 229
  materials for, adaptations of, 239–240
Adaptive aids
  creation of, 239
  for manipulation skills, 180–181
  see also Prosthetic devices
Adult responses, incorporation of time delay into, nonsymbolic communication and, 38–39
AFLR (Assessment of Functional Life Routines), 342
Age-appropriateness
  education and, 10
  functional vision programming context and, 83
Alignment, electronic travel aids and, 300
American sign language (AMESLAN), natural gestures in, 198
AMMP, 132
Anticipation, in movement-based approach, 206–210
Arms, movement of, 163–164
  see also Upper extremity movement
Assessment of Functional Life Routines (AFLR), 342
Association for Retarded Citizens, technological innovation and, 283
Atresia, hearing loss and, 101
Attention, visual, training of, 79
Attitudinal adaptations, 242–243
Attitudinal dimensions, of PQI, 336–339
Audiogram, 104–105
Audiometry
  acoustic immittance measurements in, 109–111
  auditory brainstem response measurement in, 111–117
  behavioral tests in, 104, 107–109
  graph of, 104–105
  hearing loss classification in, 105–107
  physiological tests in, 104
  purpose of, 103–104
  see also Hearing impairments
Auditory brainstem response (ABR), 104, 111–117
  characteristics of, 111–113
  general nature of, 111
  latency in, 113
  technique of, 113–115
  use of, in audiometric assessment, 115–117
Auditory impairments, *see* Deaf-blind *entries;* Dual sensory impairments; Hearing impairments
Auditory pathways, 101
Auditory prompts, for visual behaviors, 87
Awareness, nonsymbolic communication and, 27–28
Awareness level training, 318

BAER (brainstem auditory evoked responses), *see* Auditory brainstem response
BEH (Bureau of Education for the Handicapped), 4
Behavior
  changes in, goals for, 341–342
  learner-initiated, 259–260
Behavior checks, writing ICS and, 270–271
Behavioral language intervention programs, 17
Behavioral observation audiometry (BOA), 107
Binaural Sensory Aid, *see* Sonicguide™
Blindness, *see* Deaf-blind *entries;* Dual sensory impairments; Visual impairments
BOA (behavioral observation audiometry), 107
Body image, development of, 193
Body Image of Blind Children, 132
Boehm Test of Basic Concepts, Tactile Analog to, 132
Bones, middle ear, malformation of, 102
Braille, 58

Brainstem auditory evoked responses, *see* Auditory brainstem response
Bureau of Education for the Handicapped (BEH), 4

Callier-Azusa Scale (H) Scales for the Assessment of Communicative Abilities, 22–23
Cane, "marshmallow tip" for, 152
Cane techniques, 134–136
  adaptations in, 151–152
Canterbury Babies and Child's Aid, 295
Caregiver, communication by, *see* Receptive communication
Caregiver-infant interactions, nonsymbolic development and, 21, 25–26
Causality, sense of, dual sensory impairments and, 25
Child(ren)
  environment and, interaction between, 192–195
  nonverbal, symbols and, 196
  with vision and hearing impairments, number of, 4–8
  see also Infants
Choice making
  communication skill development and, 214
  ICS model and, 258
CMV (cytomegalovirus), 102–103
Coactive movement, 197, 201, 210–211
Cochlear hearing loss, 103
Cochlear implants, 119–121
Cognitive language intervention programs, 17
Communication, 49–71
  aspects of, 51
  competence in, sequence of, 52
  dyadic interaction in, 69–71
  expressive, 51–63
    see also Expressive communication
  interventions in, background of, 49–51
  movement-based
    van Dijk methodology of, 195–199
    see also Movement-based approach
  nonsymbolic, *see* Nonsymbolic communication
  receptive, 63–69
    see also Receptive communication
  vibrotactile aids for, 121–124
Communication boards, 284
Communication media, in movement-based approach, 203
  anticipation and, 208–210
Communication Placement Assessment Manual, 22–23
Communication skills, development of, facilitation of, 212–215
Communicative input, 51
Communicative output, 51
Community functioning domain, in ecological inventory process, 232
Community intensive curriculum model, 77
Comprehensive Communication Curriculum Guide, 22–23
Computers, *see* Microcomputers; Software
Concept skills, 133–134
Concurrent imitation, 197
Conductive hearing loss, 101–102
Congenital atresia, hearing loss and, 101
Consequences, natural, in ICS model, 259
Contextual instruction, communication skill development and, 213
Contingencies, provision of, nonsymbolic communication and, 36–37
Contingency awareness training, 284
  history of, 287
Continuing education, *see* Staff development
Continuous correction procedure, in functional vision programming, 79, 88–89
Continuous loop training procedures, functional vision programming and, 88–89
Contrast effects, 78
Coordination
  eye-hand, 165
    functional reaching and, 168
  of movement, 161–162
    see also Manipulation skills; Upper extremity movement
Critical visual moment, identification of, 88–87
Cues
  manipulation skills and, 184
  movement-based approach and, 201
  natural, in ICS model, 259
  receptive, nonverbal, 64–67
  selection of, functional vision programming and, 87–88

sequences of, upper extremity movement programming and, 173
situational, anticipation in response to, 208
visual, deferred imitation and, 212
Curriculum
development of, ecological approach to, 225–249
see also Ecological curriculum approach
functional versus developmental, 10
individualized sequencing model of, *see* Individualized curriculum sequencing (ICS) model
models of, 77
see also Education; Instruction
Cytomegalovirus (CMV), 102–103

Deaf-blind
definition of, 11–12
see also Dual sensory impairments
Deaf-Blind Authorization (Title VI-C), 8
"Deaf-blind" label, 3
Deaf-blind services
current trends in, 8–10
history of, 4–8
see also Program evaluation; Program quality
Decontextualization, 51, 199
Deferred imitation, in movement-based approach, 198, 211–212
Deinstitutionalization, efforts toward, 11
Denaturalization, 51, 198–199
Developmental curriculum, functional curriculum versus, 10
Developmental skills, definition of, 162
Diagonal cane technique, 151
Direct teaching aids, 284
Discrepancy analysis, in ecological curriculum approach, 237–238
Discrepancy model, professional development needs assessment, 347–353
Distance information, electronic travel aids and, 300
Distance senses, lack of, compensation for, 32–33
Distributed trial training, 256
Domestic domain, in ecological inventory process, 231
Drawings, in movement-based approach, 204
Dual sensory impairments
children with, numbers of, 4–8
communication development and, 20
see also nonsymbolic communication
sense of causality and, 25
see also Deaf-blind *entries*
Dyadic interaction, communication training and, 69–71
Dyspraxia, 193

Ear, anatomy of, 100–101
Early intervention, current trends in, 9
Ecological curriculum approach, 225–249
activity delineation in, 229
community functioning domain inventory in, 232
curriculum domain delineation in, 228
determination of necessary adaptations in, 238–243
discrepancy analysis in, 237–238
domestic domain inventory in, 231
empirical support for, 244–247
environment delineation in, 228–229
frequency of occurrence in, 234
future research needs for, 247–249
instructional personnel preference in, 233–234
instructional program development in, 243–244
parental preference in, 230, 232
priority determination in, 229
recreation/leisure domain inventory in, 234
safety concerns in, 234–235
sample instructional program for, 251–253
sensory-developmental approach versus, 225–227
skill delineation in, 235–237
social significance in, 235
steps in, 228
student preference in, 232–233
sub-environment delineation in, 229
vocational domain inventory in, 230
Ecological language intervention programs, 17
Education
advanced technology application to, 283–307
see also Technological advances

Education—(*continued*)
  age-appropriate, 10
  continuing, *see* Staff development
  movement-based approach to, 191–216
    see also Movement-based approach
  see also Curriculum; Instruction
Education for All Handicapped Children (PL 94-142), 5
  early intervention and, 9
Educational validity, 340
Electronic technology
  communication and, 58–59
  see also Technological advances
Electronic travel aids (ETAs), 152–153, 294–306
  future of, 306–307
  historical perspective on, 294
  implementation guidelines for, 301–302, 303–305
  potential applications of, 299–301
  research on, 296–299
  types of, 294–296
Environment
  child and, interaction between, 192–195
  delineation of, in ecological curriculum approach, 228–229
  nonschool, teaching in, 258–259
  restrictiveness of, current trends in, 9
  social, cooperative, 39–41
Environmental concepts, electronic travel aids and, 300
Environmental control systems, 284
ERA (evoked response audiometry), *see* Auditory brainstem response
Error correction procedure, in functional vision programming, a 79, 88–89
Essential skills, definition of, 163
ETAs, *see* Electronic travel aids
Evaluation
  definition of, 313
  see also Program evaluation
Events/skills matrix, in ICS model, 261–266
Evoked response audiometry, *see* Auditory brainstem response
Expertise, local, development of, 322
Exploratory behavior, electronic travel aids and, 299–300
Expressive communication, 51–63
  content of, 62–63
  definition of, 51
  development of, sequence in, 52
  forms of, 54–60
    electronic, 58–59
    motor/gestural, 54–55
    selection of, 59–60
    sharing of, 60
    three-dimensional symbols, 58, 59
    two-dimensional symbols, 55
  function of, 60–62
  movement-based approach and, 200
  see also Communication
Expressive development, nonsymbolic communication and, 19, 20
Eye-hand coordination, 165
  functional reaching and, 168

Facilitation methods, manipulation skills and, 184
Facility resources, program quality and, 334–335
Federal funding, current trends in, 8
Federal reporting form, 4–5
Fonator Auditory Speech Trainer, 122
Fonator Speech Trainer, 122
Formative evaluation, 314
  see also Program evaluation
Functional competence, ICS model and, 279
Functional curriculum, developmental curriculum versus, 10
Functional life skills curriculum model, 77
Functional materials, ICS model and, 259
Functional object cues, 64, 65
Functional skills, 83
  context of, visual training strategies for, 90
  definition of, 162
  upper extremity movement and, 166, 168–172
Functional Vision Inventory, 81, 132
Functional vision programming, 77–94
  components of, 80
  context selection in, 82–85
  future of, 92–94
  historical overview of, 78–79
  instructional strategies for, 86–89
    functional skill context and, 90
  residual vision skills determination and, 81–82
  sample of, 90–92
  steps in, 80

Functional vocabulary, development of, facilitation of, 213–214
Funding, current trends in, 8–9

Gazing behaviors, dual sensory impairments and, 24–25
General case instruction, 246
Gesture cues, receptive communication with, 66–67
Gestures, 54–55
  natural, movement-based approach and, 198–199, 201–202 , 212
  preverbal, 50
Goldenhaar syndrome, 101
Graphic media, in movement-based approach, 203
Grasping skills, 164–165
  see also Manipulation skills
Groups, ICS model and, 274–277, 278

Handicaps, multiple, incidence of, 159
Hands
  movement of, coactive, 211
  skills involving, 164–165
    see also Manipulative skills
Hearing aids, 117–119
Hearing impairments, 99–126
  assessment of, 103–117
    see also Audiometry
  classification of, 105–107
  communication development and, 20
  conductive, 101–102
  ear anatomy and, 100–101
  posture and movement and, 160
  prosthetic devices for, 117–124
    cochlear implants, 119–121
    hearing aids, 117–119
    vibrotactile communication aids, 121–124
  sensorineural, 102–103
  sign language and, 198
  see also Deaf-blind *entries;* Dual sensory impairments; Multiple sensory impairments
Hearing sensitivity, prediction of, acoustic reflex measurement and, 110–111
Helen Keller National Center (HKNC), 8
Herpes, maternal, 102–103
Hill Performance Test of Selected Positional Concepts, 132
HKNC (Helen Keller National Center), 8
Hypertonus, 161
Hypotonia, 161

ICS model, *see* Individualized curriculum sequencing (ICS) model
Imitation
  concurrent, 197
  deferred, in movement-based approach, 198, 211–212
  manipulation skills and. 184
Impairment, definition of, 160
Individual preferences, sensitivity to, nonsymbolic communication and, 31–32
Individualized curriculum sequencing (ICS) model, 77, 255–280
  adaptation of, 273–274
  empirical support for, 256–258
  events/skills matrix in, 261–266
  functional vision programming and, 93
  future of, 277, 279–280
  group applications of, 274–277, 278
  instructional program development in, 273
  rationale for, 258–260
  writing format for, 266–273
Individualized education program, features of, program quality and, 328–329
Infant Sonicguide™, 297–298
Infants
  early interactional processes with, nonsymbolic communication and, 24–26
  nonsymbolic communication by
    assessment of, 18–20
    caregiver interactions and, 21
  see also Child(ren)
Inner ear, anatomy of, 101
Inservice training
  approaches to, 317
  evaluation of activities in, 319–320
  levels of, 317–319
Instruction
  consistency in, nonsymbolic communication and, 35–36
  contextual, communication skill development and, 213

Instruction—(*continued*)
general case, 246
in nonschool environment, 258–259
O&M, *see* Orientation and mobility
use of software in, 292–293
visual, *see* Functional vision programming
see also Curriculum; Education
Instructional personnel, preference of, in ecological curriculum approach, 233–234
Instructional program
in ecological curriculum approach, 243–244
in ICS model, 273
Instructional strategies, program quality and, 329–331
Integrated programming, 159–186
discrepancies in posture and movement and, 160–162
effectiveness of, 185–186
for grasp and manipulation skills, 175–185
see also Manipulation skills
for skill performance, 162–165
for upper extremity movement, 165–175
see also Upper extremity movement
Intentional behavior, 52–53
Interaction
dyadic, communication training and, 69–71
nonsymbolic communication and, 28–29
social, *see* Social interaction
Interactional model of language intervention, 17
see also Nonsymbolic communication
Interpersonal relationships, *see* Social interaction
Intervention
nonsymbolic communication facilitation and, 30–41
see also nonsymbolic communication, intervention strategies for
see also Early intervention, current trends in

Joint action, 69
Joint attention, 69

Kanievski Sound system, 123
Kinesthetic cues, in movement-based approach, 87
Knowledge level training, 318

Landmarks, electronic travel aids and, 300–301
Language acquisition, 49–71
see also Communication
Language intervention programs, types of, 17
Learner
choice making by, 258
communication skill development and, 214
communication by, *see* Expressive communication
goal identification for, 341–342
performance of, program evaluation and, 340–342
Learner preference, in ecological curriculum approach, 232–233
Learner-initiated behavior, 259–260
Learning
impact of impairments on, 192–195
opportunities for, program quality and, 326–328
scheduling of, appropriate times for, 259
Leisure domain, in ecological inventory process, 234
Limb movements
anticipation in response to, 208
coactive, 211
see also Upper extremity movement
Line drawings, in movement-based approach, 204

Manipulation skills, 164–165
programming for, 175–185
desired pattern in, 176–179
functional use of movement in, 180, 182–183
measuring results of, 185
schemes lattices for, 175–176
strategies for, 180–181, 184
Manual signals, anticipation in response to, 208

Massed trial approach, 256
  writing ICS and, 266
Meningitis, 103
Microcomputers, 286–293
  advantages of, 291
  historical perspective on, 287–288
  implementation guidelines for, 292–293
  motor skill instruction and, 288–291
  see also Software
Microswitch/electronic technology, communication and, 58–59
Microtia, 101–102
Middle ear
  anatomy of, 100
  bones of, malformation of, 102
Mini-Fonator, 123
Mobility, orientation and, *see* Orientation and mobility (O&M)
Mobility aids, 284
Mobility skills, 134–136
  definition of, 131
Modeling, manipulation skills and, 184
Moisture monitors, 284
"Most promising practices," *see* Program quality
Motivation, functional vision programming and, 83–85
Motor skills, instruction of, microcomputer in, 288–291
Motor/gestural communication, 54–55
Movement
  coactive, 197
  discrepancies in, 160–162
  impact of impairments on, 192–195
  upper extremities, 163–164
    see also Upper extremity movement
Movement cuing
  manipulation skills and, 184
  upper extremity movement and, 173
Movement-based approach, 191–216
  anticipation in, 206–210
  child-environment interaction and, 192–195
  coactive movement in, 210–211
  communication media in, 203–205
  communication modes in, 200–203
  deferred imitation in, 211–212
  facilitation of communication skill development in, 212–215
  future of, 215–216
  ICS model and, 279–280
  natural gestures in, 212
  nurturance in, 206
  van Dijk methodology of, 195–199
Mowat Sensor, 153, 295
  research on, 296
Multiple handicaps, incidence of, 159
Multiple sensory impairments
  population with, 3–4
  see also Dual sensory impairments
Multiple-channel vibrotactile devices, 123–124
Muscle tone, 161

Needs, for quality program development, 10–12
Needs assessment, staff development and, 315–316
  discrepancy model for, 347–353
Nonrepresentational reference, 197–198
Non-SLIP system, 58
Nonsymbolic communication
  assessment of, 18–20, 22–23
  components of, 26–30
  definition of, 16
  development of, 15–42
  early interactional processes and, 24–26
  facilitation of, 29–30
  intervention strategies for, 30–41
    compensation for lack of distance senses in, 32–33
    consistency in, 35–36
    contingency provisions in, 36–37
    creation of need to communicate in, 37–38
    establishment of cooperative social environment in, 39–41
    incorporation of time delay into responses in, 38–39
    increasing expectations in, 41
    responsivity in, 33–34
    sensitivity to individual preferences in, 31–32
  overview of skills for, 26–29
  rationale for, 16–18
  social interaction and, 20–21, 24
Nonverbal cues, receptive, 64–67
Nonverbal Prelinguistic Communication, 22–23

Nurion Step-Forward device, 153
Nurturance, movement-based approach and, 196–197, 206

O&M, *see* Orientation and mobility (O&M)
Object cues, receptive communication with, 64, 65
Object interventions, nonsymbolic communication and, 19, 20
Object placement, upper extremity movement programming and, 173
Objects
  body movements utilizing, coactive, 211
  in movement-based approach, 203–204
OMNIBOX, 290
Optical aids, 78
Oregon State System of Higher Education, Teaching Research Division of, 5
Orientation and mobility (O&M), 127–155
  advances in, 128
  assessment of, 131, 132
  definition of, 131
  instructional development model for, 136–153
    adaptations in, 150–153
    baseline route analysis in, 141–145
    components of, 136–137
    context instruction phase in, 145–147
    context selections in, 139–141
    current performance assessment in, 137–139
    data monitoring in, 150, 151
    implementation of, 150
    planned observations in, 139
    second baseline in, 145–147
    writing program in, 147–149
  rationale for, 129–131
  skills in, 133–136
  traditional sequence of, 132–133
  see also Electronic travel aids (ETAs)
Orientation skills, 134
  definition of, 131
Orthopaedic impairments, learning and, 194–195
Ossicular chain, bones of, malformation of, 102
Otitis media, 102
Outer ear, anatomy of, 100

Parent training programs, current trends in, 10
Parental preference, in ecological curriculum approach, 230, 232
Parsons Visual Acuity Test (PVAT), 81
Pathsounder, 152, 295
  research on, 296
Peabody Developmental Motor Scales and Activity Cards, 132
Peabody Mobility Kit, 132
Peabody Mobility Scale, 132
Personal assistance, utilization of, 242
Personnel
  preference of, in ecological curriculum approach, 233–234
  qualifications of, program quality and, 332–334
  training of, needs for, 11
  see also Staff development
Photographs, in movement-based approach, 204
  anticipation in response to, 209–210
Physical guidance, for manipulation skills, 184
Physical interactions, nonsymbolic communication and, 28–29
Physical prompts, for visual behaviors, 87
Physical signals, in movement-based approach, 202–203
Pictographs, in movement-based approach, 205
Pictures
  communication and, 55
  representational, in movement-based approach, 204–205
Polarion, 153
Population, with multiple sensory impairments, 3–4
Positioning, upper extremity movement programming and, 172
Postural tone, upper extremity movement programming and, 172
Posture, discrepancies in, 160–162
Powerpad, 288
PQI checklist, 325, 326–336
  see also Program quality
Pragmatic language intervention programs, 17
Pre-intentional behavior, 52
Prelinguistic communication, 16*n*

Presymbolic communication, 16*n,* 53
Preverbal gestures, 50
"Priming," upper extremity movement programming and, 173
Professional development, *see* Staff development
Program evaluation, 313–343
  program quality and, 322–339
    see also Program quality
  staff development and, 315–322
    see also Staff development
  student performance and, 340–342
Program quality, 322–339
  dimensions of, 336–339
  indicators of, 324–336
    checklist for, 326–336
    "criterion of least dangerous assumption," 324
    "criterion of ultimate functioning," 324
    facility resources and, 334–335
    general, 335–336
    IEP features and, 328–329
    instructional strategies and, 329–331
    learning opportunities and, 326–328
    program characteristics and, 331–332
    program philosophy and, 326
    staff qualifications and, 332–334
  "most promising practices" and, 322–323
Prompts, *see* Cues
Prosthetic devices
  cochlear implants, 119–121
  creation of, 239
  hearing aids, 117–119
  technological developments in, 284
  vibrotactile communication aids, 121–124
  see also Adaptive aids
Public Law 89-313, 5
Public Law 94-142, 5
  early intervention and, 9
Public Law 99-457, 9
PVAT (Parsons Visual Acuity Test), 81

Reaching activities, 163–164
  see also Upper extremity movement
Receptive communication, 63–69
  content of, 68–69
  definition of, 51
  forms of, 64–67
    abstract, 67
    gesture cues, 66–67
    object cues, 64, 65
    selection of, 67
    touch cues, 64–65, 66
  functions of, 67–68
  movement-based approach and, 200–201
Receptive development, assessment of, 19, 20
Recreation, technological developments and, 285
Recreation domain, in ecological inventory process, 234
Reference, nonrepresentational, 197–198
Repeated prompting procedure, 79
Replacement aids, for manipulation skills, 180–181
Representational objects, in movement-based approach, 204
Representational pictures, in movement-based approach, 204–205
Residual vision
  enhancement of, *see* Functional vision programming
  skills in, determination of, 81–82
Resonance, movement-based approach and, 197
Resources, of facility, program quality and, 334–335
Responsivity, nonsymbolic communication and, 33–34
Route analysis, 141–145
Rubella, during pregnancy, 102
Rule adaptations in generating curricular content, 241–242

Safety concerns, in ecological curriculum approach, 234–235
Sensitivity, to individual preferences, nonsymbolic communication and, 31–37
Sensorimotor impairments, technological developments related to, 284–285
  see also Technological advances
Sensorineural hearing loss, 102–103
Sensory responses, nonsymbolic communication and, 19
Sensory stimulation, anticipation in response to, 206–207

Sensory-developmental approach, 225
Service delivery
  current trends in, 8–10
  history of, 4–8
  see also Program evaluation; Program quality
Sign language, 198
Single-channel vibrotactile devices, 122–123
Situational cues, anticipation in response to, 208
Skill clusters
  relation of, 257
  writing ICS and, 266–270
Skill implementation level training, 318–319
Skill performance
  goals for, identification of, 341–342
  posture and movement and, 162
  programming for, 162–165
  visual response and, 82–83
Skill sequences, adaptation of, 241
Skills
  delineation of, in ecological curriculum approach, 235–237
  essential, definition of, 163
  functional
    age appropriateness and, 83
    visual training strategies and, 90
  isolated, writing ICS and, 271
  orientation and mobility, *see* Orientation and mobility (O&M)
Smiling behaviors, dual sensory impairments and, 25
Social environment, cooperative, establishment of, 39–41
Social interaction
  initiation of, 70
  movement and, 192
  nonsymbolic development and, 19, 20–21, 24, 28
  technological developments and, 285
  see also Communication
Social significance, in ecological approach to curriculum development, 235
Societal adaptations, 242–243
Software
  developments in, 284–285
  Switchmaster, 290–291
  teaching with, 292–293
  see also Microcomputers
Sonicguide™, 295–296
  intervention strategies for, 303–305
  research on, 296–299
Spaced trial training, 256
Spatial concepts, electronic travel aids and, 300
Staff
  preference of, in ecological curriculum approach, 233–234
  qualifications of, program quality and, 332–334
Staff development, 315–322
  inservice training activity evaluation in, 319–320
  inservice training approaches to, 317
  inservice training levels in, 317–319
  local expertise development and, 322
  long-term outcome measurement in, 320–322
  needs assessment for, 315–316
    discrepancy model for, 347–353
Staff training, needs for, 11
Stenosis, hearing loss and, 101
Stimulation, sensory, anticipation in response to, 206–207
Student, *see* Learner *entries*
Sub-environments, delineation of, in ecological curriculum approach, 229
Summative evaluation, 313–314
Switching devices, *see* Technological advances
Switchmaster, 290–291
Symbolic communication, development of, 53
Symbols
  communication and, 50–51
    see also Nonsymbolic communication
  nonverbal child and, 196
  three-dimensional, 58, 59
  two-dimensional, 55

Tactile Analog to Boehm Test of Basic, Concepts, 132
Tactile prompts
  in movement-based approach, 87
  receptive communication with, 64–65, 66
  for visual behaviors, 87

Tangible-reinforcer operant-conditioning audiometry (TROCA), 104, 108–109
TASH, *see* The Association for Persons with Severe Handicaps
Task analysis
  ecological curriculum approach and, 235–237
  writing ICS and, 271–273
Task performance
  simplification of, aids for, 181
  visual response and, 82–83
Teacher
  communication by, *see* Receptive communication
  preference of, in ecological curriculum approach, 233–234
  see also Staff *entries*
Teaching, *see* Instruction
Teaching Research Division of Oregon State System of Higher Education, 5
Teaching Research Inservice Model, 317
Teamwork, communication skill development and, 214–215
Technological advances, 283–307
  communication and, 58–59
  current trends in, 283–284
  electronic travel aids, 294–306
    see also Electronic travel aids (ETAs)
  microcomputers, 286–293
    see also Microcomputers
  pitfalls of, 286
  promises of, 286
  uses of, 285
The Association for Persons with Severe Handicaps (TASH), 8–9
  on exemplary practices, 323–324
  Technical Assistance Project of, 325
Three-dimensional symbols, communication and, 58, 59
Time delay, adult responses and, nonsymbolic communication and, 38–39
Time-out techniques, 88
Title I/Chapter 1: Aid to State Schools (Public Law 89-313), 5
Title VI-C (Deaf-Blind Authorization), 8
Total body movement
  anticipation in response to, 207–208
  coactive, 210–211
Touch cues, *see* Tactile prompts
Training, of staff, *see* Staff development
Training trials
  types of, 256–257
  see also Individualized curriculum sequencing (ICS) model
Travel, *see* Electronic travel aids (ETAs); Orientation and mobility (O&M)
Treacher Collins syndrome, 101
Trisensor, 295
TROCA (tangible-reinforcer operant-conditioning audiometry), 108–109
Two-channel vibrotactile devices, 123
Two-dimensional symbols, communication and, 55
Tympanometry, 110

Upper extremity movement, 163–164
  programming for, 165–175
    desired pattern in, 166
    functional reach lattice for, 168, 170–171
    functional use of movement in, 166, 168–172
    measuring results of, 174–175
    steps in, 167
    strategies for, 172–173
Usher's syndrome, 102

Validity, educational, 340
Van Dijk methodology of movement-based education, 195–199
Vibrotactile communication aids, 121–124
Viral infection, hearing loss and, 103
Vision stimulation, 78
Visual acuity test, 81
Visual assessment, 81–82
Visual attention behaviors, training of, 79
Visual cues, deferred imitation and, 212
Visual function, responses and, 82
Visual impairments
  communication development and, 20
  early interactional processes and, 24
  posture and movement and, 160–161
  travel and, *see* Electronic travel aids (ETAs); Orientation and mobility (O&M)
  see also Deaf-blind *entries;* Dual sensory impairments; Functional vision programming; Multiple sensory impairments

Visual reinforcer audiometry (VRA), 107–108
Visual signals, in movement-based approach, 201
Visual stimulation, augmentation of, 87
Vocabulary, functional, development of, 213–214
Vocal development, nonsymbolic communication and, 19, 20
Vocal signals, in movement-based approach, 201, 202
Vocational domain, in ecological inventory process, 230
Vocoders, 123–124
VRA (visual reinforcer audiometry), 107–108